Advances in Percutaneous Coronary Interventions

Advances in Percutaneous Coronary Interventions

Edited by Eva Barnes

hayle medical
New York

Hayle Medical,
750 Third Avenue, 9th Floor,
New York, NY 10017, USA

Visit us on the World Wide Web at:
www.haylemedical.com

ISBN: 978-1-63241-927-9

Cataloging-in-Publication Data

Advances in percutaneous coronary interventions / edited by Eva Barnes.
p. cm.
Includes bibliographical references and index.
ISBN 978-1-63241-927-9
1. Coronary heart disease--Surgery. 2. Angioplasty. 3. Cardiovascular system--Diseases--Treatment.
4. Cardiac catheterization--Complications. 5. Heart--Surgery. I. Barnes, Eva.
RD598.35.A53 A38 2020
617.413--dc23

Table of Contents

Preface

This book has been an outcome of determined endeavour from a group of educationists in the field. The primary objective was to involve a broad spectrum of professionals from diverse cultural background involved in the field for developing new researches. The book not only targets students but also scholars pursuing higher research for further enhancement of the theoretical and practical applications of the subject.

Percutaneous coronary intervention (PCI) is a clinical procedure that is performed to treat stenosis of the coronary arteries of the heart. It involves the visualization of the blood vessels using coronary catheterization and X-ray imaging, followed by a coronary angioplasty using a balloon catheter. This ensures that the obstructed artery is inflated to relieve the narrowing. Stents are then deployed to keep the opening of the vessel intact. PCI is appropriate in case of stable coronary artery disease, or when coronary stenosis is more than 50%, or when angina symptoms are unresponsive to therapy. Percutaneous coronary angioplasty is a common procedure with no major complications. Mostly after three months of the procedure, the artery sufficiently heals and no longer requires the stent. This book contains some path-breaking studies in the field of coronary interventions. It outlines the procedures and practices of percutaneous coronary intervention in detail. This book includes contributions of experts and scientists which will provide innovative insights into cardiology.

It was an honour to edit such a profound book and also a challenging task to compile and examine all the relevant data for accuracy and originality. I wish to acknowledge the efforts of the contributors for submitting such brilliant and diverse chapters in the field and for endlessly working for the completion of the book. Last, but not the least; I thank my family for being a constant source of support in all my research endeavours.

Editor

1

Impact of renal insufficiency on mortality in patients with ST-segment elevation myocardial infarction treated with primary percutaneous coronary intervention

Jonas Emil Sabroe, Per Thayssen, Lisbeth Antonsen, Mikkel Hougaard, Knud Nørregaard Hansen and Lisette Okkels Jensen*

Abstract

Background: Chronic kidney disease is associated with increased risk of mortality. We examined the impact of moderate and severe renal insufficiency (RI) on short- and long-term mortality among unselected patients with ST-segment elevation myocardial infarction (STEMI) treated with primary percutaneous coronary intervention (PCI).

Methods: From January 1, 2002 to December 31, 2010 all patients with STEMI treated with primary PCI were identified. The hazard ratio (HR) for death was estimated using a Cox regression model, controlling for potential confounders. RI was defined as creatinine clearance (CrCl) < 60 mL/min (moderate RI: CrCl ≤30 < 60 mL/min and severe RI: CrCl < 30 mL/min).

Results: The study cohort consisted of 4,116 patients of whom 898 (21.8%) had RI and 3,218 (78.2%) had a CrCl ≥ 60 mL/min. Compared to patients without RI, patients with RI were older, more often female and more likely to have diabetes mellitus, hypertension and to present with a higher Killip class.
Among patients with a preserved kidney function and patients with RI, 30-day all-cause mortality was 3.5% vs. 20.9% (log-rank p < 0.001); 1-year all-cause mortality was 5.7% vs. 29.4% (log-rank p < 0.001); 5-year all-cause mortality was 13.4% vs. 47.4% (log-rank p < 0.001). Moderate and severe RI were associated with higher 1-year mortality compared to patients with a preserved renal function (CrCl ≤30 < 60 mL/min: adjusted HR 2.71 [95% CI 2.09-3.51], p < 0.001), and (CrCl < 30 mL/min: adjusted HR 7.09 [4.82-10.44], p < 0.001).

Conclusion: In unselected STEMI patients treated with primary PCI, moderate and severe RI were associated with increased risk of mortality.

Keywords: ST-segment elevation myocardial infarction, Renal insufficiency, Mortality

Background

Cardiovascular disease (CVD) is a leading cause of death in the western countries [1]. Studies have shown that impaired renal function is to be considered a risk factor in relation to CVD and patients suffering from renal disease have a higher risk of CVD [2-4]. Also, chronic kidney disease (CKD) is found to be strongly associated with an increased risk of myocardial infarction (MI) and CVD mortality [5,6]. Furthermore, CKD is found to affect patients on a global scale and with an increasing incidence and prevalence [7]. After ST-segment elevation MI (STEMI) and non-STEMI the mortality has been reported to be significantly higher among patients with renal disease compared to patients with preserved renal function [8-10]. Today primary PCI is the recommended reperfusion strategy when treating patients with STEMI, which also applies to STEMI patients with renal dysfunction [11]. Limited data are available on the outcome after primary PCI in STEMI patients with RI, because they have been underrepresented in randomized trials, as renal failure is a commonly used exclusion criterion [12].

* Correspondence: okkels@dadlnet.dk
Department of Cardiology, Odense University Hospital, Sdr. Boulevard 29, 5000 Odense, Denmark

In our study, data from the Western Denmark Heart Registry (WDHR) were used in order to assess the impact of moderate and severe renal insufficiency (RI) on short- and long-term mortality among unselected STEMI patients treated with primary PCI. Primary PCI has been the recommended treatment for STEMI after publication of the results of the DANish trial in Acute Myocardial Infarction-2 (DANAMI-2) in 2003 [13].

Methods

Setting and design

The study was conducted using WDHR for patients treated at Odense University Hospital. A detailed description of the databases has been reported previously [14]. The study was a registry study and ethical approval was not required.

Patients and procedures

To be eligible for primary PCI, patients must meet the following criteria: 1) symptoms present less than 12 hours from onset of pain to time of catheterization, and 2) ST-segment elevation (at least 0.1 mV in two or more standard leads or at least 0.2 mV in two or more contiguous pre-cordial leads) or a new left bundle-branch block (LBBB). Patient with cardiogenic shock were not excluded. We used the WDHR to identify all primary PCIs performed from January 1, 2002 through December 31, 2010. Drug eluting stent (DES), bare metal stent (BMS), glycoprotein IIb/IIIa receptor blocker, and intra-aortic balloon pump was administered at the operator's discretion. All patients received antiplatelet regimen including a bolus of 10,000 IU heparin, lifelong acetylsalicylic acid (75–150 mg once daily), and clopidogrel with a loading dose of 300 mg followed by maintenance with 75 mg daily. The recommended duration of clopidogrel treatment was 3 to 12 months until November 2002 and 12 months thereafter.

Blood samples were taken from the arterial sheath before the first contrast injection and serum creatinine - concentration was assessed in the hospital laboratory. Estimation of renal function is commonly based on estimated creatinine clearance (CrCl). Different methods are available. Studies have shown that The Modification of Diet in Renal Disease (MDRD) formula gives a reliable estimated CrCl [15-17], representing estimated glomerular filtration ratio (eGFR). Therefore the MDRD formula was used in this study: eGFR = estimated CrCl = 186 × standardized $\text{S-Cr}^{-1.154} \times \text{age}^{-0.203} \times 0.742$ [if female] [18]. The unit of this equation is expressed as mL/min per 1.73 m^2 body surface area. An eGFR less than 60 mL/min per 1.73 m^2 was considered equivalent to RI. Based on eGFR the study population was divided into three groups, a group with eGFR ≥ 60 mL/min per 1.73 m^2, a group with moderate RI: CrCl ≤30 < 60 mL/min per 1.73 m^2, and a group with severe RI: CreaCl < 30 mL/min per 1.73 m^2. This classification of patients into different stages of CKD is identical with those universally endorsed and based on the National Kidney Foundation data [7] where patients with an eGFR ≥ 60 mL/min per 1.73 m^2 is STAGE I/II, patients with 30 ≤ eGFR < 60 mL/min per 1.73 m^2 are in STAGE III, and patients with eGFR < 30 mL/min per 1.73 m^2 are in STAGE IV/V.

Endpoints

Primary end-point of the study was all cause-mortality rate. Data on mortality were obtained from the Danish Civil Registration System [19,20], which has kept electronic records on the gender, date of birth, changes in address, date of emigration, and changes in vital status of the entire Danish population since 1968.

Statistics

Continuous variables were presented as medians with inter quartile range (IQR 25th, 75th) or mean ± 1 standard deviations (SD). Medians were compared using the Mann–Whitney *U* test, and means were compared using the unpaired *t* test. Categorical variables were presented as numbers and percentages. Distributions of categorical variables were compared using the Chi-square test.

We counted end-point events that occurred during the follow-up period and compared rates for the two groups (CrCl ≥60 mL/min per 1.73 m^2 vs. CrCl <60 mL/min per 1.73 m^2). Follow-up began on the date of primary PCI procedure and continued until date of death, December 31, 2010 or after 5 years follow-up (to ensure at least 10% of the study population at risk), whichever came first. Kaplan-Meier curves for all-cause mortality according to kidney function (CrCl ≥ 60 mL/min per 1.73 m^2, CrCl ≤30 < 60 mL/min per 1.73 m^2 and CrCl <30 mL/min per 1.73 m^2) were obtained.

Cox proportional hazards regression analysis was used to estimate the hazard ratio (HR) mortality. Crude and adjusted hazard ratios (HRs) with 95% confidence intervals (CIs) were computed. Potential confounders associated with time to death in the univariable Cox regression analysis were included in the multivariable Cox regression model. Thus, in the final model, we adjusted for RI, age diabetes mellitus, hypertension, previous myocardial infarction, treatment with glycoprotein IIb/IIIa receptor blocker, Killip class and duration of procedure. All data analyses were carried out using SPSS software version 20. A two-sided P value <0.05 was considered significant.

Results

A total of 4,676 consecutive patients were treated with primary PCI for STEMI or new onset LBBB MI at Odense University Hospital between January 1, 2002 and

December 31, 2010. Mortality data was not available for 83 patients, who were foreign citizens. Patients undergoing a later acute MI after the first index procedure (n = 223) were excluded. In 254 patients the creatinine values were not available. Thus, the final study population consisted of 4,116 patients; of these were 898 patients diagnosed with RI, defined as CrCl < 60 mL/min per 1.73 m^2, and 3,218 patients had a preserved kidney function (Figure 1).

Baseline characteristics of patients with RI and patients with a preserved kidney function are listed in Table 1. Patients with RI were older and more likely to be female, to have diabetes, hypertension, previous MI, hypercholesterolemia and less likely to be smokers. Among patients with RI, patients with severe RI (CrCl < 30 mL/min per 1.73 m^2) more often had diabetes. Characteristics of angiographic findings, lesions and treatment procedures also differed between patients with normal and reduced CrCl, respectively. Patients with RI were more likely to have multi-vessel disease, a higher Killip class, left main culprit lesion, more complex lesions and longer duration of procedure. Patients with RI were less often treated with DES (Table 2).

The median follow-up interval was 3.3 years (25th – 75th percentile: 1.4-5.0 years), with a 1-year mortality of 10.7% (n = 441) and 5-year mortality of 17.2% (n = 707). Among patients with a preserved kidney function and patients with RI, 30-day all-cause mortality was 3.5% (n = 112) and 20.9% (n = 188), respectively (log-rank $p < 0.001$); 1-year all-cause mortality was 5.7% (n = 179) and 29.4% (n = 262), respectively (log-rank $p < 0.001$); 5-year all-cause mortality was 13.4% (n = 328) and 47.4% (n = 379), respectively (log-rank $p < 0.001$). Figure 2 shows the 5-year all-cause survival of the

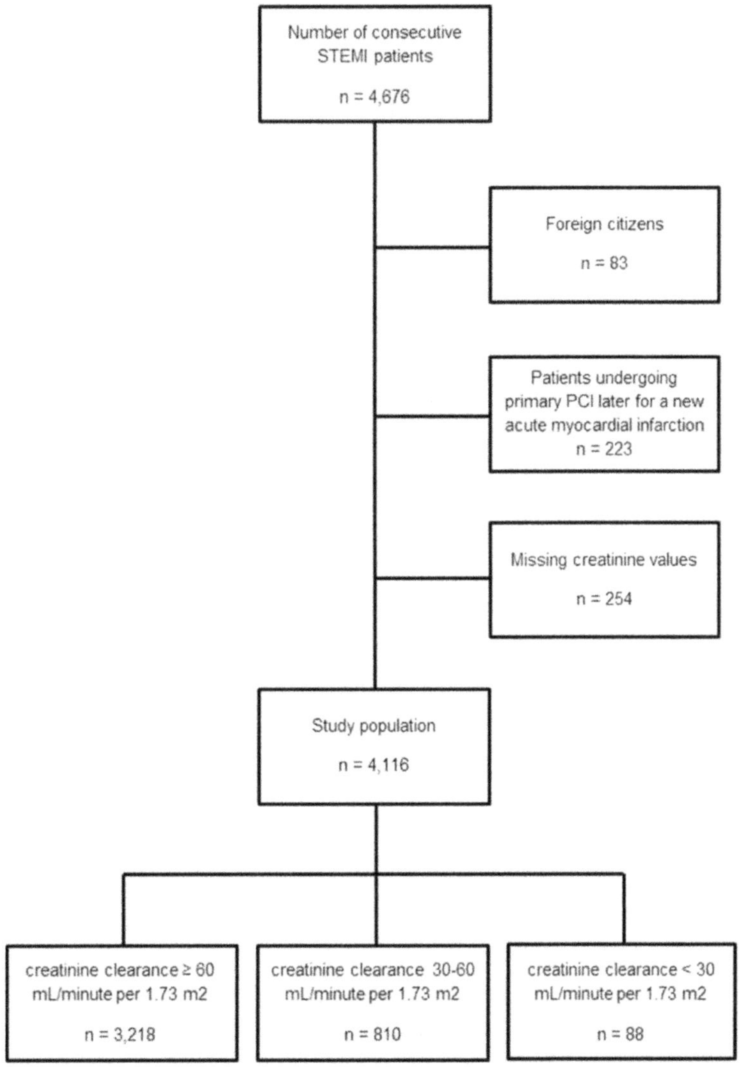

Figure 1 Flow diagram of participant selection.

Table 1 Baseline clinical characteristics according to kidney function

	CrCl ≥ 60	Valid cases	CrCl < 60	Valid cases	*P* value (CrCl ≥ 60 vs. CrCl < 60)	CrCl ≤30 < 60	CrCl < 30	*P* value (CrCl < 30 vs. CrCl ≤30 < 60)
Number of patients - no.	3,218	3,218	898	898		810	88	
Male gender - no. (%)	2,486 (77.3)	3,218	524 (58.4)	898	<0.001	471 (58.1)	53 (60.2)	0.707
Age – (year)	61.5 ± 12.1	3,218	73.5 ± 11.0	898	<0.001	73.5 ± 10.8	72.8 ± 12.8	0.532
Family history - no. (%)	1,235 (39.8)	3103	194 (23.5)	824	<0.001	178 (23.8)	16 (20.8)	0.548
Smoking - no. (%)	1,712 (57.2)	2991	290 (39.1)	741	<0.001	257 (38.1)	33 (49.3)	0.075
Body Mass Index – (kg/m^2)	26.8 (4.4)	2,132	26.6 (4.6)	507	0.256	26.7 (4.6)	24.9 (4.2)	0.009
Diabetes - no. (%)	272 (8.5)	3218	120 (13.4)	898	<0.001	101 (12.5)	19 (21.6)	0.017
Hypertension - no. (%)	930 (29.2)	3,180	404 (46.6)	867	<0.001	358 (45.8)	46 (54.1)	0.143
Previous coronary artery bypass grafting - no. (%)	64 (2.0)	3,214	23 (2.6)	893	0.283	21 (2.6)	2 (2.3)	1.000
Previous percutaneous coronary intervention - no. (%)	203 (6.4)	3,164	58 (6.7)	868	0.778	48 (6.1)	10 (11.8)	0.048
Previous myocardial infarction - no. (%)	330 (10.4)	3,168	127 (14.5)	875	0.001	108 (13.7)	19 (13.7)	0.31
Lipid lowering therapy - no. (%)	617 (19.4)	3,173	201 (23.2)	866	0.015	173 (22.2)	28 (32.9)	0.025
Glycoprotein IIb/IIIa receptor blocker – no. (%)	1,445 (48.2)	2,998	285 (34.4)	828	<0.001	263 (35.8)	22 (26.5)	0.110
Systolic blood pressure - (mmHg)	122.9 ±24.9	2,467	118.1 ±30.5	662	<0.001	118.7 ±30.3	112.4 ±32.0	0.118
Diastolic blood pressure - (mmHg)	71.8 ±13.9	2,449	66.0 ± 15.1	654	<0.001	66.4 ± 15.1	62.3 ± 15.9	0.043

Table 2 Angiographic and procedural characteristics according to kidney function

	CrCl ≥ 60	Valid cases	CrCl < 60	Valid cases	*P* value (CreaCl ≥ 60 vs. CreaCl < 60)	CrCl ≤30 < 60	CrCl < 30	*P* value (CrCl < 30 vs. CrCl ≤30 < 60)
Number of patients - no.	3,218	3,218	898	898		810	88	
Multivessel disease no. (%)	1,304 (41.6)	3,135	520 (59.4)	876	<0.001	464 (58.7)	56 (65.9)	0.198
Infarct related artery –no. (%)		3,144		867	<0.001			0.230
Left anterior descending artery - no. (%)	1,383 (44.0)		340 (39.2)			314 (40.2)	26 (30.6)	
Left circumflex artery - no. (%)	451 (14.3)		109 (12.6)			100 (12.6)	9 (10.6)	
Right coronary artery - no. (%)	1,252 (39.8)		374 (43.1)			329 (42.1)	45 (52.9)	
Left main - no. (%)	58 (1.8)		44 (5.1)			39 (5.0)	5 (5.9)	
Anterior STEMI or LBBB – no. (%)	1,401 (45.2)	3,100	372 (43.1)	864	<0.001	343 (43.8)	29 (35.8)	0.100
Killip class – no. (%)		3,152		878	<0.001			0.001
I	2,925 (92.8)		676 (77.0)			624 (78.5)	52 (62.7)	
II	135 (4.3)		62 (7.1)			55 (6.9)	7 (8.4)	
III	51 (1.6)		51 (5.8)			46 (5.8)	5 (6.0)	
IV	41 (1.3)		89 (10.1)			70 (8.8)	19 (22.9)	
Preintervention TIMI flow – no. (%)		3,143		863	0.248			0.891
Grade 0	2,198 (54.2)		2,794 (58.7)			438 (56.2)	49 (59.9)	
Grade 1	265 (6.5)		282 (5.9)			51 (6.5)	4 (4.8)	
Grade 2	597 (14.7)		623 (13.1)			117 (15.0)	11 (13.3)	
Grade 3	978 (24.1)		1,052 (22.1)			174 (22.3)	19 (22.9)	
Final TIMI flow - no. (%)		3,143		863	<0.001			0.097
Grade 0	73 (2.3)		50 (5.8)			41 (5.3)	9 (10.8)	
Grade 1	28 (0.9)		20 (2.3)			20 (2.6)	0 (0.0)	
Grade 2	166 (5.3)		78 (9.0)			70 (9.0)	8 (9.6)	
Grade 3	2,876 (91.5)		715 (82.9)			649 (83.2)	66 (79.5)	
Lesion length – mm median (IQR)	15.00 (10.0-20.0)	3,110	15.0 (10.0-20.0)	855	0.676	15.00 (10.0-20.0)	15.00 (10.0-20.0)	0.318
Reference segment – mm median (IQR)	3.3 (3.0-3.6)	3,120	3.2 (3.0-3.5)	851	0.007	3.2 (3.0-3.5)	3.2 (2.8-3.5)	0.320
Minimum lumen diameter – mm median (IQR)	0.0 (0.0-0.2)	3,134	0.0 (0.0-0.2)	859	0.749	0.0 (0.0-0.2)	0.0 (0.0-0.2)	0.625
Sapheneous vein graft – no. (%)	10 (0.3)	3,145	4 (0.5)	867	0.526	2 (0.3)	2 (2.4)	0.007
Lesion type B2/C	1,012 (32.9)	3,082	338 (40.3)	838	<0.001	302 (39.7)	36 (46.2)	0.041
Stent length – mm median (IQR)	18.0 (14.0-23-0)	2,963	18.0 (14.0-24.0)	754	0.913	18.0 (14.0-24.0)	18.0 (13.0-24.0)	0.830

Table 2 Angiographic and procedural characteristics according to kidney function *(Continued)*

Stent number - no. (%)		3,218		898	<0.001			0.007
0	255 (7.9)		144 (16.0)			120 (14.8)	24 (27.3)	
1	2,578 (80.1)		643 (71.6)			591 (73.0)	52 (59.1)	
2+	385 (12.0)		111 (12.4)			99 (12.2)	12 (13.6)	
Drug-eluting stent – no. (%)	1,962 (62.4)	3,146	366 (41.4)	885	<0.001	338 (42.3)	28 (32.6)	0.007
Max balloon pressure – atm median (IQR)	16.0 (14.0-18.0)	3,075	15.5 (14.0-17.3)	814	0.086	15.5 (14.0-17.0)	15.5 (14.0-18.0)	0.899
Max balloon diameter – mm median (IQR)	3.6 (3.2-3.8)	3,073	3.4 (3.2-3.8)	814	0.012	3.4 (3.2-3.8)	3.3 (3.0-3.7)	0.126
Duration of procedure - minutes median (IQR)	16.0 (10.0-26.0)	3,205	17.0 (11.0-28.0)	895	0.008	17.0 (11.0-28.0)	20.0 (12.0-30.8)	0.238
Flouro time - minutes median (IQR)	6.4 (4.0-11.2)	3,174	7.7 (4.5-13.0)	878	< 0.001	7.5 (4.4-13.0)	9.0 (6.0-13.3)	0.077
Contrast – ml median (IQR)	120.0 (75.0-180.0)	877	100.0 (75.0-175.0)	3,159	0.007	120.0 (75.0-185.0)	110.0 (80.0-174.0)	0.572

STEMI: ST-segment elevation myocardial infarct.
LBBB: new onset left bundle branch block.
IQR: Interquartile range.

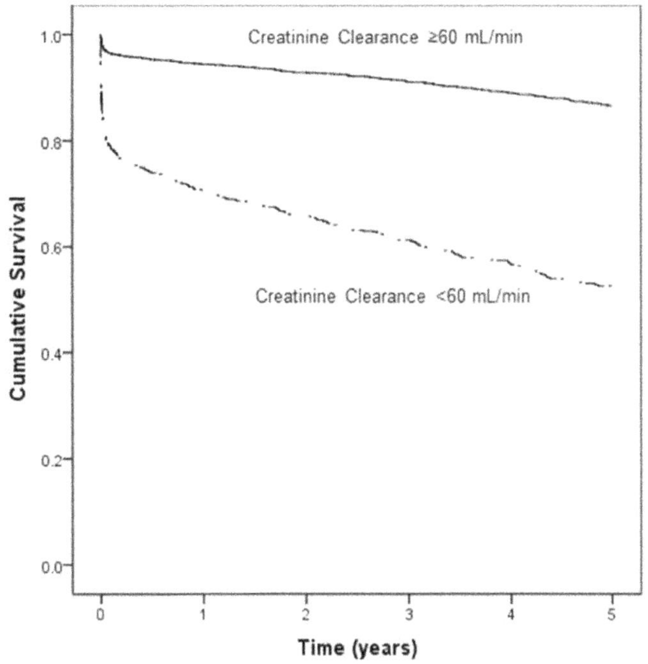

Number at risk	0 year	1 year	2 years	3 years	4 years	5 years
CrCl ≥ 60	3,218	2,678	2,269	1,843	1,392	1,016
CrCl < 60	898	588	494	395	295	206

Figure 2 Kaplan-Meier curves for all-cause mortality in patients with CrCl < 60 mL/min per 1.73 m^2 and CrCl ≥ 60 mL/min per 1.73 m^2.

study population when stratified into two groups with CrCl < 60 mL/min per 1.73 m^2 and CrCl ≥ 60 mL/min per 1.73 m^2 respectively.

Among patients with RI (group 1: CrCl <30 mL/min per 1.73 m^2 and group 2: CrCl ≤30 < 60 mL/min per 1.73 m^2) the all-cause mortality rates were: at 30-day, 40.9% (n = 36) group 1 vs. 18.8% (n = 152) group 2 (log rank $p < 0.001$); at 1-year, 57.5% (n = 50) group 1 vs. 26.4% (n = 212) group 2 (log rank $p < 0.001$) and at 5-year, 71.3% (n = 58) group 1 and 44.8% (n = 321) group 2 (log rank $p < 0.001$). Figure 3 shows the 5-year all-cause survival of STEMI patients when stratified into three groups based on CrCl.

Table 3 shows the crude HR associated with 1-year mortality. CrCl < 60 mL/min, diabetes, hypertension, previous myocardial infarction and increasing Killip class were associated with an increased mortality. Male gender and treatment with glycoprotein IIb/IIIa receptor blocker were associated with a lower mortality.

After adjustment for potential confounders (Table 3) we found CrCl, diabetes, age, hypertension and Killip class to be associated with increased 1-year mortality. After adjustment for covariates associated with mortality, RI was associated with increased mortality at 30-day (adjusted HR 2.38, 95% CI 1.34-4.21), 1-year (adjusted HR 2.29, 95% CI 1.50-3.50) and 5-year mortality (adjusted HR 2.02, 95% CI 1.50-2.72) compared to patients with preserved kidney function.

Discussion

Based on an unselected cohort of STEMI patients this study aimed to explore the impact of renal disease on all-cause mortality among 4,116 STEMI patients treated with primary PCI. In this real-world setting we found, that RI was associated with increased short- and long-term mortality. The strength of the present study is that the patients are unselected, all-comer and consecutive. Today guidelines suggest, that patients with STEMI and renal dysfunction is treated in the same way as other STEMI patients with the exception of administration of contrast dye and some medications [11]. However, as primary PCI in STEMI patients is an emergent therapy; neither the kidney function nor the creatinine clearance level will be known in these patients at the time of the primary PCI. In our registry, most of the patients were diagnosed prehospital in the ambulance and referred directly to the catheterization laboratory, where the first blood sample was collected from the arterial sheath

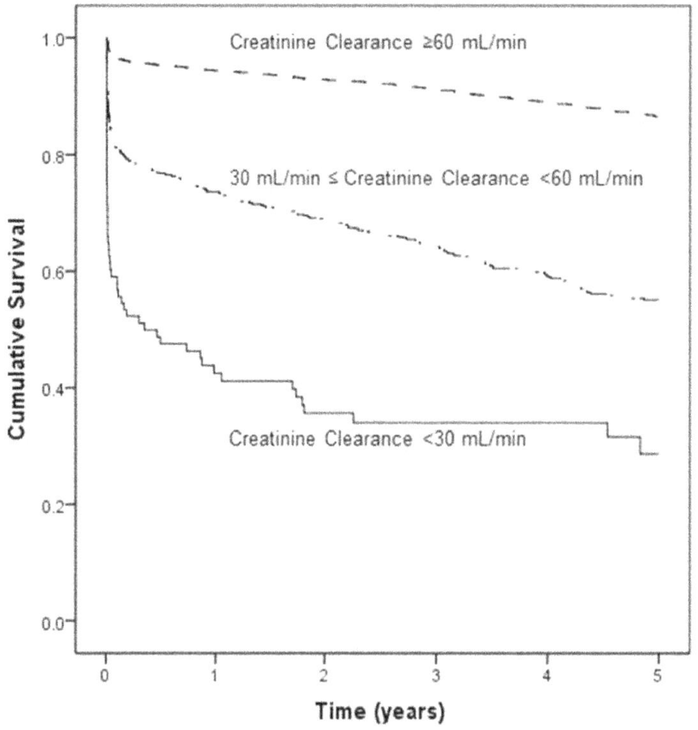

Number at risk

	0 years	1 year	2 years	3 years	4 years	5 years
CrCl≥60	3,218	2,678	2,269	1,843	1,392	1,016
30≤CrCl<60	810	556	469	375	281	199
CrCl<30	88	32	25	20	14	7

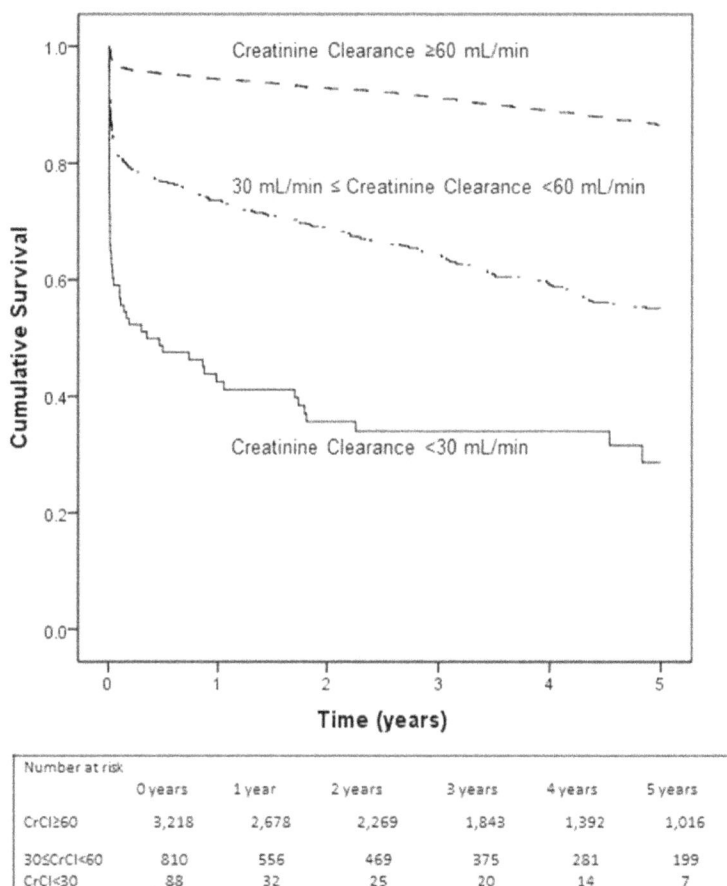

Figure 3 Kaplan-Meier curves for all-cause mortality in patients with CrCl <30 mL/min per 1.73 m^2 vs. CrCl ≤30 < 60 mL/min per 1.73 m^2 and CrCl ≥60 mL/min per 1.73 m^2.

before contrast injection. In a recent study Fox et al. [12] showed from the Acute Coronary Treatment and Intervention Outcome Network (ACTION) registry, that one third of patients with STEMI had an eGFR < 60 mL/min per 1.73 m^2. This is a higher number than the 22% of patients with RI we found in our study, which may be related to the patient population, as patients in the ACTION registry had a different comorbidity risk, as the rate of diabetes mellitus and hypertension were 2 to 3 times higher in the ACTION registry compared to our registry data. In contrast to our study, Fox et al. described that information about kidney function were available to the treating physicians when therapeutic decisions were made, and only 90% of patients with STEMI received reperfusion therapy (80% as primary PCI and 10% were treated with fibrinolysis). In our study patients with RI were more likely to receive primary PCI without stent implantation and less likely to receive treatment with glycoprotein IIb/IIIa receptor blocker compared to patients without RI. Among 2,597 STEMI and non-STEMI patients Medi et al. [21] found, that patients with RI and comorbidity were less likely to undergo coronary angiography, despite having the same frequency of primary PCI treatment as non-RI patients after angiography.

In our real-world setting registry we found, that RI was associated with increased short- and long-term mortality. This is in accordance with previous studies where RI also has been found to be associated with a higher 30-days mortality and long term mortality [22-25]. Seyfarth et al. [26] found an increase in adjusted hazard ratio after one year follow-up of 1.20 per 10-mL/min decrease in eGFR. In a study of Morel et al. [27] STEMI and non-STEMI patients were found to have a higher 9-month all-cause mortality when diagnosed with renal disease. Sadeghi et al. [28] studied 1,933 patients from the "Controlled Abciximab and Device Investigation to Lower Late Angioplasty Complications (CADILLAC)" trial, where baseline creatinine levels were obtained before angiography, including 350 patients with RI defined as CrCl < 60 mL/min per 1.73 m^2. In our registry cohort, both short-term and 1-year mortality rate was more than twice as high as in the study from Sadeghi et al. [28]. This difference is probably caused by (1) an increased

Table 3 crude and adjusted hazard ratio of covariates associated with 1-year mortality in Cox regression analysis

	Valid cases	Crude hazard ratio (95% CI)	*P* value	Adjusted hazard ratio (95% CI)	*P* value
Male gender	4,116	0.68 (0.56-0.83)	<0.001	1.11 (0.88-1.41)	0.354
Creatinine clearance	4,116		<0.001		<0.001
Creatinine clearance ≥ 60 mL/min		Reference		Reference	
Creatinine clearance ≤30 < 60 mL/min		5.31 (4.35-6.49)		2.71 (2.09-3.51)	
Creatinie clearance < 30 mL/min		15.37 (11.27-21.04)		7.09 (4.82-10.44)	
Age – years	4,116	1.07 (1.06-1.08)	<0.001	1.04 (1.03-1.06)	<0.001
Diabetes mellitus	4,116	2.47 (1.95-3.13)	<0.001	1.77 (1.33-2.35)	<0.001
Hypertension	4,047	1.26 (1.03-1.53)	0.025	1.40 (1.11-1.76)	0.004
Previous myocardial infarction	4,043	1.99 (1.57-2.53)	<0.001	1.53 (1.14-2.07)	0.006
Glycoprotein IIb/IIIa receptor blocker	3,826	0.49 (0.40-0.61)	<0.001	0.68 (0.53-0.86)	<0.001
Multivessel disease	4,011	2.32 (1.91-2.83)	<0.001	1.15 (0.90-1.46)	0.265
Infarct related artery	4,011		<0.001		0.023
Right coronary artery		Reference		Reference	
Left anterior descending artery		1.19 (0.96-1.48)		1.31 (1.03-1.68)	
Left circumflex artery		1.02 (0.74-1.40)		1.24 (0.88-1.74)	
Left main		4.02 (2.73-5.92)		1.92 (1.20-3.08)	
Killip class	4,030		<0.001		<0.001
I		Reference		Reference	
II		2.32 (1.64-3.30)		1.20 (1.20-2.69)	
III		4.54 (3.17-6.51)		1.68 (1.68-3.79)	
IV		9.55 (7.32-12.46)		1.86 (2.86-5.75)	
Duration of procedure - minutes	4,100	1.01 (1.01-1.02)	<0.001	1.01 (1.00-1.01)	0.007

mortality risk in non-randomized and all-comer patients compared to results from a randomized controlled study and (2) that patients with cardiogenic shock were not excluded in our study. Bertomeu-Gonzales et al. [29] studied the relationship between Killip class and impact of renal disease on mortality and found, that renal disease was stronger associated with mortality in STEMI patients with Killip I compared to patients with a higher Killip class. In our study, patients with RI were more likely to be older and female and they were more likely to have diabetes, hyperlipidemia, and hypertension. The finding of women representing a large proportion of STEMI patients with RI is consistent with findings from other studies [10,28,30,31]. RI was found to be an independent predictor of 1-year mortality whereas we did not find gender to be an independent risk factor for 1-year mortality when adjusted for confounders. Similar findings have been made by Damman et al. [32] where 3-year mortality was found to be associated with a decrease in renal function, whereas gender difference was not proven to be a predictor of mortality after adjustment for confounders.

Limitations

The validity of our findings depends on data quality and the ability to control for potential confounding. Like all observational studies, our study is prone to biases related to unmeasured factors. Bias due to unknown variables cannot be eliminated. Patients with cardiogenic shock were not excluded from the present study. We did not have systematically access to creatinine values taken in the following days after the primary PCI or information about contrast-induced nephropathy. Patients with RI were more often treated with balloon dilatation without stent implantation or bare metal stent. One explanation for this treatment strategy may be related to the more common finding of severely calcified lesions, which are known to limit complete DES expansion. We also lacked data on causes of mortality, however, in a previous STEMI cohort from Western Denmark Heart Registry, we found that especially the early causes of death was caused by a cardiac reason: the 1-year mortality reason was cardiac in 75% of the patients, whereas the 3-year mortality reason is cardiac death in 60% of the patients [33].

Conclusion

In unselected STEMI patients treated with primary PCI, RI was associated with increased short- and long-term mortality compared to patients with a preserved kidney function.

Competing interests

The authors declare that they have no competing interests.

Authors' contributions

JES and LOJ designed the study and were responsible for data management and for design and implementation of the statistical analysis. All other authors enrolled patients or contributed to data collection. JES and LOJ drafted the report, which was subsequently reviewed by all authors. All authors have seen the final submitted report and agree with its contents.

References

1. Mendis S: **Cardiovascular risk assessment and management in developing countries.** *Vasc Health Risk Manag* 2005, **1**:15–18.
2. Ichikawa K, Konta T, Ikeda A, Fujimoto S, Iseki K, Moriyama T, Yamagata K, Tsuruya K, Yoshida H, Asahi K, Kurahashi I, Ohashi Y, Watanabe T: **Significance of past history of renal failure for the detection of high-risk individuals for cardiovascular and end-stage renal disease: analysis of data from a nationwide health checkup.** *Clin Exp Nephrol* 2011, **15**:841–847.
3. Furuhashi T, Moroi M, Joki N, Hase H, Masai H, Kunimasa T, Nakazato R, Fukuda H, Sugi K: **The impact of chronic kidney disease as a predictor of major cardiac events in patients with no evidence of coronary artery disease.** *J Cardiol* 2010, **55**:328–336.
4. Go AS, Chertow GM, Fan D, McCulloch CE, Hsu CY: **Chronic kidney disease and the risks of death, cardiovascular events, and hospitalization.** *N Engl J Med* 2004, **351**:1296–1305.
5. Meisinger C, Doring A, Lowel H: **Chronic kidney disease and risk of incident myocardial infarction and all-cause and cardiovascular disease mortality in middle-aged men and women from the general population.** *Eur Heart J* 2006, **27**:1245–1250.
6. Manjunath G, Tighiouart H, Ibrahim H, Macleod B, Salem DN, Griffith JL, Coresh J, Levey AS, Sarnak MJ: **Level of kidney function as a risk factor for atherosclerotic cardiovascular outcomes in the community.** *J Am Coll Cardiol* 2003, **41**:47–55.
7. Levey AS, Coresh J, Balk E, Kausz AT, Levin A, Steffes MW, Hogg RJ, Perrone RD, Lau J, Eknoyan G, National Kidney F.: **National kidney foundation practice guidelines for chronic kidney disease: evaluation, classification, and stratification.** *Ann Intern Med* 2003, **139**:137–147.
8. Wright RS, Reeder GS, Herzog CA, Albright RC, Williams BA, Dvorak DL, Miller WL, Murphy JG, Kopecky SL, Jaffe AS: **Acute myocardial infarction and renal dysfunction: a high-risk combination.** *Ann Intern Med* 2002, **137**:563–570.
9. Menon V, Sarnak MJ, Lessard D, Goldberg RJ: **Recent trends in hospital management practices and prognosis after acute myocardial infarction in patients with kidney disease.** *Am J Cardiol* 2004, **94**:1290–1293.
10. Seyfarth M, Kastrati A, Mann JF, Ndrepepa G, Byrne RA, Schulz S, Mehilli J, Schomig A: **Prognostic value of kidney function in patients with st-elevation and non-st-elevation acute myocardial infarction treated with percutaneous coronary intervention.** *Am J Kidney Dis* 2009, **54**:830–839.
11. Steg PG, James SK, Atar D, Badano LP, Blömstrom-Lundqvist C, Borger MA, Di Mario C, Dickstein K, Ducrocq G, Fernandez-Aviles F, Gershlick AH, Giannuzzi P, Halvorsen S, Huber K, Juni P, Kastrati A, Knuuti J, Lenzen MJ, Mahaffey KW, Valgimigli M, van 't Hof A, Widimsky P, Zahger D: **Task Force on the management of ST-segment elevation acute myocardial infarction of the European Society of Cardiology (ESC).** *Eur Heart J* 2012, **33**:2569–2619.
12. Fox CS, Muntner P, Chen AY, Alexander KP, Roe MT, Cannon CP, Saucedo JF, Kontos MC, Wiviott SD: **Use of evidence-based therapies in short-term outcomes of st-segment elevation myocardial infarction and non-st-segment elevation myocardial infarction in patients with chronic kidney disease: a report from the national cardiovascular data acute coronary treatment and intervention outcomes network registry.** *Circulation* 2010, **121**:357–365.
13. Andersen HR, Nielsen TT, Rasmussen K, Thuesen L, Kelbaek H, Thayssen P, Abildgaard U, Pedersen F, Madsen JK, Grande P, Villadsen AB, Krusell LR, Haghfelt T, Lomholt P, Husted SE, Vigholt E, Kjaergard HK, Mortensen L: **A comparison of coronary angioplasty with fibrinolytic therapy in acute myocardial infarction.** *N Engl J Med* 2003, **349**:733–742.
14. Jensen LO, Maeng M, Kaltoft A, Thayssen P, Hansen HH, Bottcher M, Lassen JF, Krussel LR, Rasmussen K, Hansen KN, Pedersen L, Johnsen SP, Soerensen HT, Thuesen L: **Stent thrombosis, myocardial infarction, and death after drug-eluting and bare-metal stent coronary interventions.** *J Am Coll Cardiol* 2007, **50**:463–470.
15. Michels WM, Grootendorst DC, Verduijn M, Elliott EG, Dekker FW, Krediet RT: **Performance of the cockcroft-gault, mdrd, and new ckd-epi formulas in relation to gfr, age, and body size.** *Clin J Am Soc Nephrol* 2010, **5**:1003–1009.
16. Rigalleau V, Lasseur C, Perlemoine C, Barthe N, Raffaitin C, Chauveau P, Combe C, Gin H: **Cockcroft-gault formula is biased by body weight in diabetic patients with renal impairment.** *Metabolism* 2006, **55**:108–112.
17. Fesler P, Mimran A: **Estimation of glomerular filtration rate: what are the pitfalls?** *Curr Hypertens Rep* 2011, **13**:116–121.
18. Hallan S, Asberg A, Lindberg M, Johnsen H: **Validation of the modification of diet in renal disease formula for estimating gfr with special emphasis on calibration of the serum creatinine assay.** *Am J Kidney Dis* 2004, **44**:84–93.
19. Pedersen CB, Gotzsche H, Moller JO, Mortensen PB: **The danish civil registration system. A cohort of eight million persons.** *Dan Med Bull* 2006, **53**:441–449.
20. Epidemiology FL: **When an entire country is a cohort.** *Science* 2000, **287**:2398–2399.
21. Medi C, Chew DP, Amerena J, Coverdale S, Soman A, Astley C, Rankin J, Brieger D: **An invasive management strategy is associated with improved outcomes in high-risk acute coronary syndromes in patients with chronic kidney disease.** *Intern Med J* 2011, **41**:743–750.
22. Campbell NG, Varagunam M, Sawhney V, Ahuja KR, Salahuddin N, De PR, Rothman MT, Wragg A, Yaqoob MM, Knight CJ: **Mild chronic kidney disease is an independent predictor of long-term mortality after emergency angiography and primary percutaneous intervention in patients with st-elevation myocardial infarction.** *Heart* 2012, **98**:42–47.
23. Gibson CM, Pinto DS, Murphy SA, Morrow DA, Hobbach HP, Wiviott SD, Giugliano RP, Cannon CP, Antman EM, Braunwald E: **Association of creatinine and creatinine clearance on presentation in acute myocardial infarction with subsequent mortality.** *J Am Coll Cardiol* 2003, **42**:1535–1543.
24. Wilson WM, Andrianopoulos N, Clark D, Duffy SJ, Brennan A, Harries I, New G, Sebastian M, Loane P, Reid C, Ajani AE: **Long-term predictors of mortality after percutaneous coronary intervention in the era of drug-eluting stents.** *Am J Cardiol* 2011, **108**:936–942.
25. de Mulder M, van der Ploeg T, de Waard GA, Boersma E, Umans VA: **Admission glucose does not improve grace score at 6 months and 5 years after myocardial infarction.** *Cardiology* 2011, **120**:227–234.
26. Pinkau T, Mann JF, Ndrepepa G, Mehilli J, Hadamitzky M, Braun S, Kastrati A, Schomig A: **Coronary revascularization in patients with renal insufficiency: restenosis rate and cardiovascular outcomes.** *Am J Kidney Dis* 2004, **44**:627–635.
27. Morel O, El GS, Jesel L, Radulescu B, Meyer N, Wiesel ML, Caillard S, Campia U, Moulin B, Gachet C, Ohlmann P: **Cardiovascular mortality in chronic kidney disease patients undergoing percutaneous coronary intervention is mainly related to impaired p2y12 inhibition by clopidogrel.** *J Am Coll Cardiol* 2011, **57**:399–408.
28. Sadeghi HM, Stone GW, Grines CL, Mehran R, Dixon SR, Lansky AJ, Fahy M, Cox DA, Garcia E, Tcheng JE, Griffin JJ, Stuckey TD, Turco M, Carroll JD: **Impact of renal insufficiency in patients undergoing primary angioplasty for acute myocardial infarction.** *Circulation* 2003, **108**:2769–2775.
29. Bertomeu-Gonzalez V, Nunez J, Nunez E, Facila L, Sanchis J, Bodi V, Pellicer M, Bosch MJ, Martinez A, Chorro FJ, Llacer A: **Prognostic effect of renal dysfunction after st-segment elevation myocardial infarction with and without heart failure.** *Int J Cardiol* 2006, **112**:159–165.
30. Heer T, Schiele R, Schneider S, Gitt AK, Wienbergen H, Gottwik M, Gieseler U, Voigtlander T, Hauptmann KE, Wagner S, Senges J: **Gender differences in acute myocardial infarction in the era of reperfusion (the mitra registry).** *Am J Cardiol* 2002, **89**:511–517.

2

Impact of impaired fractional flow reserve after coronary interventions on outcomes

Mathias Wolfrum[1†], Gregor Fahrni[1†], Giovanni Luigi de Maria[1], Guido Knapp[2], Nick Curzen[3], Rajesh K. Kharbanda[1], Georg M. Fröhlich[4] and Adrian P. Banning[1*]

Abstract

Background: FFR is routinely used to guide percutaneous coronary interventions (PCI). Visual assessment of the angiographic result after PCI has limited efficacy. Even when the angiographic result seems satisfactory FFR after a PCI might be useful for identifying patients with a suboptimal interventional result and higher risk for poor clinical outcome who might benefit from additional procedures. The aim of this meta-analysis was to investigate available data of studies that examined clinical outcomes of patients with impaired vs. satisfactory fractional flow reserve (FFR) after percutaneous coronary interventions (PCI).

Methods: This meta-analysis was carried out according to the Cochrane Handbook for Systematic Reviews. The Mantel-Haenszel method using the fixed-effect meta-analysis model was used for combining the results. Studies were identified by searching the literature through mid-January, 2016, using the following search terms: fractional flow reserve, coronary circulation, after, percutaneous coronary intervention, balloon angioplasty, stent implantation, and stenting. Primary endpoint was the rate of major adverse cardiac events (MACE). Secondary endpoints included rates of death, myocardial infarction (MI), repeated revascularisation.

Results: Eight relevant studies were found including a total of 1337 patients. Of those, 492 (36.8 %) had an impaired FFR after PCI, and 853 (63.2 %) had a satisfactory FFR after PCI. Odds ratios indicated that a low FFR following PCI was associated with an impaired outcome: major adverse cardiac events (MACE, OR: 4.95, 95 % confidence interval [CI]: 3.39–7.22, p <0.001); death (OR: 3.23, 95 % CI: 1.19–8.76, $p = 0.022$); myocardial infarction (OR: 13.83, 95 % CI: 4.75–40.24, p <0.0001) and repeated revascularisation (OR: 4.42, 95 % CI: 2.73–7.15, p <0.0001).

Conclusions: Compared to a satisfactory FFR, a persistently low FFR following PCI is associated with a worse clinical outcome. Prospective studies are needed to identify underlying causes, determine an optimal threshold for post-PCI FFR, and clarify whether simple additional procedures can influence the post-PCI FFR and clinical outcome.

Keywords: Coronary artery disease, Percutaneous coronary interventions, Fractional flow reserve, Intracoronary imaging, Outcome, Meta-analysis

Abbreviations: ACS, Acute coronary syndrome; AUC, Area under curve; BMS, Bare metal stent; CAD, Coronary artery disease; CI, Confidence interval; DES, Drug eluting stent; FFR, Fractional flow reserve; iFR, Instantaneous wave-free ratio; IVUS, Intravascular ultrasound; MACE, Major adverse cardiac events; MSA, Minimal stent area; OCT, Optical coherence tomography; PCI, Percutaneous coronary intervention; POBA, Plain old balloon angioplasty; ROC, Receiver operating characteristic curve; TLR, Target lesion revascularisation; TVF, Target vessel failure; TVR, Target vessel revascularisation

* Correspondence: adrian.banning@ouh.nhs.uk
†Equal contributors
[1]Oxford Heart Centre, Oxford University Hospitals, Headley Way, Oxford OX39DU, UK
Full list of author information is available at the end of the article

Background

Fractional flow reserve (FFR) is the established gold standard used in the cardiac catheterisation laboratory to assess the ischemic burden associated with an atheromatous lesion of the coronary arteries. Evidence from various clinical scenarios has shown that an FFR-guided PCI strategy reduces the need for stenting and improves clinical outcomes. Therefore, FFR has been incorporated in current revascularisation guidelines [1–3]. With improved wire technology, it is increasingly cost effective and time-saving to use the pressure wire for diagnosis and as the platform for any subsequent PCI [4]. Nevertheless, post-PCI FFR measurement has not yet become part of established clinical practice and only a minority of operators (22 %) consider FFR to evaluate the post-stenting result [5].

Visual assessment, by angiography and quantitative coronary angiography (QCA), has limited efficacy with respect to identifying patients with suboptimal PCI results and subsequent worse clinical outcomes [6, 7]. Even with an angiographic satisfactory result after PCI 19–32 % of these patients experience an adverse cardiovascular event during a 2-year follow-up [8]. Post-PCI FFR measurement might be a useful indicator for the identification of a suboptimal PCI result and, if so, would be beneficial to both operator and patient. Of note, a recent small prospective interventional study provides evidence that the post-PCI FFR helps to identify patients that might benefit from further optimisation procedures in order to improve clinical outcome [9].

However, the value of post-PCI FFR might be confounded by several factors, such as gender [10] and comorbidities [11]. The subsequent cut-off for a satisfactory post-PCI FFR might differ among patient populations. As the clinical impact of post-PCI FFR has not been determined in larger scale trials this meta-analysis was setup to examine existing data pertaining to post-PCI FFR measurement and its association with clinical outcome.

Methods

This study was carried according to current recommendations of the Cochrane Handbook for Systematic Reviews and the Meta-analysis of Observational Studies in Epidemiology recommendations (MOOSE checklist, Additional file 1: Table S1) [12]. Two authors (MW, GF) planned and designed this meta-analysis evaluating the association between FFR post PCI and clinical outcomes and created an electronic database with variables of interest.

Search strategy

Medline, BIOS, and ISI Web of Science databases were searched through January 14, 2016. Additionally, editorials and web-based information sources (http://www.tctmd.com, http://www.theheart.org, http://www.europcronline.com, http://www.cardiosource.com, and http://www.crtonline.com) were screened. The following search terms were used: fractional flow reserve, coronary circulation, after, percutaneous coronary intervention, balloon angioplasty, stent implantation, and stenting. Reference lists of the selected articles were checked for other relevant citations. A more detailed search strategy for Medline can be found in the Additional file 1: Table S2.

Study selection

Studies included in the meta-analysis were published in full text and in English. Only studies where it was possible to clearly categorise patients into groups with low and high post-PCI FFR were included. Two authors (MW, GF) independently identified appropriate articles. Disagreements were discussed, and a third author (GMF) was consulted in unclear cases. All included studies were approved by the local ethics committees and were in compliance with the Helsinki Declaration.

Data extraction and quality assessment

Relevant information from each study, retrieved using a dedicated standardised database, included study design, baseline clinical characteristics of the study population, and clinical outcomes. Study quality was ascertained according to the Cochrane Handbook [12], but without using a quality score, due to the limitations associated with this approach [13].

Endpoints and definitions

Primary endpoint was the rate of major adverse cardiac events (MACE) at longest follow-up. MACE was defined according to the individual study (Table 1). Secondary endpoints included rates of death, myocardial infarction (MI), repeated revascularisation (repeated PCI, target vessel revascularisation [TVR], target lesion revascularisation [TLR] and CABG) and in-stent restenosis.

Data synthesis and analysis

Odds ratio and 95 % confidence intervals (CIs) for binary outcomes were calculated. Since we mostly deal with rare events, Mantel-Haenszel method was used for combining the results [14]. The method can include single-zero and double-zeroes studies. The fixed-effect meta-analysis model was used as no relevant between-study variance was observed (see Additional file 1: Table S3). Weighted incidence of events is presented for both groups calculated according to random-effects meta-analysis for proportions with the Knapp-Hartung adjustment [14, 15]. Given the limitations for the assessment of publication bias in meta-analysis with a small study number using Funnel plots the Egger's test and Begg's rank correlation test were applied (Additional file 1: Table S4) [16, 17].

Sensitivity analyses excluded the study by Bech et al. [18], which used only plain old balloon angioplasty (POBA)

Table 1 Characteristics of included studies

First author, year of publication	Design	Indication for PCI	PCI technique	Cut-off for low FFR - group	FFR technique		Definition of MACE
					Adenosine	Pressure wire pullback	
Bech *et al.*, [18]	Retrospective	Stable angina	POBA	<0.9	i.v.	NA	MACE (death, MI, recurrent angina, CABG, repeated PTCA)
Pijls *et al.*, [31]	Prospective, observational	All comers	"stent" (type NA)	≤ 0.9	i.v. or i.c.	No	MACE (death, MI, CABG, TVR)
Klauss *et al.*, [30]	Retrospective	Stable angina	BMS	< 0.95	i.c.	Not mandatory	MACE (death, MI, TVR)
Nam *et al.*, [19]	Retrospective	2/3 ACS, 1/3 stable angina	DES	≤ 0.9	i.c.	No	MACE (death, MI, TVR)
Leesar *et al.*, [9]	Prospective, interventional	Stable angina	DES > BMS	< 0.96	i.c.	No	MACE (death, MI, TLR)
Ito *et al.*, [23]	Retrospective	92 % stable angina, 8 % unstable angina	DES plus IVUS	≤ 0.9	i.c.	No	MACE (cardiac death, MI, TVR, stent thrombosis)
Reith *et al.*, [24]	Prospective, observational	Stable angina	DES > BMS plus OCT	≤ 0.905	i.c.	No	MACE (death, MI, TLR)
Doh *et al.*, [22]	Prospective, observational	1/3 ACS, 2/3 stable angina	DES plus IVUS	< 0.89	i.v. or i.c.	Not mandatory	TVF (death and MI attributed to target vessel, TVR)

Abbreviations: *ACS* acute coronary syndrome, *AUC* area under curve, *BMS* bare metal stent, *CABG* coronary artery bypass graft, *CI* confidence interval, *DES* drug eluting stent, *i.c.* intracoronary, *i.v.* intravenous, *IVUS* intravascular ultrasound, *FFR* fractional flow reserve, *FU* follow up, *MACE* major adverse cardiac events, *MI* myocardial infarction, *Mo* months, *N* patient number, *NA* not applicable, *OCT* optical coherence tomography, *TLR* target lesion revascularisation, *TVF* target vessel failure, *TVR* target vessel revascularisation, *PCI* percutaneous coronary intervention, *POBA* plain old balloon angioplasty

for the endpoints. Because a post-PCI FFR <0.9 has been identified as an optimal predictor of a worse clinical outcome [19], one analysis considered only studies with an FFR cut-off of 0.9 between low and high FFR groups. All meta-analyses were carried out using the package metafor in the statistical software package R, version 3.2.3 [20, 21].

Results

Included studies

A total of eight studies with 1337 patients met our inclusion criteria: four prospective studies (983 patients) and four retrospective studies (354 patients), published between 1999 and 2015 (Fig. 1). Study and population characteristics are presented in Tables 1 and 2.

Main outcomes

MACE

MACE rate was defined (Table 1) and reported by all included studies. The overall weighted incidence for MACE was 21.4 (95 % CI: 17.0–25.8 %) in the low FFR group and 5.0 (95 % CI: 3.5–6.4 %) in the high FFR group (Fig. 2a). A low FFR after PCI was associated with significantly higher odds for MACE (OR: 4.95, 95 % CI: 3.39–7.22, p <0.001).

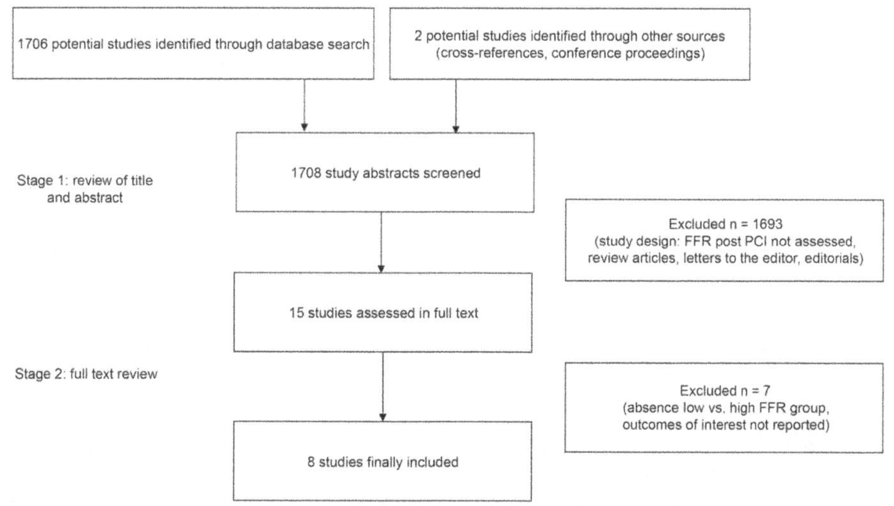

Fig. 1 Study selection process. FFR - fractional flow reserve, PCI - percutaneous coronary intervention

Table 2 Patient characteristics

	Bech *et al.*		Pijls *et al.*		Klauss *et al.*		Nam *et al.*		Leesar *et al.*		Ito *et al.*		Reith *et al.*		Doh *et al.*		Combined	
FFR group	Low	High	Low	High	Low	High	Low	High	Low	High	Low	High	Low	High	Low	High	Low	High
N	32	26	237	507	53	66	40	40	31	35	53	44	26	40	20	95	492	853
Age (years) (SD)	61.5		62 (11)		62 (10)		62 (10)	63 (8)	63 (11)	60 (12)	71 (9)		69 (10)	69 (10)	64 (9)		65 (4) 64 (4)	64 (4)
Male (%)	69		NA		75		78	70	77	70	75		88	75	83		80 77	77
HTN (%)	33		51		79		58	43	68	94	92		65	88	82		63 61	74
Diabetes (%)	17		24		26		20	8	32	23	37		58	53	51		34 28	28
HC (%)	31		61		83		10	15	58	74	85		54	60	68		37 61	49
Smoking (%)	24		48		38		28	48	32	46	54		15	23	30		26 41	38
FHx (%)	41		38		38		NA		NA		NA		39	63	NA		40	
Prior MI (%)	17		NA		56		10	13	NA		NA		NA		5.6		25	
MVD (%)	NA		NA		67		63	60	NA		NA		73	68	63		67 65	64
LAD (%)	66		52		39		83	55	39	34	56		NA		100	71	71 54	59
Complex lesion[a] (%)	NA		NA		65		90	78	NA		NA		NA		95	67	92 72	70
FU (months)	24		6		6		12		24		18		20		23		16	

Separate data provided for low FFR group and high FFR group if available from respective study, otherwise overall value

Abbreviations: *FHx* family history, *FFR* fractional flow reserve, *FU* follow up, *HC* hypercholesterolemia, *HTN* Hypertension, *LAD* left anterior descending artery, *MI* myocardial infarction, *MVD* multi-vessel-disease, *N* patient number, *SD* standard deviation

[a]Complex lesion is defined as B2 or C category according to American College of Cardiology/American Heart Association (ACC/AHA) lesion classification

Death

Overall rate of death was reported by seven studies involving 1230 patients. The weighted incidence for overall death was 1.7 % (95 % CI: 0.6–2.9 %) in the low FFR group and 0.8 % (95 % CI: 0.0–1.7 %) in the high FFR group (Fig. 2b). A low FFR after PCI was associated with significantly higher risk of death (OR: 3.23, 95 % CI: 1.19–8.76, $p = 0.022$).

Myocardial infarction

The event rate for MI was reported by all included studies. The weighted incidence for MI was 3.3 (95 % CI: 1.1–5.6 %) in the low FFR group and 0.8 % (95 % CI: 0.2–1.4 %) in the high FFR group (Fig. 2c). A low FFR after PCI was associated with significantly higher risk of MI during follow-up (OR: 13.83, 95 % CI: 4.75–40.24, $p < 0.0001$).

Repeated revascularisation

Data for repeated revascularisation was available for repeated PCI from three studies, and for CABG from 5 studies. There was an increased risk for repeated revascularisation for patients in the low FFR group, compared to patients in the high FFR group (OR: 4.42, 95 % CI: 2.73–7.15, $p < 0.0001$, Fig. 2d): repeated PCI (OR: 3.81, 95 % CI: 2.26–6.43, $p < 0.0001$), CABG (OR: 6.35, 95 % CI: 1.96–20.54, $p = 0.002$,). Four studies included data about TVR [9, 19, 22, 23], and two studies about TLR [9, 24], and these indicated that the risk for both endpoints was higher for patients with impaired FFR after PCI: TVR (OR: 3.40, 95 % CI: 1.44–8.03, $p = 0.005$), TLR (OR: 5.48, 95 % CI: 1.12–26.78, $p = 0.036$). Two studies reported the rate of in-stent restenosis [9, 19]. The weighted incidence for in-stent restenosis was 16.9 % (95 % CI: 8.2–25.6 %) in the low FFR group and 3.4 % (95 % CI: 0.0–7.5 %) in the high FFR group. A low FFR after PCI was associated with significantly higher risk of in-stent restenosis (OR: 4.93, 95 % CI: 1.32–18.37, $p = 0.018$).

Sensitivity analysis

After excluding the study by Bech et al. [18], the results still demonstrated that patients with a low post-PCI FFR

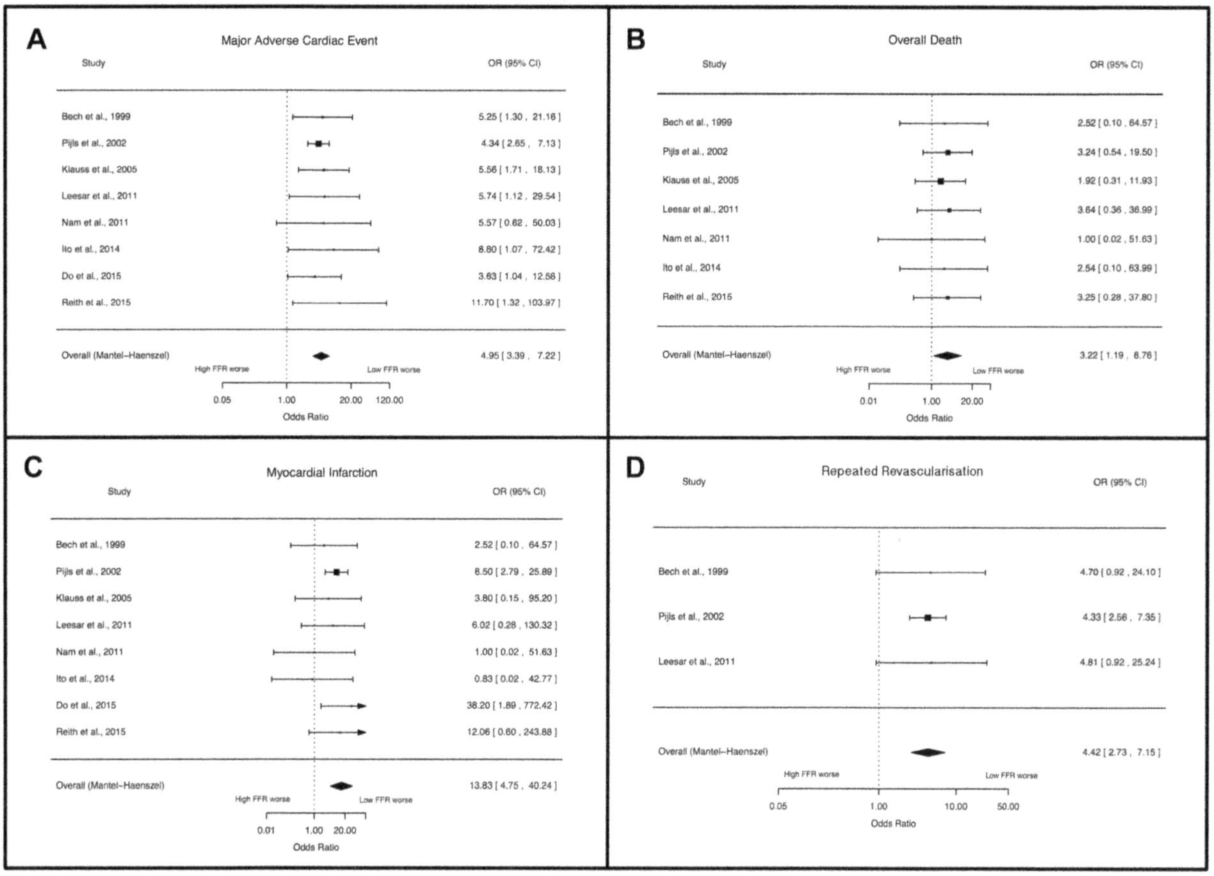

Fig. 2 Forest plots of odds ratios (OR) for major adverse cardiac events (MACE, Panel **a**), death (Panel **b**), myocardial infarction (Panel **c**) and repeated revascularisation (Panel **d**). Markers represent point estimates of odds ratios, marker size represents study weight. *Horizontal bars* indicate 95 % confidence intervals (CI). FFR - fractional flow reserve

had a significantly higher risk for all main outcomes than patients in the high FFR group (Additional file 1: Figure S1): MACE (OR: 4.93, 95 % CI: 3.33–7.29, $p < 0.0001$), death (OR: 3.03, 95 % CI: 1.11–8.28, $p = 0.03$), MI (OR: 13.45, 95 % CI: 4.63–39.05, $p < 0.0001$) and repeated PCI (OR: 3.96, 95 % CI: 2.29–6.85, $p < 0.0001$). When only studies with an FFR cut-off of 0.9 were included (Additional file 1: Figure S2), the results showed that patients in the low FFR group had significantly higher risk than the high FFR group for MACE (OR: 4.92, 95 % CI: 3.11–7.78, $p < 0.0001$), myocardial infarction (OR: 10.02, 95 % CI: 3.33–30.12, $p < 0.0001$), and a statistical trend towards higher risk for overall death (OR: 3.70, 95 % CI: 0.89–15.43, $p = 0.073$). Other endpoints were not included in this analysis, as the number of appropriate studies was ≤ 2.

Discussion

Post-PCI FFR as an indicator of clinical outcome

Results of the meta-analysis reported herein, which included different clinical scenarios and data from different era of interventional cardiology, support the hypothesis that a persistently low FFR following PCI is associated with an adverse clinical outcome. We found that patients with an impaired post-PCI FFR had significantly increased risk for the primary endpoint of MACE, as well as for the secondary endpoints of death, myocardial infarction, and repeat revascularization (PCI and CABG). These results were not changed by the exclusion of data from one study that used only POBA [18], a technique known to convey a higher risk for MACE than stenting [25, 26].

Data supporting present findings of the primary endpoint of MACE comes from a study by Johnson et al. [27], which primarily studied the continuous relationship between pre-PCI FFR and clinical outcomes. A small sub-analysis of this study focused on FFR measured immediately after stenting and showed that low FFR is inversely correlated with subsequent adverse events in both continuous (Cox hazard ratio: 0.86, 95 % CI: 0.80–0.93; $P < 0.001$) and tertile (log- rank $P < 0.001$) analyses.

Causes of persistently low FFR after PCI

A number of factors can cause a post-PCI pressure drop over a treated epicardial segment, eventually leading to an impaired FFR, including incomplete stent expansion, stent malapposition, "geographical miss," plaque protrusion, edge dissection, and plaque shift at the stent edge (Fig. 3).

The pathophysiological concept is explained by the Hagen-Poiseuille law (e.g. if malapposition or plaque protrusion is present): the pressure loss is caused by viscous friction along a treated segment. Additionally, e.g. if incomplete stent-expansion or geographical miss is considered the Bernoulli's law can be applied. In this scenario residual narrowing leads to a conversion of pressure into kinetic energy. As a substantial amount of energy is lost due to the presence of turbulent flow not the entire coronary pressure can be recovered at the exit of the target lesion. Even without a significant narrowing a suboptimal PCI result can cause turbulent flow within and beyond the treated coronary segment (stent malapposition, plaque protrusion, edge dissection, plaque shift at the stent edge), especially during the hyperaemic phase of FFR assessment, when high flow rates of blood are induced. The switch from laminar to turbulent flow results in the formation of eddies and a dramatic increase in flow resistance, leading to a pressure drop downstream from the treated coronary segment. The total pressure loss during hyperaemia causes the impaired FFR.

The first study to establish a link between a persistent pressure gradient and a suboptimal stent result was published by Hanekamp et al., who used quantitative coronary angiography, intravascular ultrasound, and coronary pressure measurement to assess deployment of coil stents [28]. They found a close relationship between poor PCI results, such as stent underexpansion and/or malapposition, and suboptimal stent symmetry, and in-stent gradients. Another study using slotted-tube stents found that a post-stent FFR <0.96 predicted a suboptimal stent result identified by IVUS [29]. In 70 % of those patients, a low post-stent FFR was linked to incomplete stent expansion. Studies using drug eluting stents confirmed a substantial rate of under-expanded stents in patients with low post-stent FFR, despite reasonable angiographic results [22, 30]. One of these studies found that low post-stent FFR correlated with adverse clinical outcomes at three years [22].

A number of additional factors can affect the final results of stent implantation and account for the relationship between post-PCI FFR and clinical outcome. Ito et al. suggested a link between high residual plaque volume, identified by IVUS, and impaired post-stent FFR after DES implantation [23]. Patients with high residual plaque had a significantly higher rate of MACE after 18 months.

Lesion complexity may also affect the final result of stent-implantation. Two included studies of our meta-analysis reported a significant lower FFR in patients with complex lesions [19, 22]. In both studies a low FFR post PCI was associated with a significantly higher rates of MACE rates (Table 2). Stent dimensions were also reported to influence post-stent FFR and clinical outcome [19, 22, 31]. Stents with greater length or smaller diameter were significantly correlated with a low post-stent FFR and higher MACE rates. These observations might

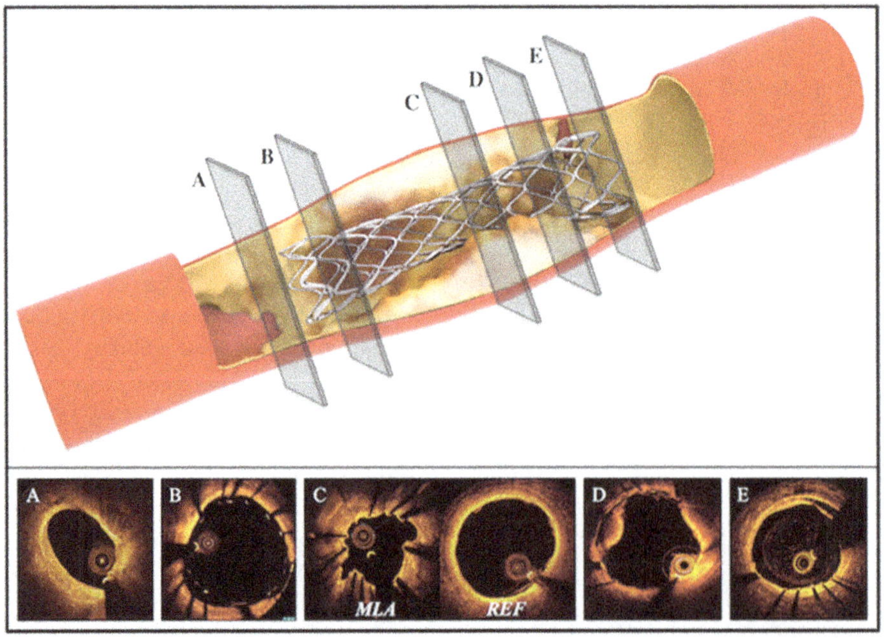

Fig. 3 Potential causes of suboptimal FFR after percutaneous coronary interventions. Panel **a** 'geographical miss' (diseased reference segment). Panel **b** stent mal-apposition. Panel **c** stent under-expansion. Panel **d** intrastent plaque-protrusion/thrombus. Panel **e** edge dissection. MLA - minimal lumen area, REF - proximal reference segment

help to explain the previously described association between these characteristics in BMS and DES procedures and higher subsequent event rates [32–34].

Variations in post-PCI FFR and ultimately outcome seem to be linked to different coronary arteries. A suboptimal post-stent FFR was more frequent in patients with a PCI to the left anterior descending (LAD) artery than to the right coronary artery or left circumflex [19, 22]. This finding presumably reflects the larger myocardial territory subtended by the LAD, leading to greater peak flow and lower post-stent FFR for any given residual stenosis in this vessel. Interestingly, in the aforementioned studies an impaired post-PCI FFR was associated with higher rate of MACE.

Potential clinical application of the results

Based on the results of our meta-analysis, use of a pressure wire to check the PCI result seems to be a promising concept, even after PCI with an apparently satisfactory angiographic result. Measurement of post-PCI FFR is especially appropriate when a pressure wire was used before PCI to guide the treatment strategy. If FFR remains low after PCI and a pressure wire pullback manoeuvre during maximal hyperaemia demonstrates a step increase of pressure within or close to the stent edges subsequent intravascular imaging might provide the ability to identify causes of suboptimal post-PCI FFR (Fig. 3). Based on the result of imaging, simple additional procedures could improve the interventional result. However, only one small previous study has prospectively examined whether additional interventions can reduce the risk of future MACE in patients with low post-PCI FFR [9]. Their results suggested that consistent postdilatation after coronary stenting in patients with a post-stent FFR ≥0.96 could achieve consequently favourable clinical outcomes in 53 % of patients.

In contrast, a continuous gradual reduction in FFR during pressure wire pullback manoeuvre along the course of the coronary artery suggests diffuse CAD. The observation of diffuse CAD may not be evident from an angiographic examination, but can lead to severely impaired FFR (<0.75), with myocardial ischemia and high rates of MACE [35]. For example, diffuse CAD is more common in patients with diabetes mellitus and, in these patients, is often associated with impaired post-stent FFR, despite an angiographically optimal PCI [36]. Thus, low post-stent FFR without a notable point of decrease could indicate advanced diffuse CAD, associated with a relatively high MACE rate. This is an important finding as further interventional optimisation of PCI is not a promising option for diffuse CAD and should be deferred. Patients with diffuse CAD might benefit from a stronger medical secondary prevention or from prolonged dual antiplatelet therapy. However, at current stage these strategies are only hypothetical and need validation in large scale randomised clinical trials.

Study limitations

Most of the studies included in the meta-analysis were retrospective or observational and, therefore, were subject to patient selection bias, lack of independent event adjudication, heterogeneity in event definitions, and differences in the duration of follow-up (Tables 1 and 2). With the exception of one large multicenter registry [31], most of the studies had small sample sizes, ranging from 60 to 119 patients. Most studies had no restrictions with regard to co-morbidities, which led to a generally heterogeneous patient population (Table 2).

The existing data on post-PCI FFR covers a wide range of coronary interventions, including POBA, BMS, and first and second generation DES (Table 1). Because different stent designs differentially affect blood flow and post-stent FFR, the results must be considered hypothesis-generating. Furthermore, induction of hyperaemic FFR was accomplished by intracoronary adenosine in the majority of trials, so the results cannot entirely be compared to cases using intravenous adenosine, especially in combination with pressure wire pullback.

Some of the studies included in the meta-analysis used different cut-off points to distinguish between low and high FFR groups. Therefore, we included a sensitivity analysis that considered only studies with an FFR cut-off of 0.9, the value identified as an optimal predictor for a worse clinical outcome following PCI [19]. The results demonstrated a significantly higher risk for patients in the low FFR group for MACE and myocardial infarction, and a trend towards a higher risk for overall death. However, prospective validation of this cut-off is an important future challenge. It is conceivable that the optimal cut-off will vary among different coronary arteries and different clinical scenarios, similar to results of FFR assessment before PCI [27].

Furthermore, current data provides evidence only for the use of conventional FFR. However, alternative modes of physiological assessment are promising such as the instantaneous wave-free ratio (iFR). iFR assess the severity of a coronary stenosis using a pressure wire without the need for potent vasodilators. This might be an advantage over FFR as it obviates the need for adenosine, which is contraindicated in some patients and could safe time and costs in the cathlab. Especially with the introduction of iFR pullback (iFR Scout™, Volcano Corporation, San Diego, California) it seems to be a promising concept for the assessment of the PCI result. However, no data exists on this topic yet and further research is strongly warranted.

Conclusion

Results of the meta-analysis presented herein provide evidence that a persistently low FFR following PCI is associated with an adverse clinical outcome. Prospective studies are warranted to determine an optimal threshold (or thresholds, in different scenarios) for post-PCI FFR. Observational studies using intra-coronary imaging, such as IVUS and OCT, have suggested different underlying causes for a suboptimal FFR. Large prospective studies are needed to confirm that these are the responsible mechanisms and to examine whether additional simple procedures can influence post-stent FFR and potentially improve clinical outcome.

Acknowledgements
Not applicable.

Funding
GF was supported by fellowship grants from the Bangerter- Rhyner-Stiftung, Freiwillige Akademische Gesellschaft Basel, and NIHR Oxford Biomedical Research Centre.

Authors' contributions
AB, NC and MW had the original idea for the study. The protocol was designed and refined by AB, NC, RK, MW, GMF and GM. The literature search and data collection was performed by MW, GF and GMF. GK led the statistical analysis. All authors contributed to the interpretation of the data. MW and GF wrote the initial draft of the manuscript. All authors contributed to this paper significantly and approved the final version of the manuscript.

Competing interests
Professor Banning has received an unrestricted research funding from Boston Scientific. No other authors have relationships relevant to the contents of this paper.

Author details
[1]Oxford Heart Centre, Oxford University Hospitals, Headley Way, Oxford OX39DU, UK. [2]Department of Statistics, TU University Dortmund, Dortmund, Germany. [3]University Hospital Southampton NHS Foundation Trust, Southampton, UK. [4]Department of Cardiology, Charité Universitätsmedizin Berlin (Campus Benjamin Franklin), Berlin, Germany.

References

1. Fihn SD, Gardin JM, Abrams J, Berra K, Blankenship JC, Dallas AP, Douglas PS, Foody JM, Gerber TC, Hinderliter AL, King III SB, Kligfield PD, Krumholz HM, Kwong RY, Lim MJ, Linderbaum JA, Mack MJ, Munger MA, Prager RL, Sabik JF, Shaw LJ, Sikkema JD, Smith Jr CR, Smith Jr SC, Spertus JA, Williams SV, Anderson JL. CCF/AHA/ACP/AATS/PCNA/SCAI/STS guideline for the diagnosis and management of patients with stable ischemic heart disease: a report of the American College of Cardiology Foundation/American Heart Association task force on practice guidelines, and the American College of Physicians, American Association for Thoracic Surgery, Preventive Cardiovascular Nurses Association, Society for Cardiovascular Angiography and Interventions, and Society of Thoracic Surgeons. Circulation. 2012;126(25):e354–471.
2. Fihn SD, Blankenship JC, Alexander KP, Bittl JA, Byrne JG, Fletcher BJ, Fonarow GC, Lange RA, Levine GN, Maddox TM, Naidu SS, Ohman EM, Smith PK. ACC/AHA/AATS/PCNA/SCAI/STS focused update of the guideline for the diagnosis and management of patients with stable ischemic heart disease: a report of the American College of Cardiology/American Heart Association Task Force on Practice Guidelines, and the American Association for Thoracic Surgery, Preventive Cardiovascular Nurses Association, Society for Cardiovascular Angiography and Interventions, and Society of Thoracic Surgeons. Circulation. 2014;130(19):1749 67
3. Windecker S, Kolh P, Alfonso F, Collet JP, Cremer J, Falk V, Filippatos G, Hamm C, Head SJ, Juni P, Kappetein AP, Kastrati A, Knuuti J, Landmesser U, Laufer G, Neumann FJ, Richter DJ, Schauerte P, Sousa Uva M, Stefanini GG, Taggart DP, Torracca L, Valgimigli M, Wijns W, Witkowski A. 2014 ESC/EACTS Guidelines on myocardial revascularization: The Task Force on Myocardial Revascularization of the European Society of Cardiology (ESC) and the European Association for Cardio-Thoracic Surgery (EACTS)Developed with the special contribution of the European Association of Percutaneous Cardiovascular Interventions (EAPCI). Eur Heart J. 2014;35(37):2541–619.
4. Fearon WF, Bornschein B, Tonino PA, Gothe RM, Bruyne BD, Pijls NH, Siebert U. Economic evaluation of fractional flow reserve-guided percutaneous coronary intervention in patients with multivessel disease. Circulation. 2010;122(24):2545–50.
5. Tebaldi M, Biscaglia S, Pecoraro A, Fineschi M, Campo G. Fractional flow reserve implementation in daily clinical practice: A European survey. Int J Cardiol. 2016;207:206–7.
6. Rensing BJ, Hermans WR, Vos J, Tijssen JG, Rutch W, Danchin N, Heyndrickx GR, Mast EG, Wijns W, Serruys PW. Luminal narrowing after percutaneous transluminal coronary angioplasty. A study of clinical, procedural, and lesional factors related to long-term angiographic outcome. Coronary Artery Restenosis Prevention on Repeated Thromboxane Antagonism (CARPORT) Study Group. Circulation. 1993;88(3):975–85.
7. Strauss BH, Escaned J, Foley DP, di Mario C, Haase J, Keane D, Hermans WR, de Feyter PJ, Serruys PW. Technologic considerations and practical limitations in the use of quantitative angiography during percutaneous coronary recanalization. Prog Cardiovasc Dis. 1994;36(5):343–62.
8. Valgimigli M, Tebaldi M, Borghesi M, Vranckx P, Campo G, Tumscitz C, Cangiano E, Minarelli M, Scalone A, Cavazza C, Marchesini J, Parrinello G. Two-year outcomes after first- or second-generation drug-eluting or bare-metal stent implantation in all-comer patients undergoing percutaneous coronary intervention: a pre-specified analysis from the PRODIGY study (PROlonging Dual Antiplatelet Treatment After Grading stent-induced Intimal hyperplasia studY). JACC Cardiovasc Interv. 2014;7(1):20–8.
9. Leesar MA, Satran A, Yalamanchili V, Helmy T, Abdul-Waheed M, Wongpraparut N. The impact of fractional flow reserve measurement on clinical outcomes after transradial coronary stenting. EuroIntervention. 2011;7(8):917–23.
10. Fineschi M, Guerrieri G, Orphal D, Palmerini E, Münzel T, Warnholtz A, Pierli C, Gori T. The impact of gender on fractional flow reserve measurements. EuroIntervention. 2013;9(3):360–6.
11. Tebaldi M, Biscaglia S, Fineschi M, Manari A, Menozzi M, Secco GG, Di Lorenzo E, D'Ascenzo F, Fabbian F, Tumscitz C, et al. Fractional flow reserve evaluation and chronic kidney disease: Analysis from a multicenter Italian registry (the FREAK study). Catheter Cardiovasc Interv. 2015 [Epub ahead of print].
12. Higgins JPT, Green S. Cochrane Handbook for Systematic Reviews of Interventions Version 5.1.0 [updated March 2011]. The Cochrane Collaboration; 2011. http://training.cochrane.org/handbook. Access 12 Jan 2016
13. Juni P, Witschi A, Bloch R, et al. The hazards of scoring the quality of clinical trials for meta-analysis. JAMA. 1999;282(11):1054–60.
14. Bohning D, Mylona K, Kimber A. Meta-analysis of clinical trials with rare events. Biom J. 2015;57(4):633–48.
15. Veroniki AA, Jackson D, Viechtbauer W, Bender R, Knapp G, Kuss O, Langan D. Recommendations for quantifying uncertainty in the summary intervention effect and estimating between-study heterogeneity variance in random-effects meta-analysis. Cochrane Database Syst Rev. 2015;Supplement 1:25–7.
16. Begg CB, Mazumdar M. Operating characteristics of a rank correlation test for publication bias. Biometrics. 1994;50(4):1088–101.
17. Egger M, Davey Smith G, Schneider M, Minder C. Bias in meta-analysis detected by a simple, graphical test. BMJ. 1997;315(7109):629–34.
18. Bech GJ, Pijls NH, De Bruyne B, Peels KH, Michels HR, Bonnier HJ, Koolen JJ. Usefulness of fractional flow reserve to predict clinical outcome after balloon angioplasty. Circulation. 1999;99(7):883–8.
19. Nam CW, Hur SH, Cho YK, Park HS, Yoon HJ, Kim H, Chung IS, Kim YN, Kim KB, Doh JH, Koo BK, Tahk SJ, Fearon WF. Relation of fractional flow reserve after drug-eluting stent implantation to one-year outcomes. Am J Cardiol. 2011;107(12):1763–7.
20. R Core Team. R: A Language and Environment for Statistical Computing. R Founda- tion for Statistical Computing 2015, Vienna, Austria. URL http://www.R-project.org.

21. Viechtbauer W. Conducting meta-analyses in R with the metafor package. J Stat Softw. 2010;36:1–48.
22. Doh JH, Nam CW, Koo BK, Lee SY, Choi H, Namgung J, Kwon SU, Kwak JJ, Kim HY, Choi WH, Lee WR. Clinical Relevance of Poststent Fractional Flow Reserve After Drug-Eluting Stent Implantation. J Invasive Cardiol. 2015;27(8):346–51.
23. Ito T, Tani T, Fujita H, Ohte N. Relationship between fractional flow reserve and residual plaque volume and clinical outcomes after optimal drug-eluting stent implantation: insight from intravascular ultrasound volumetric analysis. Int J Cardiol. 2014;176(2):399–404.
24. Reith S, Battermann S, Hellmich M, Marx N, Burgmaier M. Correlation between OCT-derived intrastent dimensions and fractional flow reserve measurements after coronary stent implantation and impact on clinical outcome. J Invasive Cardiol. 2015;27(5):222–8.
25. Fischman DL, Leon MB, Baim DS, Schatz RA, Savage MP, Penn I, Detre K, Veltri L, Ricci D, Nobuyoshi M, Cleman M, Heuser R, Almond D, Teirstein PS, Fish RD, Colombo A, Brinker J, Moses J, Shaknovich A, Hirshfeld J, Bailey S, Ellis S, Rake R, Goldberg S. A randomized comparison of coronary-stent placement and balloon angioplasty in the treatment of coronary artery disease. Stent Restenosis Study Investigators. N. Engl J Med. 1994;331(8):496–501.
26. Serruys PW, de Jaegere P, Kiemeneij F, Macaya C, Rutsch W, Heyndrickx G, Emanuelsson H, Marco J, Legrand V, Materne P, Belardi J, Sigwart U, Colombo A, Goy JJ, van den Heuvel P, Delcan J, Morel A. A comparison of balloon-expandable-stent implantation with balloon angioplasty in patients with coronary artery disease. Benestent Study Group. N Engl J Med. 1994; 331(8):489–95.
27. Johnson NP, Toth GG, Lai D, Zhu H, Acar G, Agostoni P, Appelman Y, Arslan F, Barbato E, Chen SL, Di Serafino L, Dominguez-Franco AJ, Dupouy P, Esen AM, Esen OB, Hamilos M, Iwasaki K, Jensen LO, Jimenez-Navarro MF, Katritsis DG, Kocaman SA, Koo BK, Lopez-Palop R, Lorin JD, Miller LH, Muller O, Nam CW, Oud N, Puymirat E, Rieber J, Rioufol G, Rodes-Cabau J, Sedlis SP, Takeishi Y, Tonino PA, Van Belle E, Verna E, Werner GS, Fearon WF, Pijls NH, De Bruyne B, Gould KL. Prognostic value of fractional flow reserve: linking physiologic severity to clinical outcomes. J Am Coll Cardiol. 2014;64(16):1641–54.
28. Hanekamp CE, Koolen JJ, Pijls NH, Michels HR, Bonnier HJ. al. Comparison of quantitative coronary angiography, intravascular ultrasound, and coronary pressure measurement to assess optimum stent deployment. Circulation. 1999;99(8):1015–21.
29. Fearon WF, Luna J, Samady H, Powers ER, Feldman T, Dib N, Tuzcu EM, Cleman MW, Chou TM, Cohen DJ, Ragosta M, Takagi A, Jeremias A, Fitzgerald PJ, Yeung AC, Kern MJ, Yock PG. Fractional flow reserve compared with intravascular ultrasound guidance for optimizing stent deployment. Circulation. 2001;104(16):1917–22.
30. Stempfle HU, Konig A, Drescher E, Siebert U, Klauss V. Discrepancy between morphologic and functional criteria of optimal stent deployment using intravascular ultrasound and pressure derived myocardial fractional flow reserve. Int J Cardiovasc Intervent. 2005;7(2):101–7.
31. Pijls NH, Klauss V, Siebert U, Powers E, Takazawa K, Fearon WF, Escaned J, Tsurumi Y, Akasaka T, Samady H, De Bruyne B. Coronary pressure measurement after stenting predicts adverse events at follow-up: a multicenter registry. Circulation. 2002;105(25):2950–4.
32. Applegate RJ, Sacrinty MT, Kutcher MA, Santos RM, Gandhi SK, Little WC. Effect of length and diameter of drug-eluting stents versus bare-metal stents on late outcomes. Circ Cardiovasc Interv. 2009;2(1):35–42.
33. Caputo RP, Goel A, Pencina M, Cohen DJ, Kleiman NS, Yen CH, Waksman R, Tolerico P, Dhar G, Gordon P, Bach RG, Lopez JJ. Impact of drug eluting stent length on outcomes of percutaneous coronary intervention (from the EVENT registry). Am J Cardiol. 2012;110(3):350–5.
34. Kobayashi Y, De Gregorio J, Kobayashi N, Akiyama T, Reimers B, Finci L, Di Mario C, Colombo A. Stented segment length as an independent predictor of restenosis. J Am Coll Cardiol. 1999;34(3):651–9.
35. De Bruyne B, Hersbach F, Pijls NH, Bartunek J, Bech JW, Heyndrickx GR, Gould KL, Wijns W. Abnormal epicardial coronary resistance in patients with diffuse atherosclerosis but 'Normal' coronary angiography. Circulation. 2001;104(20):2401–6.
36. Rieber J, Schiele TM, Erdin P, Stempfle HU, Konig A, Erhard I, Segmiller T, Baylacher M, Theisen K, Haufe MC, Siebert U, Klauss V. Fractional flow reserve predicts major adverse cardiac events after coronary stent implantation. Z Kardiol. 2002;91 Suppl 3:132–6.

3

Long-term clinical outcomes of everolimus-eluting stent versus paclitaxel-eluting stent in patients undergoing percutaneous coronary interventions

Min Meng[1], Bei Gao[1], Xia Wang[1], Zheng-gang Bai[2], Ri-na Sa[1] and Bin Ge[1*]

Abstract

Background: Everolimus -eluting stent (EES) is common used in patients undergoing percutaneous coronary interventions (PCI). Our purpose is to evaluate long-term clinical outcomes of everolimus -eluting stent (EES) versus paclitaxel-eluting stent (PES) in patients undergoing percutaneous coronaryinterventions (PCI) in randomized controlled trials (RCTs).

Methods: We searched Medline, EMBASE, Cochrane Library, CNKI, VIP and relevant websites (https://scholar-google-com.ezproxy.lib.usf.edu/) for articles to compare outcomes between everolimus-eluting stent and paclitaxel-eluting stent without language or date restriction. RCTs that compared the use of everolimus -eluting stent and paclitaxel-eluting stent in PCI were included. Variables relating to patient, study characteristics, and clinical endpoints were extracted. Meta-analysis was performed using RevMan 5.2 software.

Results: We identified 6 published studies (from three randomized trials) more on everolimus-eluting stent ($n = 3352$) than paclitaxel-eluting ($n = 1639$), with follow-up duration ranging from 3, 4 and 5 years. Three-year outcomes of everolimus-eluting stent compared to paclitaxel-eluting were as following: the everolimus-eluting stent significantly reduced all-cause death (relative risk [RR]:0.63; 95 % confidence interval [CI]: 0.46. to 0.82), MACE (RR: 0.56; 95 % CI: 0.41 to 0.77), MI (RR: 0.64; 95 % CI: 0.48 to 0.86), TLR (RR: 0.72; 95 % CI: 0.59 to 0.88), ID-TLR (RR: 0.74; 95 % CI: 0.59 to 0.92) and ST (RR: 0.54; 95 % CI: 0.32 to 0.90). There was no difference in TVR between the everolimus-eluting and paclitaxel-eluting (RR: 0.76; 95 % CI: 0.58 to 1.10); Four-year outcomes of everolimus-eluting compared to paclitaxel-eluting: the everolimus-eluting significantly reduced MACE (RR: 0.44; 95 % CI: 0.18 to 0.98) and ID-TLR (RR: 0.47; 95 % CI: 0.23 to 0.97). There was no difference in MI (RR: 0.48; 95 % CI: 0.16 to 1.46), TLR (RR: 0.46; 95 % CI: 0.20 to1.04) and ST ((RR: 0.34; 95 % CI: 0.05 to 2.39). Five-year outcomes of everolimus-eluting stent compared to paclitaxel-eluting: There was no difference in ID-TLR (RR: 0.67; 95 % CI: 0.45 to 1.02) and ST (RR: 0.71; 95 % CI: 0.28 to1.80).

Conclusions: In the present meta-analysis, everolimus-eluting appeared to be safe and clinically effective in patients undergoing PCI in comparison to PES in 3-year clinical outcomes; there was similar no difference in reduction of ST between EES and PES in long-term(≥4 years) clinical follow-ups. Everolimus-eluting is more safety than paclitaxel-eluting in long-term clinical follow-ups, whether these effects can be applied to different patient subgroups warrants further investigation.

Keywords: Everolimus-eluting stent, Paclitaxel-eluting stent, Percutaneous coronary interventions, Systematic review, Meta-analysis

* Correspondence: 550313937@qq.com
[1]Department of Pharmacy, Gansu Provincial Hospital, Donggang West Road No. 204, Lanzhou, Gansu 730000, China
Full list of author information is available at the end of the article

Background

Acute coronary syndrome (ACS) is a major public health concern worldwide. Coronary artery disease is a leading cause of morbidity and mortality in adults around the world, and accounts for an even higher proportion of deaths in developed countries. The WHO estimates that 7.3 million people died of coronary heart disease in 2008. Moreover, the number of people who die from cardiovascular diseases, mainly from heart disease and stroke, will increase and accounts for 23.3 million by the year of 2030 [1, 2]. Furthermore, ACS bears a heavy economic burden for government and society in developed countries [3, 4], which has also drawn attention of the experts in developing countries due to the increased risk factors of cardiovascular disease, including the prevalence of hypercholesterolemia [5] and more smokers [6] etc.

Currently, percutaneous coronary intervention (PCI) is another important means of reperfusion therapy in treatment of patients with ACS, especially for patients with ST-segment elevation myocardial infarction (STEMI), with the additional drug therapies such as antiplatelet drugs, anticoagulants, stains and thrombolytic therapy etc. [7]. Compared with thrombolytic therapy, PCI is more effective in restoring coronary blood flow. Numerous studies, including a large meta-analysis showed that PCI have shown the superiority in reducing mortality, recurrent myocardial infarction and stroke compared with thrombolytic therapy while the lower risk of bleeding caused by PCI. Therefore, reperfusion therapy is regarded as the standards and is recommended for patients with STEMI [8].

Stents become more and more popular used to PCI. Since the advent of the first use of stents—Palmaz stents in the last century [9], bare metal stents (BMS) were widely used in balloon angioplasty which was the most popular method of treating heart disease and was recommended by the American Medical Association as the standard treatment [10]. But a long-term study for patients who received a single Palmaz stents showed that the incidence of restenosis was 30.2 %, while the incidence ranged from 28 % to 41 % in patients who received angioplasty alone [11]. Arterial wall damage response mechanism triggered by Balloon angioplasty and stenting, resulting in intimal hyperplasia was an important cause of restenosis [10]. In order to reduce tissue proliferation, first-generation drug-eluting stents (DES) were being designed and coated with a polymer allowing controlled local delivery of a pharmaceutical agent with antineoplastic and anti-inflammatory properties [12]. Now, recommendations of the European Society of Cardiology call for the use of drug-eluting stents for PCI if the patient has no contraindication to extended treatment with dual-antiplatelet therapy [13].

Paclitaxel-eluting stent was one of the first-generation drug eluting stents. Comparing with BMS, Paclitaxel-Eluting Stent reduced the rates of restenosis significantly. However, some studies have shown that some type of stent thrombosis occurs [14], the two large researches in first-generation DES showed that an annual rate of late stent thrombosis was 0.4–0.6 % for up to 4 years after stent implantation [15–17]. Thus, the second-generation DES was designed to reduce the incidence of late stent thrombosis and solve the problem of restenosis by replacing the coating drug.

Everolimus-eluting stent (EES) was a second generation DES approved by the FDA in July 2008 with its cobalt chromium stent design, high deliverability, and everolimus drug coating used to prevent abnormal tissue growth [18]. Due to its lipophilic chemical structure, it is more rapidly absorbed into the arterial wall, potentially making it a better drug for local intravascular delivery following stent implantation [19, 20]. The FUTURE Trail, EXAMINATION Trail [21] and SPIRIT FIRST Trail showed the EES to be safe, feasible, and efficient [14, 22–26]. The studies showed the superiority of PES to EES for short time [27–30]. Despite this, the long-term efficacy of EES use should be investigated to reduce the individual trails and the limitations of short-term studies.

Similarly, the TAXUS trials assessed the safety and efficacy of paclitaxel-eluting stent (PES) in the treatment of coronary artery disease [31–34]. Large randomized clinical trials such as SPIRIT Trail and COMPARE Trails designed to compare EES with PES have shown reduced rates of repeat revascularization, major adverse cardiac events, myocardial infarction and stent thrombosis [35–38]. Hence, it is necessary to carry out a new meta-analysis including RCTs only and to update the prior meta-analyses on the basis of the preferred reporting items for systematic reviews and meta-analysis (PRISMA) items [39].

A comprehensive network meta-analysis had displayed that cobalt-chromium everolimus eluting stents (CoCr-EES) has the lowest rate of baremetal stents, paclitaxel-eluting stents(PES), sirolimus-eluting stents, phosphorylcholine-based zotarolimuseluting stentss-tent thrombosis, and Resolute zotarolimus-eluting stents within 2 years of implantation. However, the study only inculed 6 stduies with one and 2 years follow ups. The aim of this meta-analysis was to compare the efficacy and safety of EES versus PES especially with regards to the patient of all-cause death, major adverse cardiac events, stent thrombus, and myocardial infarction as primary outcomes, and of target lesion revascularization, ischemia-driven target lesion revascularization, and target vessel revascularization as secondary outcomes over long-term (followed up 3, 4 and 5 years), and to provide much more reliable evidences for clinical decision-making and to guide future research [40].

Methods

Protocol and registration

No protocol has been registered in public, however draft related to the study already exists.

Search strategy and selection criteria

We searched Medline, EMBASE, Cochrane Library, CNKI, VIP, and relevant websites (https://scholar-google-com.ezproxy.lib.usf.edu/) by two researchers (Min.M. and Bei.G.). Disagreements were resolved by consensus. The reference list of relevant studies was further scanned. No restrictions of language, publication date or publication status were imposed. The last search was run on October 2014.

The following search terms were used: "percutaneous coronary intervention", "randomized trial", "everolimus-eluting stent", "Xience", "drug-eluting stent", "paclitaxel-eluting stent" and "TAXUS". To be included in this study, the citation had to meet the following criteria: randomized controlled trials that compared the use of EES and PES in percutaneous coronary intervention (PCI). Exclusion criteria were: (1) ongoing studies; (2) irretrievable data; (3) Follow up duration of less than 3 years; (4) non randomized studies; (5) animal studies; (6) case reports; (7) related reviews; (8) protocols; (9) conference abstracts. The Flow Diagram was shown in Fig. 1.

Data extraction and risk of bias assessment

Two investigators (MENG.M. and GAO.B.) independently included reports at title and/or at abstract level, disagreement was resolved with a third reviewer (GE.B.), and studies that met inclusion criteria were selected for further analysis. Furthermore, we e-mailed authors of trials for supplemental data which were partially published.

Data extraction included:

1. General information: title, authors, publication date, and article sources;
2. Study characteristics: subject characteristics, purpose, sites, study period, comparability of baseline, research results;
3. Primary Outcomes: major adverse cardiac events (MACE), myocardial infarction (MI), cardiac death, stent thrombus (ST); Secondary outcomes: target lesion revascularization (TLR), target vessel revascularization (TVR), all-cause death,, ischemia-driven target lesion revascularization (ID-TLR).

Quality of included studies was appraised by two investigators (M.M. and G.B.), and the assessment is shown in Fig. 2. The risk of selection, performance, detection, attrition, and reporting bias (expressed as low risk of bias, high risk or unclear risk of bias, the underlying risk of bias can't be determined due to incomplete reporting) were evaluated separately [41].

Data analysis

We used Review Manager (5.2) software for Meta analysis, and calculated the relative risk (RR) from the abstracted data. The average effects for the outcomes and 95 % confidence intervals (CI) were obtained using a random effects mode. Heterogeneity of RR across trials was assessed using the Cochrane Q statistic (P value ≤ 0.05 was considered significant) and the I2 statistic.

For the primary endpoint, small-study effects were analyzed by constructing a funnel plot, in which the standard error of the lnRR was plotted against RR for 3–5 years follow ups as minimize the publication bias. The absence of any asymmetric distribution suggested no publication bias. The funnel plots of primary outcomes were shown in Fig. 3(a-g).

Results

Search results

One thousand three hundred twenty articles were accessed through searching, and 734 articles were retrieved after duplicate were removed by Endnote X4 software, then abstracts and full texts were reviewed again with excluding duplicate papers and articles that do not meet the inclusion criteria. Finally, six published studies [42–47] from 3 randomized controlled trials were included in the present meta-analysis.

Characteristics of the included reviews

There were more patients randomized to EES ($n = 3352$) than to PES ($n = 1639$), resulted from imbalanced randomization in certain studies. The mean age ranged from 62 to 65 years with the majority of patients being male. Diabetes were not excluded. The frequency of diabetes mellitus ranged from 23.67 % to 32.14 %. Follow-up period ranged from 3.4 to 5 years. General characteristics of the included studies are shown in Table 1.

Results of meta-analysis

Three-year outcomes of EES compared to PES [42, 44, 45]

Primary outcomes

MACE SPIRIT IV Trail [45] did not publish the MACE data of 3-year outcomes of EES compared to PES. Therefore, the incidence of MAGE at all follow-ups was 9.10 % (75 of 824) among patients treated with the EES and 16.31 % (61 of 374) among patients treated with the PES (RR: 0.56, 95 % CI: 0.41–0.77; $P < 0.05$) [42, 44], with no significant study heterogeneity (Chi2 = 0.43; $P = 0.51$;

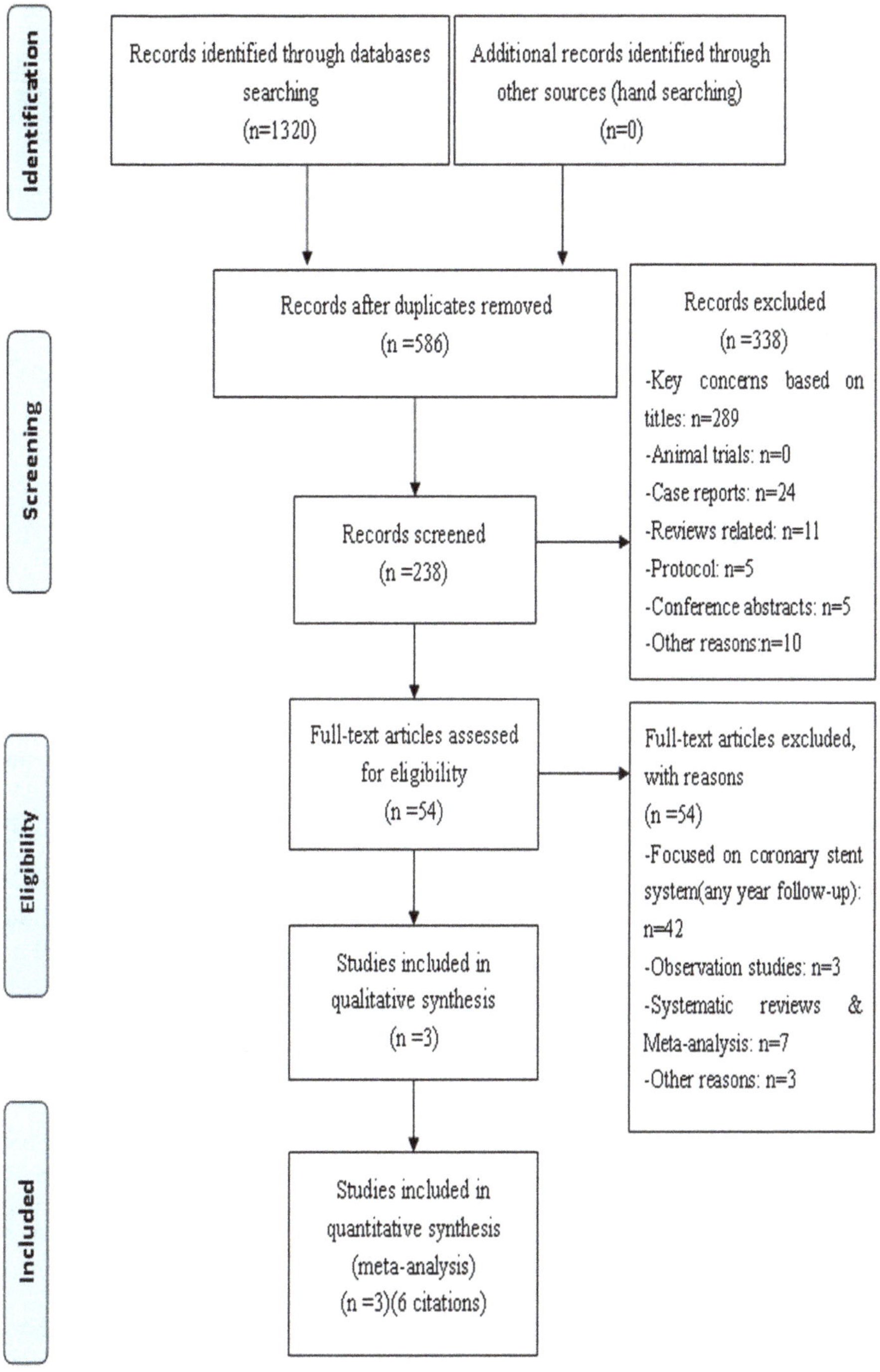

Fig. 1 Data source flow chart diagram

I2 = 0 %) (Fig. 4(a)). There was a statistically significant difference between EES and PES.

MI The incidence of MI at all follow-ups was 3.14 % (103 of 3282) among patients treated with the EES and 4.86 % (78 of 1603) among patients treated with the PES (RR: 0.64, 95 % CI: 0.48–0.86; $P < 0.05$) [42, 44, 45], with no significant study heterogeneity (Chi2 = 2.26; $P = 0.88$; I2 = 0 %) (Fig. 4(b)). There was a statistically significant difference between EES and PES.

All-cause death The incidence of all-cause death at all follow-ups was 3.12 % (103 of 3297) among patients treated with the EES and 5.02 % (81 of 1614) among patients treated with the PES (RR: 0.63, 95 % CI: 0.46–0.82; $P < 0.05$) [42, 44, 45], with no significant study

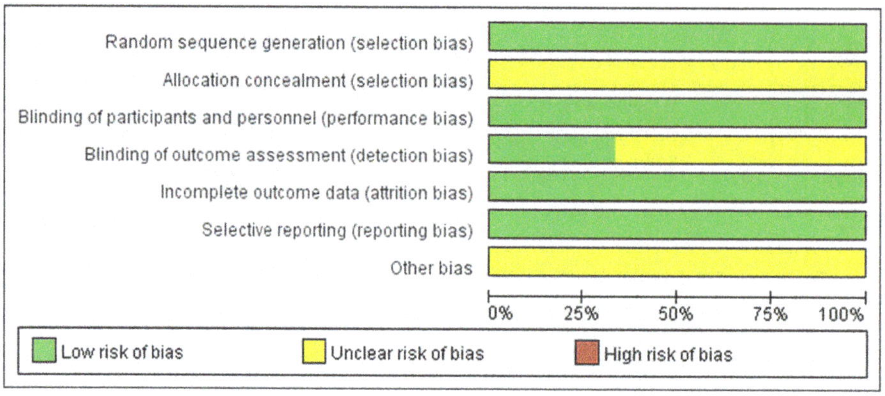

Fig. 2 Risk of bias graph

heterogeneity (Chi2 = 0.38; $P = 0.83$; I2 = 0 %) (Fig. 4(c)). There was a statistically significant difference between EES and PES.

ST The Academic Research Consortium's (ARC) consensus definite/probable ST were totally included for analysis. The incidence of all STs at all follow-ups was 0.73 % (24 of 3270) among patients treated with the EES and 1.63 % (26 of 1596) among patients treated with the PES (RR: 0.44, 95 % CI: 0.26–0.97; $P < 0.05$) [42, 44, 45], with no significant study heterogeneity (Chi2 = 1.30; $P = 0.52$; I2 = 0 %) (Fig. 4(d)). There was a statistically significant difference between EES and PES.

Secondary outcomes

TLR The incidence of TLR at all follow-ups was 6.46 % (213 of 3297) among patients treated with the EES and 8.98 % (145 of 1614) among patients treated with the PES (RR: 0.66, 95 % CI: 0.47–0.92; $P < 0.05$) [42, 44, 45], with no significant study heterogeneity (Chi2 = 3.68; $P = 0.16$; I2 = 46 %) (Fig. 4(e)). There was a statistically significant difference between EES and PES.

TVR The incidence of TVR at all follow-ups was 9.28 % (306 of 3297) among patients treated with the EES and 10.90 % (176 of 1614) among patients treated with the PES (RR: 0.82, 95 % CI: 0.57–1.19; $P > 0.05$) [42, 44, 45], with a significant study heterogeneity (Chi2 = 5.59; $P = 0.06$; I2 = 64 %) (Fig. 4(f)). There was no statistically significant difference between EES and PES.

ID-TLR The incidence of ID-TLR at all follow-ups was 5.68 % (187 of 3289) among patients treated with the EES and 7.76 % (125 of 1610) among patients treated with the PES (RR: 0.74, 95 % CI: 0.59–0.92; $P < 0.05$) [42, 44, 45], with no significant study heterogeneity (Chi2 = 1.56; $P = 0. 46$; I2 = 0 %) (Fig. 4(g)). There was a statistically significant difference between EES and PES.

Four-year outcomes of EES compared to PES [47]

In all included studies, only SPRIT II Trail reported 4-year follow-up clinical outcomes. We extracted the data of 4 year-end points and analyzed as following.

Primary outcomes

MACE The incidence of MAGE at all follow-ups was 7.62 % (15 of 195) among patients treated with the EES and 16.42 % (11 of 67) among patients treated with the PES (RR: 0.47, 95 % CI: 0.23–0.97; $P < 0.05$) [47] (Fig. 5(a)). There was a statistically significant difference between EES and PES.

MI The incidence of MI at all follow-ups was 3.59 % (7 of 195) among patients treated with the EES and 7.46 % (5 of 67) among patients treated with the PES (RR: 0.48, 95 % CI: 0.16–1.46; $P > 0.05$) [47] (Fig. 5(b)). There was no statistically significant difference between EES and PES.

ST The incidence of ST at all follow-ups was 1.02 % (2 of 195) among patients treated with the EES and 2.98 % (2 of 67) among patients treated with the PES (RR: 0.34, 95 % CI: 0.05–2.39; $P > 0.05$) [47] (Fig. 5(c)). There was no statistically significant difference between EES and PES.

Secondary outcomes

TLR The incidence of TLR at all follow-ups was 6.15 % (12 of 195) among patients treated with the EES and 13.43 % (9 of 67) among patients treated with the PES (RR: 0.46, 95 % CI: 0.20–1.04; $P > 0.05$) [47] (Fig. 5(d)). There was no statistically significant difference between EES and PES.

ID-TLR The incidence of ID-TLR at all follow-ups was 7.69 % (15 of 195) among patients treated with the EES and 16.42 % (11 of 67) among patients treated with the

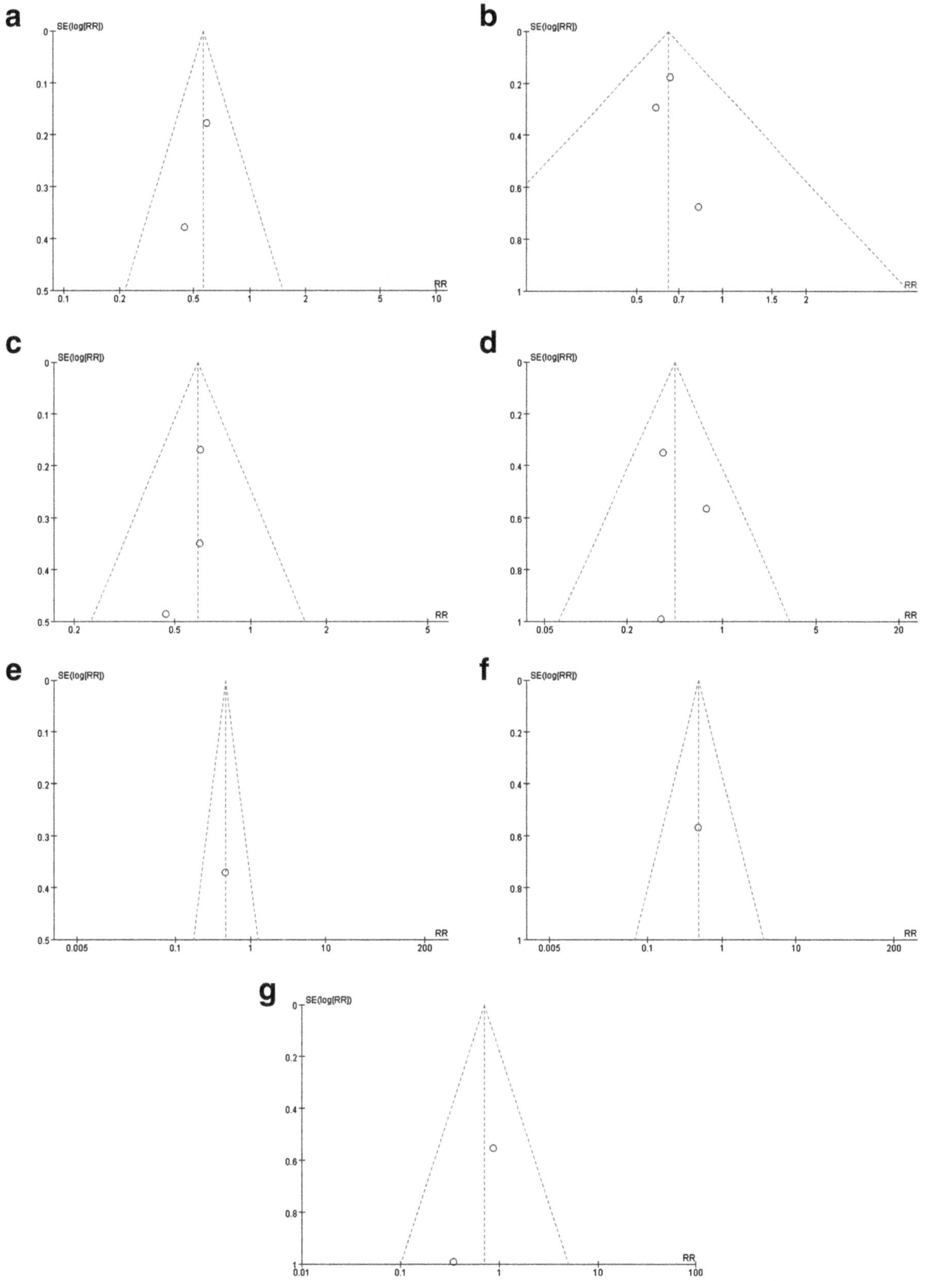

Fig. 3 (See legend on next page.)

(See figure on previous page.)
Fig. 3 Funnel plot of primary outcomes included in the meta-analysis. The funnel plot of (**a**: 3-year MACE, **b**: 3-year MI, **c**: 3-year death, **d**: 3-year ST, **e**: 4-year MACE, **f**: 4-year MI, **g**: 5-year ST). the standard error (SE) of the ln relative risk (RR) was plotted against the relative risk for (**a**:3-year MACE, **b**: 3-year MI, **c**: 3-year death, **d**: 3-year ST, **e**: 4-year MACE, **f**: 4-year MI, **g**: 5-year ST) 3-year MACE. The absence of any asymmetric distribution suggested no publication bias

PES (RR: 0.47, 95 % CI: 0.23–0.97; $P < 0.05$) [47] (Fig. 5(f)). There was a statistically significant difference between EES and PES.

Five-year outcomes of EES compared to PES [43, 46]

In all included studies, only SPRIT II, III and IV Trail reported 4-year follow-up clinical outcomes, SPRIT III Trail did not publish relevant data, so we extracted the reported data of 5 year-end points and analyzed as following.

Primary outcomes

ST The incidence of definite/probable ARC ST at all follow-ups was 1.30 % (11 of 844) among patients treated with the EES and 1.86 % (7 of 377) among patients treated with the PES (RR: 0.71, 95 % CI: 0.28–1.80; $P >$ 0.05) [43, 46], with no significant study heterogeneity (Chi2 = 0.66; $P = 0.42$; I2 = 0 %) (Fig. 6(a)). There was no statistically significant difference between EES and PES.

Secondary outcomes

ID-TLR The incidence of ID-TLR at all follow-ups was 7.53 % (53 of 704) among patients treated with the EES and 11.50 % (33 of 287) among patients treated with the PES (RR: 0.67, 95 % CI: 0.45–1.02; $P > 0.05$) [43, 46], with no significant study heterogeneity (Chi2 = 0.42; $P =$ 0. 52; I2 = 0 %) (Fig. 6(b)). There was no statistically significant difference between EES and PES.

Discussions

Characteristic and quality of included studies

For this meta-analysis, we screened 1320 articles, only 6 studies (three trails) [42–47] which met the inclusion criteria were considered. The randomized trials in our meta-analysis included patients with PCI, and two of which described a method of generating randomness. SPRIT Trails were all single-blinded, but it was not clear whether allocation concealment was used, and reported failing in follow-ups. Risk of bias graph is shown in Fig. 2.

SPIRIT Trails included a proportion of the diabetic population, especially SPIRIT IV trail, which included 32.14 % diabetics [45]. The baseline characteristic of SPRIT Trails were consistent, described safety of eluting stent using the dangers of endpoints such as MACE, MI, TLR,ID-TLR, instead of beneficial indicators, in order to avoid biases in outcome evaluation.

Clinical significance of this meta-analysis

In recent years, drug-eluting stents have revolutionized interventional cardiology and become an important part of interventional cardiology. New stents through large RCT trials has been verified to be effective, but it should be a long-term follow-up of clinical indicators to evaluate the difference of long-term efficacy and safety of new stents and old stents. Meta-analysis and RCT trials showed that EES could reduce dangerous endpoints, such as MACE, MI, TLR, ID-TLR in ≤ 3 year follow-ups when compared with PES.

The present meta-analysis of RCTs compared EES to PES for PCI with clinical follow-ups from three to 5 years, using multiple endpoints. Based on results of the 3-year clinical follow-up [42, 44, 45] combined dataset, significant reductions with EES compared with PES were observed for the safety endpoints of all-cause death and MACE, MI, and ST, and improved efficacy with reducing rates of TLR, ID-TLR, but similar rates in the two groups of TVR. Only one trail (SPIRIT IV) [47] was included for analyzing 4-year clinical follow-up results, which demonstrated EES could reduce MACE and ID-TLR, which is better than PES, but couldn't reduce MI, TLR and ST.

The main finding of our meta-analysis is that we demonstrated EES was superior clinical efficacy to the PES in the reduction of ID-TLR and ST by the four [47] and 5-year clinical follow-up [43, 46] combined dataset. However, the differences were not statistically significant. A meta-analysis reported by Ashraf Alazzoni [29] demonstrated that EES was superior to PES in reducing early (0–30 days), late (31–365 days), and very late ST (>365 days) with statistically significant difference, but the very late ST group had not to subgroup analysis. It might imply a non-significant trend for reducing ST at a very long term clinical follow up, and that might be related to sample size problem.

Study limitations

First, the 3-year follow-up clinical trial [42, 44, 45] comparing outcomes demonstrated that a consistent heterogeneity was observed for the TVR endpoints(I2 ≥ 50 %), even when Odds Ratio were used for analysis. A source of heterogeneity might be due to the reported inconsistency in patients' number of TVR. for example, SPIRIT II Trail [42, 46, 47] clearly illustrated all of TVR numbers included all the numbers of TLR, but SPIRIT III [43, 44] and SPIRIT IV Trail [46] did not clearly state whether the occurrence of

Table 1 Baseline of characteristics of the included trials

Source		Number of patents	Age	Male	Diabetes	Diameter stenosis (%)	Vessel diameter (mm)	Lesion length (mm)	Inclusion criteria	Exclusion criteria	Primary outcomes	Secondary outcomes	Other outcomes	Follow-up duration, year	Funding
SPIRIT II [45–47]	EES*	223	62 ± 10	158	51	61 ± 12	2.70 ± 0.52	13.0 ± 5.7	1. Ischemia and vessel size 2.5–4.25 mm and lesion length ≤ 28 mm; 2. A percentage diameter stenosis (DS) 50 %–99 %	1. Recent MI‡,LVEF× ≤ 30 %; 2. LM§ heavily calcified lesion; 3. Visible thrombus	.MI‡ST††	ID-TLR# ID-MACE‖	CABG**	3,4,5	Abbott vascular
	PES†	77	62 ± 9	61	20	59 ± 10	2.82 ± 0.58	13.2 ± 6.4							
SPIRIT III [48, 49]	EES*	669	63.2 ± 10.5	469	198	70.0 ± 13.3	2.77 ± 0.45	14.7 ± 5.6	1. Stable, unstable angina; 2. Ischemia with vessel size 2.5–3.75 mm and lesion length ≤ 28 mm	1. Recent MI‡,LVEF× < 30 %; 2. LM§ bifurcation; 3. BG; 4. Calcification; 5. Thrombus	MAGE‡‡ Cardiac death MI‡ST††	TLR×× TVR§§	TLF‖‖	3.5	Abbott vascular
	PES†	332	62.8 ± 10.2	218	92	69.4 ± 13.6	2.76 ± 0.46	14.7 ± 5.7							
SPIRIT IV[50]	EES*	2460	63.3 ± 10.5	1664	787	72.3 ± 12.6	—	—	1. Stable, unstable angina; 2. Ischemia with vessel size 2.5–4.25 mm and lesion length ≤ 28 mm	1. Recent MI‡,LVEF× < 30 %; 2. LM§ bifurcation; 3. Icomplex lesions; 4. Totally occluded vessels; 5. Large bifurcations; 6. Excessive calcification; 7. Tortuosity; 8. Angulation; 9. Thrombus	MAGE‡‡ Cardiac death MI‡.ST††	TLR×× ID-TLR#	TLF‖‖	3	Abbott vascular
	PES†	1230	63.3 ± 10.2	833	399	72.0 ± 12.8	—	—							

Abbreviations: *:everolimus-eluting stent; †:paclitaxel-eluting stent; ‡:myocardial infarction; ×LVEF: left ventricular ejection fraction; §:left main; ‖:major adverse cardiac events; #:ischemia-driven target lesion revascularization; **:coronary artery bypass graft; ††:sent thrombus ; ‡‡ :major adverse cardiac events; ××:target lesion revascularization; §§:target vessel revascularization; ‖‖:Target lesion failure

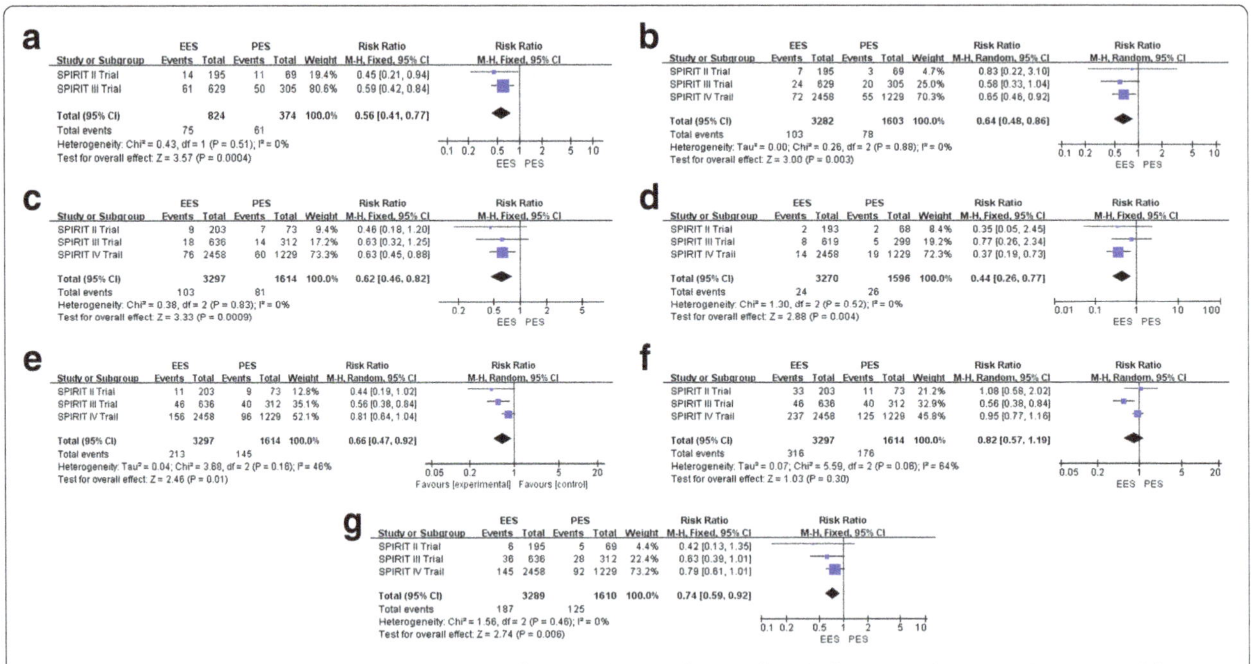

Fig. 4 Risk Ratio of 3-year clinical outcomes: the Risk Ratio of (**a**: MACE, **b**: MI, **c**: all cause of death; **d**: ST; **e**: TLR, **f**: TVR, **g**: ID-TLR) at 3-year follow-up associated with EES versus PES

TVR number included all TLR patients. However, other key indicators clearly demonstrated that EES had certain superiority to PES by the 3-year clinical follow-up combined dataset.

Second, Spirit Trails were all sponsored by Abbott Vascular, therefore there might be a certain risk of results' bias.

Third, this meta-analysis of RCT trials were from the same series, due to the relatively limitation of probably same inclusion standard and same researchers, there is a certain risk of results' bias for long-term efficacy and safety with EES and PES. Therefore, we should include outcomes data of Compare Trail for 3–5 years clinical follow-up, in order to avoid results' bias mentioned above. Unfortunately, the relevant data of Compared Trail has not been reported so far [37, 38].

Finally, limited databases were searched and only published articles were included, as a result, there is the possibility of no comprehensive trails. As clinical significance of this meta-analysis might be uncertain, larger sample size will be needed to collect, and higher quality of research will be needed.

Future research directions

It has been reported that elderly, women and types of vascular of Sprite III Trial were analyzed for evaluating a

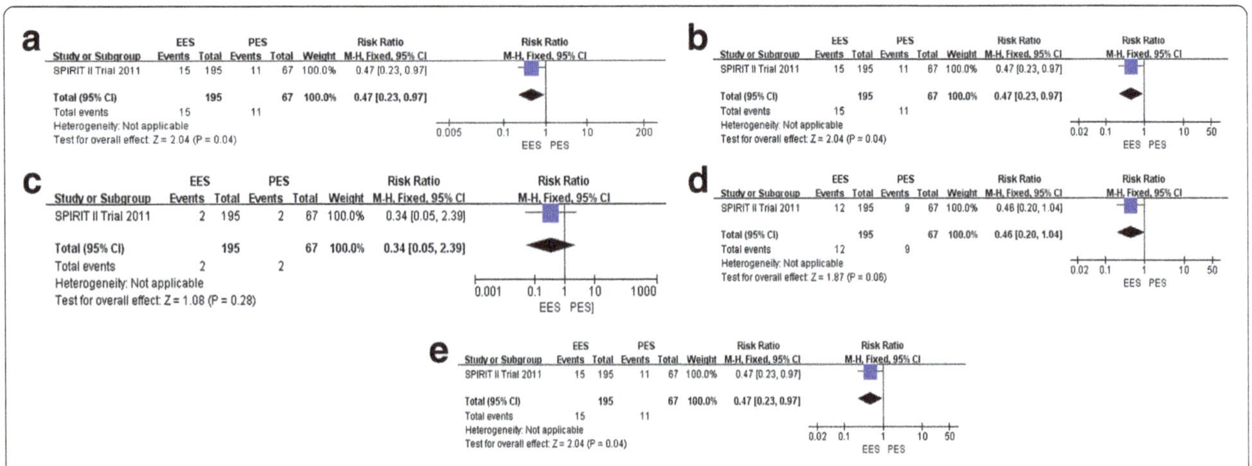

Fig. 5 Risk Ratio of 4-year clinical outcomes: the Risk Ratio of **a**: MACE, **b**: MI; **c**: ST; **d**: TLR; **e**: ID-TLR) at 4-year follow-up associated with EES versus PES

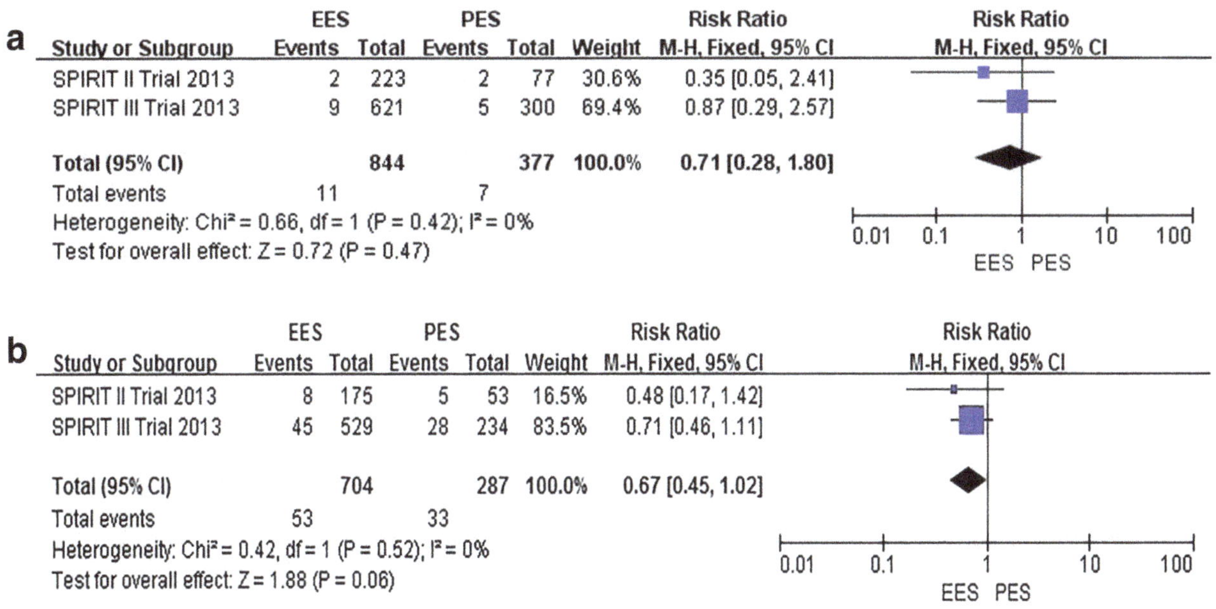

Fig. 6 Risk Ratio of 5-year clinical outcomes: the Risk Ratio of **a**: ST, **b**: ID-TLR) at 5-year follow-up associated with EES versus PES

long term clinical endpoints [48, 49]. Considering the bias of present study, it is recommended that future large, randomized clinical trials for diabetic patients should be carried out, and then diabetes will be included for sub-analysis respectively in order to evaluate significance safety of EES and PES in diabetes, which do not continue to further at moment for few original research data. The risk of stent fracture in EES has not been assessed [50], therefore, further studies should focus on that as well.

Conclusions

The current evidence showed that EES appeared to be safe and clinically effective in patients undergoing PCI comparing to PES in long-term clinical outcomes. However, more randomized data are needed, especially on 4-year follow-ups.

Role of the funding source

There was no funding source for this study. The corresponding author had full access to all the data in the study and had final responsibility for the decision to submit for publication.

Abbreviations

EES: everolimus-eluting stent; PES: paclitaxel-eluting stent; PCI: percutaneous coronary interventions; RCT: randomized controlled trial; RR: relative risk; CI: confidence interval; ACS: acute coronary syndrome; BMS: bare metal stents; DES: drug-eluting stents; MACE: major adverse cardiac events; MI: myocardial infarction; TLR: target lesion revascularization; TVR: target vessel revascularization; TLR: target lesion failure; ID-TLR: ischemia-driven target lesion revascularization; ST: stent thrombus.

Competing interests

The authors declare that the research was conducted in the absence of any commercial or financial relationships that could be construed as a potential conflict of interests.

Authors' contributions

Ge B and Meng M conceived of the study and its design. Gao B, Wang X and Sa R N helped with the acquisition and preparation of data. Bai Z G, Ge B and Meng M carried out the study, performed the statistical analysis, drafted, and revised the manuscript. All authors read and approved the final manuscript.

Author details

[1]Department of Pharmacy, Gansu Provincial Hospital, Donggang West Road No. 204, Lanzhou, Gansu 730000, China. [2]Evidence-Based Medicine Center, Lanzhou University, Lanzhou, Gansu 730000, China.

References

1. Mathers CD, Loncar D. Projections of global mortality and burden of disease from 2002 to 2030. PLoS Med. 2006;3:e442.
2. Peterson MC, Syndergaard T, Bowler J, Doxey R. A systematic review of factors predicting door to balloon time in ST-segment elevation myocardial infarction treated with percutaneous intervention. Int J Cardiol. 2012;157:8–23.
3. Mantovani LG, Fornari C, Madotto F, et al. Burden of acute myocardial infarction. Int J Cardiol. 2011;150:111–2.
4. Menzin J, Wygant G, Hauch O et al. One-year costs of ischemic heart disease among patients with acute coronary syndromes: findings from a multi-employer claims database*. Curr. Med. Res. Opin.® 2008; 24: 461–468.
5. Al-Lawati J, Sulaiman K, Panduranga P. The Epidemiology of Acute Coronary Syndrome in Oman: Results from the Oman-RACE study. Sultan Qaboos Univ Med J. 2013;13:43.
6. Hata J, Kiyohara Y. Epidemiology of Stroke and Coronary Artery Disease in Asia. Circ. J. 2013;77:1923–1932.
7. Makki N, Brennan TM, Girotra S. Acute Coronary Syndrome. J Intensive Care Med. 2013;18:1–15.
8. Keeley EC, Boura JA, Grines CL. Primary angioplasty versus intravenous thrombolytic therapy for acute myocardial infarction: a quantitative review of 23 randomised trials. Lancet. 2003;361:13–20.
9. Schatz RA, Palmaz J, Tio F, et al. Balloon-expandable intracoronary stents in the adult dog. Circulation. 1987;76:450–7.

10. Puranik AS, Dawson ER, Peppas NA. Recent advances in drug eluting stents. Int J Pharm. 2013;441:665–79.
11. Ellis SG, Savage M, Fischman D, et al. Restenosis after placement of Palmaz-Schatz stents in native coronary arteries. Initial results of a multicenter experience. Circulation. 1992;86:1836–44.
12. Claessen BE, Caixeta A, Henriques JP, Piek JJ. Current status of the Xience V® everolimus-eluting coronary stent system. Expert Rev Cardiovasc Ther. 2010;8:1363–74.
13. Wijns W, Kolh P, Danchin N, et al. Guidelines on myocardial revascularization the task force on myocardial revascularization of the european society of cardiology (esc) and the european association for cardio-thoracic surgery (eacts). Eur Heart J. 2010;31:2501–55.
14. Grube E, Silber S, Hauptmann KE, et al. TAXUS I six-and twelve-month results from a randomized, double-blind trial on a slow-release paclitaxel-eluting stent for de novo coronary lesions. Circulation. 2003;107:38–42.
15. McFadden EP, Stabile E, Regar E, et al. Late thrombosis in drug-eluting coronary stents after discontinuation of antiplatelet therapy. Lancet. 2004;364:1519–21.
16. Wenaweser P, Daemen J, Zwahlen M, et al. Incidence and correlates of drug-eluting stent thrombosis in routine clinical practice4-year results from a large 2-institutional cohort study. J Am Coll Cardiol. 2008;52:1134–40.
17. Daemen J, Wenaweser P, Tsuchida K, et al. Early and late coronary stent thrombosis of sirolimus-eluting and paclitaxel-eluting stents in routine clinical practice: data from a large two-institutional cohort study. Lancet. 2007;369:667–78.
18. Harris E. Industry Update: The latest developments in therapeutic delivery. Ther Deliv. 2013;4:659–65.
19. Kahan BD, Wong RL, Carter C, et al. A Phase I Study of A 4-Week Course of Sdz-Rad (Rad) in Quiescent Cyclosporine-Prednisone-Treated Renal Transplant Recipients1, 2. Transplantation. 1999;68:1100–6.
20. Allocco DJ, Joshi AA, Dawkins KD. Everolimus-eluting stents: update on current clinical studies. Medical Devices (Auckland, NZ). 2011;4:91.
21. Sabaté M, Brugaletta S, Cequier A, et al. The EXAMINATION (Everolimus-Eluting Stents Versus Bare-Metal Stents in ST-Segment Elevation Myocardial Infarction) Trial: 2-Year Results From a Multicenter Randomized Controlled Trial. J Am Coll Cardiol Intv. 2013;7:64–71.
22. Costa RA, Lansky AJ, Mintz GS, et al. Angiographic results of the first human experience with everolimus-eluting stents for the treatment of coronary lesions (the FUTURE I trial). Am J Cardiol. 2005;95:113–6.
23. Grube E, Sonoda S, Ikeno F, et al. Six-and twelve-month results from first human experience using everolimus-eluting stents with bioabsorbable polymer. Circulation. 2004;109:2168–71.
24. Tsuchiya Y, Lansky AJ, Costa RA, et al. Effect of *Everolimus*-Eluting Stents in Different Vessel Sizes (from the Pooled FUTURE I and II Trials). Am J Cardiol. 2006;98:464–9.
25. Serruys PW, Ong A, Piek JJ, et al. A randomized comparison of a durable polymer Everolimus-eluting stent with a bare metal coronary stent: The SPIRIT first trial. EuroIntervention. 2005;1:58–65.
26. Stone GW, Ellis SG, Cox DA, et al. A polymer-based, paclitaxel-eluting stent in patients with coronary artery disease. N Engl J Med. 2004;350:221–31.
27. Cassese S, Piccolo R, Galasso G, et al. Twelve-month clinical outcomes of everolimus-eluting stent as compared to paclitaxel-and sirolimus-eluting stent in patients undergoing percutaneous coronary interventions. A meta-analysis of randomized clinical trials. Int J Cardiol. 2011;150:84–9.
28. Baber U, Mehran R, Sharma SK, et al. Impact of the Everolimus-Eluting Stent on Stent ThrombosisA Meta-Analysis of 13 Randomized Trials. J Am Coll Cardiol. 2011;58:1569–77.
29. Alazzoni A, Al-Saleh A, Jolly SS. Everolimus-eluting versus paclitaxel-eluting stents in percutaneous coronary intervention: meta-analysis of randomized trials. Thrombosis. 2012;2012:1–8.
30. Dangas GD, Serruys PW, Kereiakes DJ, et al. Meta-Analysis of Everolimus-Eluting Versus Paclitaxel-Eluting Stents in Coronary Artery Disease Final 3-Year Results of the SPIRIT Clinical Trials Program (Clinical Evaluation of the Xience V Everolimus Eluting Coronary Stent System in the Treatment of Patients With De Novo Native Coronary Artery Lesions). J Am Coll Cardiol Intv. 2013;6:914–22.
31. Colombo A, Drzewiecki J, Banning A, et al. Randomized study to assess the effectiveness of slow-and moderate-release polymer-based paclitaxel-eluting stents for coronary artery lesions. Circulation. 2003;108:788–94.
32. Silber S, Colombo A, Banning AP, et al. Final 5-Year Results of the TAXUS II Trial A Randomized Study to Assess the Effectiveness of Slow-and Moderate-Release Polymer-Based Paclitaxel-Eluting Stents for De Novo Coronary Artery Lesions. Circulation. 2009;120:1498–504.
33. Stone GW, Ellis SG, Cannon L, et al. Comparison of a polymer-based paclitaxel-eluting stent with a bare metal stent in patients with complex coronary artery disease: a randomized controlled trial. JAMA. 2005;294:1215–23.
34. Tanabe K, Serruys PW, Grube E, et al. TAXUS III Trial In-stent restenosis treated with stent-based delivery of paclitaxel incorporated in a slow-release polymer formulation. Circulation. 2003;107:559–64.
35. Stone GW, Midei M, Newman W, et al. Comparison of an everolimus-eluting stent and a paclitaxel-eluting stent in patients with coronary artery disease: a randomized trial. JAMA. 2008;299:1903–13.
36. Planer D, Smits PC, Kereiakes DJ, et al. Comparison of Everolimus-and Paclitaxel-Eluting Stents in Patients With Acute and Stable Coronary SyndromesPooled Results From the SPIRIT (A Clinical Evaluation of the XIENCE V Everolimus Eluting Coronary Stent System) and COMPARE (A Trial of Everolimus-Eluting Stents and Paclitaxel-Eluting Stents for Coronary Revascularization in Daily Practice) Trials. J Am Coll Cardiol Intv. 2011;4:1104–15.
37. Smits PC, Kedhi E, Royaards K-J, et al. 2-Year Follow-Up of a Randomized Controlled Trial of Everolimus-and Paclitaxel-Eluting Stents for Coronary Revascularization in Daily PracticeCOMPARE (Comparison of the everolimus eluting XIENCE-V stent with the paclitaxel eluting TAXUS LIBERTÉ stent in all-comers: a randomized open label trial). J Am Coll Cardiol. 2011;58:11–8.
38. Smits PC, Sheikjoesoef K, Royaards K-J, et al. Final Five Year Results From The All-comer COMPARE Trial: A Prospective, Randomized Trial of Everolimus-Eluting vs. Paclitaxel-Eluting Stents. J Am Coll Cardiol. 2013;62:B5–5.
39. Moher D, Liberati A, Tetzlaff J, Altman DG. Preferred reporting items for systematic reviews and meta-analyses: the PRISMA statement. Ann Intern Med. 2009;151:264–9.
40. Palmerini T, Biondi-Zoccai G, Riva DD, et al. Stent thrombosis with drug-eluting and bare-metal stents: evidence from a comprehensive network meta-analysis. Lancet. 2012;379:1393–402.
41. Higgins JP, Green S. Cochrane handbook for systematic reviews of interventions. Wiley Online Library 2008.
42. Garg S, Serruys P, Onuma Y, et al. 3-Year Clinical Follow-Up of the XIENCE V Everolimus-Eluting Coronary Stent System in the Treatment of Patients With De Novo Coronary Artery LesionsThe SPIRIT II Trial (Clinical Evaluation of the Xience V Everolimus Eluting Coronary Stent System in the Treatment of Patients with de novo Native Coronary Artery Lesions). J Am Coll Cardiol Intv. 2009;2:1190–8.
43. Gada H, Kirtane AJ, Newman W, et al. 5-Year Results of a Randomized Comparison of XIENCE V Everolimus-Eluting and TAXUS Paclitaxel-Eluting StentsFinal Results From the SPIRIT III Trial (Clinical Evaluation of the XIENCE V Everolimus Eluting Coronary Stent System in the Treatment of Patients With De Novo Native Coronary Artery Lesions). J Am Coll Cardiol Intv. 2013;6:1263–6.
44. Hermiller JB, Nikolsky E, Lansky AJ, et al. Clinical and angiographic outcomes of elderly patients treated with everolimus-eluting versus paclitaxel-eluting stents: three-year results from the SPIRIT III randomised trial. EuroIntervention. 2011;7:307–13.
45. Brener SJ, Kereiakes DJ, Simonton CA, et al. Everolimus-eluting stents in patients undergoing percutaneous coronary intervention: Final 3-year results of the Clinical Evaluation of the XIENCE V Everolimus Eluting Coronary Stent System in the Treatment of Subjects With de Novo Native Coronary Artery Lesions trial. Am Heart J. 2013;166:1035–42.
46. Onuma Y, Miquel-Hebert K, Serruys PW. Five-year long-term clinical follow-up of the XIENCE V everolimus-eluting coronary stent system in the treatment of patients with de novo coronary artery disease: the SPIRIT II trial. EuroIntervention. 2013;8:1047–51.
47. Garg S, Serruys PW, Miquel-Hebert K. Four-year clinical follow-up of the XIENCE V everolimus-eluting coronary stent system in the treatment of patients with de novo coronary artery lesions: The SPIRIT II trial. Catheter Cardiovasc Interv. 2011;77:1012–7.
48. Ng VG, Lansky AJ, Hermiller JB, et al. Three-Year Results of Safety and Efficacy of the *Everolimus*-Eluting Coronary Stent in Women (from the SPIRIT III Randomized Clinical Trial). Am J Cardiol. 2011;107:841–8.
49. Lansky AJ, Brar SS, Yaqub M, et al. Impact of routine angiographic follow-up after percutaneous coronary intervention with drug-eluting stents in the SPIRIT III randomized trial at three years. Am J Cardiol. 2012;110:21–9.
50. Almasood AS, Freixa X, Khan SQ et al. Stent Fracture after Everolimus-Eluting Stent Implantation. Cardiol. Res. Pract. 2011;2011:1–5.

4

Safety of the primary percutaneous coronary intervention strategy combining pre-hospital prasugrel, enoxaparin and in-hospital bivalirudin in acute ST-segment elevation myocardial infarction

Juho Viikilä[1*], Tuomo Nieminen[2], Ilkka Tierala[2] and Mika Laine[2]

Abstract

Backround: The optimal antithrombotic treatment during a primary percutaneous coronary intervention (pPCI) is not known. This single center registry study aims to assess the safety of a novel antithrombotic regimen combining enoxaparine and prasugrel at presentation, followed by bivalirudin at the catheterisation laboratory.

Methods: All consecutive patients who underwent a pPCI were collected prospectively. The primary endpoint was major bleeding within 30 days. The secondary endpoints were a composite of major adverse cardiovascular events (MACE) consisting of cardiovascular death, non-fatal myocardial infarction, non-fatal stroke, a new target vessel revascularisation and all-cause mortality at 30 days.

Results: Ninety-nine out of the total of 390 patients were treated according to the new regimen (protocol-treated group). The rest received other antithrombotic treatment (non-protocol-treated group). The protocol-treated group had a lower risk than the non-protocol-treated group according to the GRACE ischaemic (112 vs. 124, $p = 0.002$) and CRUSADE bleeding scores (21 vs. 28, $p < 0.0001$). The incidences of bleeding were similar: severe GUSTO or TIMI bleeding occurred in 0 % of the protocol-treated group and in 1.0 and 0.3 %, respectively, of the other group ($p = 0.311$ for GUSTO and $p = 0.559$ for TIMI). The incidence of MACE in the groups was 6.1 and 10.7 %, respectively ($p = 0.178$). The respective incidences of all-cause mortality were 5.1 and 9.6 % ($p = 0.158$).

Conclusions: Administration of the novel antithrombotic regimen seems to be safe.

Background

Primary percutaneous coronary intervention (pPCI) is the preferred first-line treatment for acute ST- segment elevation myocardial infarction (STEMI) [1]. Antithrombotic treatment is an essential part of the pPCI procedure in enhancing the opening of the occluded coronary artery as well as preventing peri- and post-procedural thrombotic complications and late recurrent ischaemic events. Peri-procedural stroke, for example, has been recognised as an important life-limiting complication [2]. The development of new antithrombotic agents has been rapid over the last decade. The application of clopidogrel and glycoprotein (GP) IIb/IIIa inhibitors in addition to heparin and aspirin has been shown to decrease early and late adverse cardiac events with a concomitant and undesired increase in bleeding events [3–6]. Bleeding has been recognised as a major determinant of cardiovascular death and adverse events in acute coronary syndrome (ACS) patients [7].

Prasugrel is a novel thrombocyte receptor P2Y12 inhibitor, which has a more rapid, efficacious and consistent antithombotic effect than clopidogrel [8, 9]. In the TRITON TIMI-38 trial, prasugrel was more effective than clopidogrel in reducing adverse cardiac events in

* Correspondence: juho.viikila@phsotey.fi
[1]Department of Cardiology, Päijät-Häme Central Hospital, Keskussairaalankatu 7, 15850 Lahti, Finland

both acute non-ST-elevation myocardial infarction and STEMI patients [10]. However, the incidence of severe bleeding events, especially in elderly and low-weight patients as well as those with prior ischaemic cerebrovascular events was raised with prasugrel when compared to clopidogrel.

Bivalirudin is an intravenously administered direct, short-acting thrombin inhibitor [11]. In the HORIZONS-AMI trial, it reduced severe bleeding events as well as early and late net adverse events in STEMI patients when compared to heparin plus GPIIb/IIIa-inhibitor, with an increase in the incidence of early stent thromboses [12]. In the EUROMAX study, bivalirudin started during transport for pPCI was similarily associated with a reduction in major bleeding events and an increase in early stent thrombosis compared to heparin or enoxaparin with optional GPIIb/IIIa inhibitor [13]. The recent HEAT-PPCI compared heparin and bivalirudin in a randomised settings; heparin reduced the incidence of major ischaemic events with equal safety profile [14]. Importantly, the other antithrombotic drugs used differed between the studies.

Enoxaparine is an alternative to unfractionated heparin. In the ATOLL trial, intravenous enoxaparine, in comparison to heparin, was associated with fewer ischaemic events with similar bleeding rates for acute STEMI patients undergoing pPCI [15].

No previous study has combined prehospital prasugrel and enoxaparine with bivalirudin. We hypothesized that using this combination of drugs might balance the risk of early stent thrombosis and bleeding events in pPCI patients. Thus, we report the results of our new antithrombotic pPCI regimen including aspirin, a low-dose enoxaparine i.v. bolus and prasugrel loading upon first medical contact (FMC) combined with a bivalirudin infusion initiated in the catheterisation laboratory.

Methods

Study patients and data collection

The present study took place in the Meilahti hospital, responsible of all PCIs for STEMI in the Helsinki-Uusimaa Hospital District of 1.5 million inhabitants. According to the new local STEMI guidelines launched on 1 November 2010, all acute STEMI patients referred to pPCI should receive aspirin 250 mg, enoxaparine 30 mg intravenously and prasugrel 60 mg upon FMC. The bivalirudin infusion (a bolus of 0.75 mg/kg followed by an infusion of 1.75 mg/kg/h) should be started in the catheter laboratory. After PCI, aspirin 100 mg daily should be continued indefinitely and prasugrel 10 mg daily for 12 to 15 months. A lower prasugrel dosage of 5 mg daily, or clopidogrel 75 mg daily instead of prasugrel, is recommended for patients weighing under 60 kg or aged over 75 years. Those with a previous stroke or transient ischemic attack are recommended to continue with clopidogrel 75 mg daily. When switching to clopidogrel, it is advised to load the new drug at 300–600 mg the day after prasugrel loading.

In order to assess the efficacy and safety of the new antithrombotic regimen, we examined all acute STEMI patients treated with pPCI in the Meilahti hospital between 1 January 2011 and 30 April 2012. The patients were prospectively collected into a local STEMI registry. All hospital files regarding the index STEMI hospitalisation and the following 30-day period were searched to receive detailed data on patients risk profile, treatments and clinical outcome. Mortality data was available for all patients from the National Population Register Centre. This was a registry study, which did not need an approval from the ethics committee. An informed consent was not needed; no contact to the patient was taken in this registry study and the data was anonymized and de-identified prior to analysis. The study protocol was approved by the Helsinki-Uusimaa Hospital District. The study was performed in accordance with the Declaration of Helsinki.

The inclusion criteria were acute STEMI treated with pPCI within the first 12 hours after symptom onset. The criteria for a STEMI diagnosis were acute chest pain (or equivalent) and 1) ST elevations of ≥ 2 mm (≥ 1.5 mm for women) in at least two of the leads V1–3, or 2) ST elevations of ≥ 1 mm in at least two other leads (V4–6, V8–9, V4R, I, aVL, II, III, aVF), or 3) a new left bundle branch block in ECG. Patients who received fibrinolysis were excluded from the study.

Definitions of study endpoints

The primary endpoint was major bleeding within 30 days. Bleedings were classified and reported according to GUSTO and TIMI criteria [16, 17]. The secondary endpoints were 1) a composite of major adverse cardiovascular events (MACE) consisting of cardiovascular death, non-fatal myocardial infarction, non-fatal stroke and a new target vessel revascularisation procedure, and 2) all-cause mortality at 30 days. Myocardial infarction was defined according to current international guidelines [18]. Stroke was defined as any focal neurological deficit of ischaemic or haemorrhagic origin lasting for longer than 24 hours.

Statistical analysis

The follow-up of the acute STEMI patients who received the guideline-defined adjuvant treatment was analysed primarily without a control group. Secondarily, a comparison with pPCI patients who had received other adjuvant treatment was performed. Continuous variables are described using medians, means and standard deviations (SD). Categorical variables are described with absolute (number) and relative (percentage) frequency distribution. Statistical analyses across the groups were done with a chi-square test for categorical variables and ANOVA for continuous variables. A Cox regression survival analysis was performed for MACE using age, sex, access site, thrombectomy, antithrombotic treatment as well as GRACE and CRUSADE scores as covariates. IBM SPSS Statistics version 19.0 was used for all analyses.

Results

In total, 390 acute STEMI patients fulfilling the study criteria were identified within the study period. Ninety-nine patients (25 %) received the complete guideline-defined antithrombotic treatment with aspirin, a bolus of i.v. enoxaparine and a loading dose of prasugrel at presentation followed by a bivalirudin infusion at the catheter laboratory (protocol-treated group). The remaining 291 patients received some other combination of antithrombotic agents (non-protocol treated group).

The patients in the protocol-treated group were significantly younger and less likely to be on warfarin treatment at presentation than the patients in the non-protocol-treated group (Table 1). There was a trend towards a higher prevalence of diabetes and prior coronary artery bypass operations in the non-protocol-treated group. Smoking was more common in the protocol-treated group. Other cardiovascular risk factors or prior cardiovascular disease did not vary significantly across the groups (Table 1). At presentation, according to the GRACE and CRUSADE score calculations, the predicted risk of short- and long-term adverse cardiovascular events and in-hospital bleeding events was significantly higher in the non-protocol-treated group (Table 2). The proportion of patients presenting with acute heart failure was also significantly higher in the non-protocol-treated group.

Sixteen percent of patients in the non-protocol-treated group had normal coronary arteries or only modest coronary artery lesions, whereas all patients in the protocol-treated group had significant coronary artery disease. Consequently, normal coronary artery flow before PCI was more frequent in the non-protocol-treated group (Table 2). However, the prevalence of left-main or tree-vessel disease did not vary significantly across the

Table 1 Baseline characteristics, cardiovascular risk factors, prior cardiovascular diseases, revascularisations and medications in the protocol and non-protocol treated groups

	Protocol $n = 99$	Non-protocol $n = 291$	*p*
Mean age, years, mean (SD)	59.5 (14)	66.1 (14)	<0.001
Age > 75 years, *n* (%)	11 (11.1)	97 (33.3)	<0.001
Male sex, *n* (%)	74 (74.7)	198 (68.0)	0.210
Diabetes, *n* (%)	13 (13.1)	64 (22.0)	0.056
Current smoker, *n* (%)	50 (50.5)	95 (32.6)	0.001
Hypertension, *n* (%)	49 (49.5)	158 (54.3)	0.408
Dyslipidaemia, *n* (%)	39 (39.4)	123 (42.3)	0.616
Renal dysfunction[a], *n* (%)	3 (3.0)	11 (3.8)	0.729
Peripheral vascular disease, *n* (%)	4 (4.0)	14 (4.8)	0.752
Previous myocardial infarction, *n* (%)	9 (9.1)	32 (11.0)	0.593
Previous stroke, *n* (%)	4 (4.0)	21 (7.2)	0.265
Previous CABG, *n* (%)	1 (1.0)	15 (5.2)	0.073
Previous PCI, *n* (%)	10 (10.1)	39 (13.4)	0.392
Aspirin, *n* (%)	21 (21.2)	81 (27.8)	0.195
P2Y12-receptor inhibitor, *n* (%)	2 (2.0)	11 (3.8)	0.399
Warfarin, *n* (%)	2 (2.0)	37 (12.7)	0.002

CABG coronary artery by-pass intervention, *PCI* percutaneous coronary intervention
[a]estimated glomerular filtration rate <60 ml/min/1.73 m^2

Table 2 Clinical characteristics at presentation, coronary angiography and revascularisation procedures in the protocol and non-protocol treated groups

	Protocol $n = 99$	Non-protocol $n = 291$	*p*-value
Anterior STEMI, *n* (%)	43 (43.4)	138 (47.4)	0.492
GRACE score, mean (SD)	112 (31)	124 (36)	0.002
CRUSADE score, mean (SD)	21 (13)	28(16)	<0.0001
Killip class > I, *n* (%)	8 (8.1)	62 (21.5)	0.003
Killip class IV, *n* (%)	2 (2.0)	13 (4.5)	0.270
eGFR ml/min, mean (SD)	103 (40)	90 (41)	0.009
Hemoglobin g/l, mean (SD)	135 (15)	133 (18)	0.283
Weight kg, mean (SD)	81 (16)	80 (17)	0.644
Angiography			
Radialis access, *n* (%)	33 (33.3)	77 (26.6)	0.196
3VD, *n* (%)	14 (14.1)	56 (19.2)	0.253
LMD, *n* (%)	2 (2.0)	16 (5.5)	0.154
TIMI flow grade 0–1, *n* (%)	68 (70.1)	119 (57.2)	0.031
TIMI flow grade 3, *n* (%)	15 (15.5)	58 (27.9)	0.018
Normal findings or modest coronary artery disease	0 (0)	46 (16.0)	<0.0001
PCI, *n* (%)	99 (100)	205 (70.4)	<0.0001
Use of stents (of all PCI), *n* (%)	91 (91.9)	187 (91.2)	0.838
Use of DES (of stents), *n* (%)	13 (14.3)	24 (12.8)	0.738
Thrombectomy (of all PCI), *n* (%)	53 (53.5)	68 (33.2)	0.001
TIMI flow grade 0–1 post PCI, *n* (%)	0 (0)	8 (3.8)	0.053
TIMI flow grade 3 post PCI, *n* (%)	89 (91.8)	182 (85.8)	0.143
CABG, *n* (%)	2 (2.0)	17 (5.8)	0.127

eGFR glomerular filtration rate estimated by Cockcroft-Gault formula, *3VD* three vessel coronary artery disease, *LMD* left main coronary artery disease, *LAD-PCI* percutaneous coronary intervention to left anterior descending artery, *DES* drug-eluting stent, *CABG* coronary artery bypass graft surgery groups. A percutaneous coronary intervention was performed more often in the protocol-treated group. The use of bare metal or drug-eluting stents among the PCI-treated patients did not vary significantly across the groups. However, thrombectomy was more common in the protocol-treated group. There were no significant differences in post-PCI coronary artery flow between the groups. The median total ischaemic time (delay from symptom onset to PCI) was 300 min. and 264 min. in the protocol-treated and non-protocol-treated groups, respectively ($p = 0.165$ between the groups).

The use of glycoprotein-inhibitors was uncommon in the protocol-treated group, whereas they were used in approximately one quarter of the patients in the non-protocol-treated group (Table 3). Clopidogrel was used frequently in the non-protocol-treated group.

Bleeding events were rare in the overall population, and their occurrence did not differ between the groups (Table 4). None of the patients suffered intracranial or fatal bleedings during the study period. Major adverse cardiac events and deaths were observed more frequently in the non-protocol-treated group, but the difference across the groups was not statistically significant (Table 4). In the multivariable Cox analysis for MACE, high GRACE and CRUSADE scores were the only variables associated with worse prognosis (data not shown).

At discharge, prasugrel was used in 77 and 26 % of the patients in the protocol-treated and non-protocol-treated groups, respectively, ($p < 0.0001$ between the groups) and clopidogrel in 17 and 46 % of the patients, respectively ($p < 0.001$). Statins were used in 94 and 82 % ($p = 0.004$), beta blockers in 89 and 78 % ($p = 0.04$) and angiotensin convertase inhibitors or angiotensin II receptor blockers in 81 and 65 % of the patients ($p = 0.003$), respectively.

Table 3 Antithrombotic treatment in the protocol ($n = 99$) and non-protocol ($n = 291$) treated groups

	Protocol, *n* (%)	Non-protocol, *n* (%)	*P*-value
First medical contact			
Aspirin	99 (100)	257 (88.3)	<0.0001
Prasugrel loading dose	99 (100)	139 (47.8)	<0.0001
Clopidogrel loading dose	1(1.0)	116 (39.9)	<0.0001
Enoxaparin bolus i.v.	99 (100)	192 (66.0)	<0.0001
Glycoprotein IIb/IIIa inhibitor	0 (0)	15 (5.2)	0.021
Catheter laboratorio			
Bivalirudin	99 (100)	36 (12.4)	<0.0001
Glycoprotein IIb/IIIa inhibitor	6 (6.1)	79 (27.1)	<0.0001
Enoxaparin i.v.	9 (9.1)	56 (19.2)	0.019
Unfractionated heparin	0 (0)	7 (2.4)	0.119

Table 4 Major adverse cardiac events, mortality and bleeding events at 30 days in the protocol ($n = 99$) and non-protocol ($n = 291$) treated groups

	Protocol *n* (%)	Non-protocol *n* (%)	*p*-value
MACE	6 (6.1)	31 (10.7)	0.178
Cardiovascular death	4 (4.0)	26 (8.9)	0.114
Non-fatal myocardial infarction	0 (0)	1 (0.3)	0.559
Non-fatal stroke	1 (1.0)	4 (1.4)	0.781
Target vessel revascularisation	1 (1.0)	3 (1.0)	0.986
Death from any cause	5 (5.1)	28 (9.6)	0.158
Severe GUSTO bleeding	0 (0)	3 (1.0)	0.311
Mild or minor GUSTO bleeding	3 (3.0)	6 (2.1)	0.579
Major TIMI bleeding	0 (0)	1 (0.3)	0.559
Minor or minimal TIMI bleeding	2 (2.0)	4 (1.4)	0.652

Discussion

Bleeding events

In this paper, we report the results on STEMI patients treated with a novel antithrombotic regimen combining aspirin, an i.v. enoxaparine bolus and a prasugrel loading dose at presentation, followed by bivalirudin infusion at the catheterisation laboratory. To the best of our knowledge, no previous study has used the same adjuvant therapy. Our principal finding is that the administration of the new regimen is safe. None of the protocol-treated patients suffered a severe bleeding event during the 30-day follow-up. The incidence of mild to moderate bleeding events was only 3 % in that group. This outcome was favourable compared to the CRUSADE-score-based estimation of 5.5 % in-hospital incidence of bleeding events in the protocol treated group. On the other hand, the incidence of severe bleeding events was low also in the non-protocol-treated group as well, and there were no significant differences in bleeding events between the groups. Therefore, our findings support the concept that bivalirudin can be combined to low-dose low-molecular heparin without increasing bleeding complications.

The safety of bivalirudin compared to heparin plus GP IIb/IIIa-inhibitors in pPCI-patients is supported by two major trials: HORIZONS-AMI and EUROMAX [12, 13]. The incidence of net adverse and severe bleeding events was reduced with bivalirudin in both trials. In HORIZONS-AMI, bivalirudin was compared to heparin plus GP-inhibitors with almost all patients having a clopidogrel loading at the time of admission. Heparin was given in 68 % in the bivalirudin group. In the Euromax study, 51 % of the patients had a clopidogrel loading as soon as possible and the rest received either prasugrel (30 %) or ticagrelor (19 %). Heparin was used in only 2.2 % in the bivalirudin group.

Adverse events

None of the protocol-treated patients suffered from stent thrombosis or recurrent myocardial infarction. The non-protocol group presented one stent thrombosis and one myocardial infarction within a month. The incidence of MACE and all-cause death in the protocol-treated group was 6.1 and 5.1 percent, respectively. These numbers are comparable to MACE and mortality figures recently published based on the French and Swedish STEMI registries [19, 20]. From this perspective, the new anti-thrombotic regimen also seems to be efficient.

The non-protocol group presented with a higher risk profile (older age, warfarin usage, higher GRACE and CRUSADE scores, higher Killip class at presentation, worse renal function) than those treated with the new protocol. However, the number of endpoints did not differ between the treatment groups, which is probably due to the low number of adverse events. The Cox regression analysis presented the GRACE and CRUSADE scores – which integrate patient-related information from several angles – as the only variables predicting poor prognosis.

The rate of early stent thromboses was increased with bivalirudin in both the HORIZONS-AMI and EUROMAX trials. This may be partly due to an inconsistent action of clopidogrel used widely in both trials. Importantly, in HORIZONS-AMI, those patients who had received the heparin bolus prior to randomisation had a lower risk of stent thrombosis than those without pre-randomisation heparin [21]. In EUROMAX, only 2 % of the bivalirudin treated patients were protected by heparin. However, in our study, the usage of prasugrel and enoxaparine with bivalirudin might have protected patients against stent thromboses.

The recent HEAT-PPCI study randomised STEMI patients to receive either bivalirudin or heparin infusion, with provisional GP IIb/IIIa inhibitors used in only 13-15 % of the patients in each group [14]. Only 11 % received clopidogrel, as prasugrel (27 %) and ticagrelor (62 %) were clearly more common. The rate of major adverse events during 28 day follow-up was significantly higher with bivalirudin mainly due to increased rate of stent thromboses. The bleeding rates did not differ across the groups. This might be due to low usage of GP IIb/IIIa inhibitors also in the heparin arm. Of note, the patients in the bivalirudin group were not protected with either heparin or enoxaparine.

Our hypothesis was that combining pre-hospital enoxaparine and prasugrel with bivalirudin during the pPCI procedure might balance the risk of bleeding and early stent thromboses. The observed low incidence of bleeding events and the lack of stent thromboses and recurrent myocardial infarctions in the protocol-treated patients support the hypothesis. We replaced heparin, which was widely used in the bivalirudin arm in the HORIZONS-AMI trial, by a low dose of enoxaparine at FMC without any evident rise in bleeding events.

Adoption of the new protocol

The rate of adoption of the new local guidelines in daily practice was clearly lower than we expected. The deviations were mostly due to the omission of prasugrel and, particularly, bivalirudin. Firstly, only half of the patients in the non-protocol-treated group received prasugrel at FMC. This might reflect the fact that we started the survey period relatively soon, two months after the guideline implementation. Patients were referred to our pPCI centre from a relatively large area with different emergency medical system organisations, a setting that may have compromised the early guideline implementation process. Secondly, the utilisation of bivalirudin in the catheter laboratory was low in the non-protocol-treated group. Operators seemed to prefer to see the angiographic result before deciding whether to use bivalirudin. This policy is reflected as a higher incidence of normal angiographic findings in the non-protocol-treated groups.

Limitations

We observed unexpectedly low bleeding rates in both treatment groups. Despite the differences in GRACE and CRUSADE scores the rate of adverse events did not differ across the groups. These findings might be related to the relatively small sample size and the non-randomised trial design, which are limitations to our study. Another limitation is the low penetration of the guidelines in daily practice, leaving open questions on the usability of the new regimen in unselected patient populations.

Conclusions

The present study offers preliminary findings on a new antithrombotic regimen combining low-dose enoxaparine, prasugrel and bivalirudin in STEMI patients. The data are promising and suggest that the regimen is both safe and efficient, but the results need to be confirmed in randomised studies.

Abbreviations

ACS, acute coronary syndrome; CABG, coronary artery by-pass graft surgery; FMC, first medical contact; Gp-inhibitor, glycoprotein receptor inhibitor; MACE, major adverse cardiovascular event; PCI, percutaneous coronary intervention; STEMI, ST-segment elevation myocardial infarction

Acknowledgements

We thank Eeva Parviainen who performed English language revision.

Funding

None.

Authors' contributions

JV drafted the manuscript, performed the statistical analysis and participated in the design and conception of the study, TN made main contribution to conception and design of the study, performed data collection and helped to draft the manuscript and make the statistical analysis. IT participated in the design and coordination of the study and participated in the data collection. ML participated in the design and coordination of the study and helped to draft the manuscript. All authors have read and accepted the manuscript.

Competing interests

The authors declare that they have no competing interests.

Author details

[1]Department of Cardiology, Päijät-Häme Central Hospital, Keskussairaalankatu 7, 15850 Lahti, Finland. [2]Department of Cardiology, Helsinki University Central Hospital, Helsinki, Finland.

References

1. The Task Force on the management of ST-segment elevation acute myocardial infarction of the European Society of Cardiology (ESC) Authors/ Task Force Members, Steg G, James SK, Atar D, Badano LP, Blöstrom-Lundqvist C, Bogerm, et al. ESC guidelines for the management of acute myocardial infarction in patients presenting with ST-segment elevation. Eur Heart J. 2012;33:2569–19.
2. D'Ascenzo F, Barbero U, Moretti C, Plamerini T, Della Riva D, Mariani A, et al. Percutaneous coronary intervention versus coronary artery bypass graft for stable angina: meta-regression of randomized trials. Contemp Clin Trials. 2014;28:51–8.
3. Yusuf S, Zhao F, Mehta SR, Chrolavicius S, Tognoni G, Fox KK. Clopidogrel in unstable angina to prevent recurrent events trial investigators. Effects of clopidogrel in addition to aspirin in patients with acute coronary syndromes without ST-segment elevation. N Engl J Med. 2001;345:494–502.
4. Chen ZM, Jiang LX, Chen YP, Xie JX, Pan HC, Peto R, COMMIT (ClOpidogrel and Metoprolol in Myocardial Infarction Trial) collaborative group, et al. Addition of clopidogrel to aspirin in 45,852 patients with acute myocardial infarction: randomised placebo-controlled trial. Lancet. 2005;366:1607–21.
5. Mehta SR, Tanguay JF, Eikelboom JW, Jolly SS, Joyner CD, Granger CB, et al. Double-dose versus standard-dose clopidogrel and high-dose versus low-dose aspirin in individuals undergoing percutaneous coronary intervention for acute coronary syndromes (CURRENT-OASIS 7): a randomised factorial trial. Lancet. 2010;376:1233–43.
6. De Luca G, Navarese E, Marino P. Risk profile and benefits from Gp IIb-IIIa inhibitors among patients with ST-segment elevation myocardial infarction treated with primary angioplasty: a meta-regression analysis of randomized trials. Eur Heart J. 2009;30:2705–13.
7. Eikelboom JW, Mehta SR, Anand SS, Xie C, Fox KA, Yusuf S. Adverse impact of bleeding on prognosis in patients with acute coronary syndromes. Circulation. 2006;114:774–82.
8. Niitsu Y, Jakubowski JA, Sugidachi A, Asai F. Pharmacology of CS-747 (prasugrel, LY640315), a novel, potent antiplatelet agent with in vivo P2Y12 receptor antagonist activity. Semin Thromb Hemost. 2005;31:184–94.
9. Jernberg T, Payne CD, Winters KJ, Darstein C, Brandt JT, Jakubowski JA. Prasugrel achieves greater inhibition of platelet aggregation and a lower rate of non-responders compared with clopidogrel in aspirin-treated patients with stable coronary artery disease. Eur Heart J. 2006;27:1166–73.
10. Montalescot G, Wiviott SD, Braunwald E, Murphy SA, Gibson CM, McCABE CH, et al. Prasugrel compared with clopidogrel in patients undergoing percutaneous coronary intervention for ST-elevation myocardial infarction (TRITON TIMI 38): double-blind, randomised controlled trial. Lancet. 2009;373:723–31.
11. Warkentin TE, Greinacher A, Koster A. Bivalirudin. Thromb Haemost. 2008;99:830–9.
12. Stone GW, Witzenbichler B, Guagliumi G, Peruga JZ, Brodie BR, Dudek D, et al. Bivalirudin during primary PCI in acute myocardial infarction. N Engl J Med. 2008;358:2218–30.
13. Steg PG, van't Hof A, Hamm CW, Clemmensen P, Lapostelle F, Coste P, et al. Bivalirudin started during emergency transport for primary PCI. N Engl J Med. 2013;369:2207–17.
14. Shahzad A, Kemp I, Mars C, Wilson K, Roome C, Cooper R, et al. Unfractionated heparin versus bivalirudin in primary percutaneous coronary intervention (HEAT-PPCI); an open-label, single centre, randomised controlled trial. Lancet. 2014;384:1849–58.
15. Montalescot G, Zeymer U, Silvain J, Boulanger B, Cohen M, Goldstein P, ATOLL Investigators et al. Intravenous enoxaparin or unfractionated heparin in primary percutaneous coronary intervention for ST-elevation myocardial infarction: the international randomised open-label ATOLL trial. Lancet. 2011;378:693–703.
16. The GUSTO investigators. An international randomized trial comparing four thrombolytic strategies for acute myocardial infarction. N Engl J Med. 1993;329:673–82.
17. Chesebro JH, Knatterud G, Roberts R, Borer J, Cohen LS, Dalen J, et al. Thrombolysis in Myocardial Infarction (TIMI) Trial, Phase I: a comparison between intravenous tissue plasminogen activator and intravenous streptokinase. Clinical findings through hospital discharge. Circulation. 1987;76:142–54.
18. Thygesen K, Alpert JS, Jaffe AS, Simoons ML, Chaitman BR, White HD, Joint ESC/ACCF/AHA/WHF Task Force for the Universal Definition of Myocardial, et al. Third universal definition of myocardial infarction. Eur Heart J. 2012;33:2551–67.
19. Hanssen M, Cottin Y, Khalife K, Hammer L, Goldstein P, Puymirat P, for the FAST-MI 2010 investigators et al. French registry on acute ST-elevation and non ST-elevation myocardial infarction 2010. FAST-MI 2010. Heart. 2012;98:699–705.
20. Stenestrand U, Lindback J, Wallentin L, RIKS-HIA Registry. Long-term outcome of primary percutaneous coronary intervention vs prehospital and in-hospital thrombolysis for patients with ST-elevation myocardial infarction. JAMA. 2006;296:1749–56.
21. Dangas GD, Caixeta A, Mehran R, Parise H, Lansky AJ, Cristea E, et al. Harmonizing Outcomes With Revascularization and Stents in Acute Myocardial Infarction (HORIZONS-AMI) trial investigators. Frequency and predictors of stent thrombosis after percutaneous coronary intervention in acute myocardial infarction. Circulation. 2011;123:1745–56.

5

Should a prolonged duration of dual anti-platelet therapy be recommended to patients with diabetes mellitus following percutaneous coronary intervention?

Pravesh Kumar Bundhun[1], Chandra Mouli Yanamala[2] and Feng Huang[1*]

Abstract

Background: This study aimed to compare the adverse clinical outcomes associated with a short and a prolonged duration of Dual Anti-Platelet Therapy (DAPT) in patients with Diabetes Mellitus (DM) after undergoing Percutaneous Coronary Intervention (PCI).

Methods: Medline/PubMed, EMBASE and the Cochrane library were searched for studies comparing the short and prolonged DAPT use in patients with DM. Adverse outcomes were considered as the clinical endpoints in this analysis. Odds Ratios (OR) with 95 % Confidence Intervals (CI) were used to express the pooled effect on discontinuous variables and the pooled analyses were performed with RevMan 5.3.

Results: Fifteen studies with a total number of 25,742 patients with DM were included in this current analysis which showed no significant differences in primary endpoints, net clinical outcomes, myocardial infarction and stroke with OR: 1.03, 95 % CI: 0.65–1.64; $P = 0.90$, OR: 0.96, 95 % CI: 0.69–1.34; $P = 0.81$, OR: 0.85, 95 % CI: 0.70–1.04; $P = 0.12$ and OR: 0.94, 95 % CI: 0.65–1.36; $P = 0.75$ respectively. Revascularization was also similar between these 2 groups of patients with DM. However, even if mortality favored prolonged DAPT use, with OR: 0.87, 95 % CI: 0.76–1.00; $P = 0.05$, the result only approached significance. Also, stent thrombosis insignificantly favored a prolonged DAPT duration with OR: 0.56, 95 % CI: 0.27–1.17; $P = 0.12$. Thrombolysis In Myocardial Infarction (TIMI) defined major and minor bleeding were not significantly different in these diabetic patients with OR: 0.91, 95 % CI: 0.60–1.37; $P = 0.65$ and OR: 1.08, 95 % CI: 0.62–1.91; $P = 0.78$ respectively. However, bleeding defined by the Bleeding Academic Research Consortium (BARC) classification was significantly higher with a prolonged DAPT use in these diabetic patients with OR: 1.92, 95 % CI: 1.58–2.34; $P < 0.00001$.

(Continued on next page)

* Correspondence: huangfeng7925@163.com
[1]Institute of Cardiovascular Diseases, the First Affiliated Hospital of Guangxi Medical University, Nanning, Guangxi 530021, People's Republic of China
Full list of author information is available at the end of the article

(Continued from previous page)

Conclusion: Following PCI, a prolonged DAPT use was associated with similar adverse clinical outcomes but with a significantly increased BARC defined bleeding compared to a short term DAPT use in these patients with DM. However, even if mortality and stent thrombosis favored a prolonged DAPT use, these outcomes only either reached statistical significance or were insignificant respectively, showing that a clear decision about recommending a prolonged duration of DAPT to patients with DM might not be possible at this moment, warranting further research in this particular subgroup.

Keywords: Dual antiplatelet therapy, Percutaneous coronary intervention, Diabetes mellitus, Drug eluting stents, Clopidogrel, Stent thrombosis, Bleeding events

Abbreviations: ACS, Acute coronary syndrome; BARC, Bleeding academic research consortium; DAPT, Dual antiplatelet therapy; DES, Drug eluting stents; DM, Diabetes mellitus; PCI, Percutaneous coronary intervention; TIMI, Thrombolysis in myocardial infarction

Background

According to guidelines, Dual Anti-Platelet Therapy (DAPT) with aspirin and P2Y12 inhibitors, mainly clopidogrel, is recommended for at least one year following Percutaneous Coronary Intervention (PCI) with Drug Eluting Stents (DES) [1]. However, even in this new era, several Randomized Controlled Trials (RCTs) still could not predict the exact duration of DAPT use and suggested that this issue might possibly be solved only using a larger number of randomized patients following PCI with DES [2]. To be more clear, in a previously published study comparing 6 months with 12 months DAPT use, the authors stated that larger trials would be able to completely solve this issue [3]. Even if several meta-analyses comparing the short and prolonged DAPT use in the general population following PCI showed a longer duration of DAPT to be associated with favorable clinical outcomes [4], other meta-analyses showed no benefits of a prolonged DAPT duration [5] giving rise to controversies. However, whether these results also apply to the subgroup of patients with Diabetes Mellitus (DM) have seldom been studied. Therefore, this study aimed to compare the adverse clinical outcomes associated with a short and prolonged duration of DAPT use in patients with DM following PCI.

Methods

Data sources and search strategy

Medline/PubMed, EMBASE and the Cochrane library were searched for studies comparing the short and prolonged use of DAPT in patients with Acute Coronary Syndrome (ACS) following PCI by typing the words 'dual anti-platelet therapy, diabetes mellitus and percutaneous coronary intervention'. Another search was performed using the phrase 'prolonged clopidogrel use, diabetes mellitus and percutaneous coronary intervention'. To widen this search, the abbreviations 'DAPT, DM, and PCI' as well as the term 'coronary angioplasty' were also used. In addition, reference lists of suitable studies were also reviewed for relevant articles. Only articles published in English were considered in this search process.

Inclusion and exclusion criteria

Studies were included if:

(a) They were randomized trials or observational studies.
(b) They compared short and prolonged DAPT use and included patients with DM.
(c) They reported adverse outcomes as their clinical endpoints.
(d) They were published in English.

Studies were excluded if:

(a) They were meta-analyses, case studies or editorials.
(b) They did not involve patients with DM.
(c) They did not report adverse outcomes as their clinical endpoints.
(d) They did not compare short with prolonged DAPT use, but instead, compared aspirin monotherapy with DAPT following PCI.
(e) They were duplicates or involved the same trial.

Definitions, outcomes and follow up

DM was defined as a state of high blood sugar levels observed at least on two separate occasions, with a fasting blood glucose test or an oral glucose tolerance test, with or without symptoms (asymptomatic) such as polydipsia (frequent thirst), polyuria (frequent urination) and weight loss.

Adverse clinical outcomes which were analyzed in this study included:

(a) Primary endpoint which was a composite endpoint of all-cause death, Myocardial Infarction (MI), stroke, revascularization and stent thrombosis.

(b) MI (any type or any classification of MI) was relevant including the universal definition [6].
(c) Target Lesion Revascularization (TLR).
(d) Target Vessel Revascularization (TVR).
(e) All-cause death (cardiac and non-cardiac).
(f) Stroke.
(g) Net Adverse Clinical and Cerebral Events (NACCE) were defined as a composite of all-cause death, all MI, stroke or major bleeding.
(h) Stent thrombosis which was defined by the Academic Research Consortium (ARC) [7].
(i) Bleeding:
(1) All/Any bleeding.
(2) Major and Minor bleeding defined by Thrombolysis in Myocardial Infarction (TIMI) [8].
(3) Bleeding defined according to the Bleeding Academic Research Consortium (BARC) [9] which was further divided into BARC type 2, BARC type 3 and BARC type 5.

The adverse clinical outcomes reported have been listed in Table 1.

Short and prolonged duration of DAPT

Short and prolonged duration of DAPT use were based on the following criteria:

If the short term DAPT duration period was 3 months, its corresponding prolonged duration period should be more than 3 months (6, 12, 24, or more).

If the short term duration of DAPT was 6 months, its corresponding prolonged duration period should be more than 6 months (12, 18, 24, or more).

If the short term duration of DAPT use was 12 months, its corresponding prolonged duration period should be more than 12 months.

Therefore, a prolonged duration of DAPT was defined as the use of DAPT during a period of time longer than the actual short term duration corresponding to that particular trial. Different trials had different short and prolonged duration of DAPT use. Table 2 further illustrated the short and prolonged duration periods of DAPT use in each of the studies included in this meta-analysis.

Data extraction and review

Two authors (PKB and CMY) independently assessed the studies involved and reviewed the methodological quality of each eligible trial. Information regarding the study/trial names, time period of patients' enrollment, adverse clinical outcomes reported, the follow up periods, data concerning the total number of patients with DM classified into the short and prolonged DAPT groups respectively, the total number of clinical events reported in each subgroup, as well as information concerning the baseline features of the patients were carefully extracted and cross checked. During the data extraction process, any disagreement which occurred between these two authors was carefully discussed, and if they could not reach a consensus, the disagreement was solved and a final decision was made by the third author (FH). The bias risk among the trials (low risk, moderate risk and high risk) was assessed with the components recommended by the Cochrane Collaboration [10]. The six components of the bias risk were as follow:

Table 1 Reported outcomes

Studies	Reported outcomes	Follow up period	Bias grade
Brar2008	Death, MI	9.7 months	-
I-LOVE IT 2	NACCE, death, MI, stroke, TVR, TLR, ST, all bleeding, major bleeding	12 and 18 months	B
ISAR-SAFE	Primary endpoints, death, MI, ST, stroke, TIMI major and minor bleeding, BARC bleeding	9 months	B
Tarantini2016	Death, MI, composite endpoints, stent thrombosis, BARC type 3 or 5 bleeding, stroke, revascularization	1 year	-
ARCTIC	Primary endpoints, Death, MI, ST, stroke, revascularization	17 months	B
OPTIMIZE	NACCE, death, MI, stroke, ST, major bleeding, TLR, TVR, any bleeding	1 year	B
RESET	Primary endpoints, death, MI, TVR, ST, major and minor bleeding, stroke	1 year	B
EXCELLENT	Death, MI, stroke, TVR, TLR, ST, any bleeding, TIMI major bleeding	1 year	B
PEGASUS	Death, MI, stroke, TIMI major and minor bleeding	3 years	B
DAPT	ST, MACCEs, death, stroke, MI, BARC type 2,3 or 5	12 to 30 months	B
Sardella2011	Death, MI, stroke, TIMI minor bleeding, revascularization	2 years	-
PRODIGY	Death, MI, stroke, ST, TLR, TVR, TIMI major and minor bleeding, BARC bleeding	2 years	B
Thukkani2015	Death, MI, Stroke	4 years	-
ENDEAVOR	Death, MI, ST (definite and probable), stroke, major bleeding	2 years	B
ITALIC	Primary endpoints, minor bleeding, minimal bleeding, death, MI, stroke, TVR, ST, major bleeding	1 year	B

Abbreviations: *MI* myocardial infarction, *ST* stent thrombosis, *TVR* target vessel revascularization, *TLR* target lesion revascularization, *NACCE* net adverse clinical and cerebral events, *BARC* bleeding academic research consortium, *TIMI* thrombolysis in myocardial infarction

Table 2 General features of the studies included

Features	No of DM patients in the short term group (*n*)	No of DM patients in the long term group (*n*)	Type of study	Enrollment period	Duration of DAPT use (months)
Brar2008	378	371	OB	2002–2004	<9 vs > 9
I-LOVE IT 2	211	203	RCT	2012–2015	6 vs 12
ISAR-SAFE	495	484	RCT	2008–2014	6 vs 12
Tarantini2016	206	223	RCT	2009–2014	6 vs > 12
ARCTIC	222	198	RCT	2009–2011	<12 vs >12
OPTIMIZE	554	549	RCT	2010–2015	3 vs 12
RESET	316	305	RCT	2009–2010	3 vs 12
EXCELLENT	272	278	RCT	2008–2009	6 vs 12
PEGASUS	1950	1574	RCT	2010–2013	<12 vs > 12
DAPT	1481	1556	RCT	2009–2011	12 vs 30
Sardella2011	133	139	OB	2005–2006	12 vs > 12
PRODIGY	35	36	RCT	2006–2012	6 vs 24
Thukkani2015	6568	5949	OB	2002–2006	12 vs > 12
ENDEAVOR	198	183	RCT	2005–2011	12 vs > 24
ITALIC	331	344	RCT	2011–2015	6 vs 24
Total no of patients (n)	13,350	12,392			

Abbreviations: *DM* diabetes mellitus, *DAPT* dual antiplatelet therapy, *RCT* randomized controlled trials, *OS* observational studies

A. Sequence generation
B. Allocation sequence concealment
C. Blinding of participants and personnel
D. Blinding of outcome assessment
E. Incomplete outcome data
F. Selective outcome reporting and other potential bias

The trials included in this study were analyzed according to these six components and a bias grade was given accordingly after a careful assessment. A grade ranging from A to E was considered whereby grade A was allocated if an extremely low risk of bias was reported, while a grade E was allocated if a very high risk of bias was observed. Note that these bias grades were just an approximation according to what the authors were able to assess. The bias risk grades allocated to each trial were provided in Table 1. Note that observational studies were ignored during this assessment.

Methodological and statistical analysis

Recommendations of the PRISMA (Preferred Reporting Items for Systematic Reviews and Meta-Analyses) statement were followed in this study [11]. Heterogeneity among the subgroups was assessed using the Cochrane Q-statistic test whereby a P value less than 0·05 was considered statistically significant whereas *P* value ≥ 0.05 was considered statistically insignificant. I^2-statistic test which also assessed heterogeneity, whereby an I^2 with a low percentage (<25 %) represented a low heterogeneity, an I^2 with a percentage between 25 and 50 % represented a moderate heterogeneity and an I^2 with a high percentage above 50 % denoted an increasing heterogeneity. If I^2 was less than 50 %, a fixed effect model was used during this subgroup analysis. However, if I^2 was more than 50 %, a random effect model was used. Publication bias was visually estimated by assessing funnel plots. Odds Ratios (OR) with 95 % Confidence Intervals (CIs) were calculated for categorical variables and the pooled analyses were performed with RevMan 5.3 software. Ethical committee or medical institutional board approval was not required since this is a systematic review and meta-analysis of several studies.

Results

Search result

Two thousand two hundred seventy four articles were obtained from PubMed/Medline, EMBASE, the Cochrane Library and from suitable reference lists. After a careful selection and assessment of titles and abstracts, 2168 articles were eliminated since they were not related to the topic of this research. Among the 106 remaining articles, 52 articles were further eliminated since they were duplicates. Fifty-four full-text articles were assessed for eligibility. Ten studies were further eliminated since they were meta-analyses, 11 studies were case studies, 2 studies were protocol of future ongoing trials, 6 articles were letter to editors, and 10 articles were associated with the same trial. Finally, 15 studies (Brar2008 [12], I-LOVE IT 2 [13], ISAR-SAFE [14], Tarantini2016 [15], ARCTIC [16], OPTIMIZE [17], RESET [18], EXCELLENT [3],

PEGASUS [19], DAPT [20], Sardella2011 [21], PRODIGY [22], Thukkani2015 [23], ENDEAVOR [24], ITALIC [25]) that satisfied all the inclusion and exclusion criteria of this current analysis, were included. The flow diagram representing the study selection has been illustrated in Fig. 1.

Study Tarantini2016 [15] was a sub-study of the SECURITY trial [26] including patients only with DM and trials DES LATE [27] and REAL-LATE ZEST-LATE [28] were excluded because they compared aspirin monotherapy versus DAPT, instead of prolonged DAPT use versus short term DAPT use.

General features of the studies included

A total number of 25,742 patients with DM (13,350 patients assigned to short term DAPT group whereas 12,392 patients assigned to prolonged DAPT group) were included. Patients were enrolled from the year 2002 to the year 2015. The general features of the studies included have been listed in Table 2.

Baseline features of the studies included

Table 3 summarized the baseline characteristics of the patients included in this meta-analysis.

Mean age was reported in years. Patients who were enrolled in this study had a mean age ranging from 60.0 to 70.0 years. Trials ITALIC [25], ISAR-SAFE [14] and ARCTIC [16] had a majority of males patients. Trial ISAR-SAFE [14] and study Thukkani2015 [23] involved a high number of patients with hypertension. According to the baseline features reported, no significant difference was observed among patients assigned to either a short or prolonged duration of DAPT use.

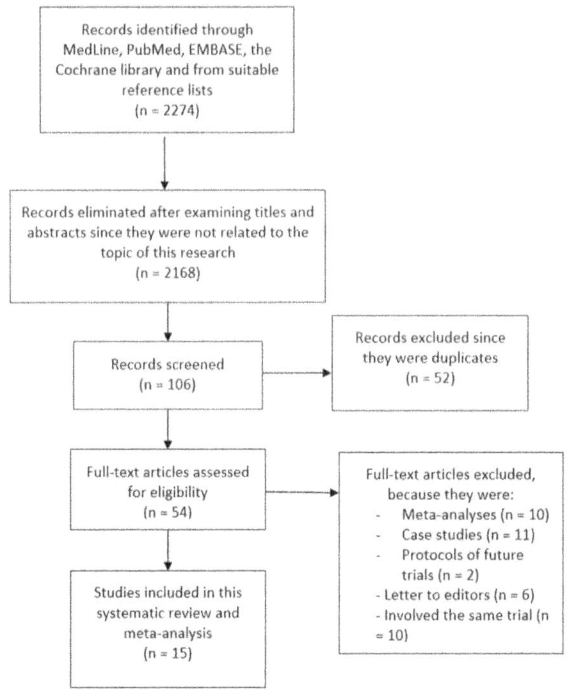

Fig. 1 Flow diagram representing the study selection

Table 3 Baseline features of the studies included

Studies	Mean age S/L	Males (%) S/L	HT (%) S/L	Ds (%) S/L	Cs (%) S/L
Brar2008	62.9/62.9	70.0/70.0	-	-	-
I-LOVE IT 2	60.4/60.0	67.2/68.7	61.0/64.8	25.3/23.4	24.2/24.9
ISAR-SAFE	67.2/67.2	80.7/80.5	90.1/91.5	87.5/87.4	24.9/25.7
Tarantini2016	65.5/66.7	71.8/74.0	82.5/80.3	69.4/70.9	18.9/20.2
ARCTIC	64.0/64.0	81.0/80.0	62.0/59.0	68.0/67.0	24.0/23.0
OPTIMIZE	61.3/61.9	63.5/63.1	86.4/88.2	63.2/63.7	18.6/17.3
RESET	62.4/62.4	64.4/62.9	62.3/61.4	57.7/59.9	25.2/22.8
EXCELLENT	63.0/62.4	65.1/63.9	72.7/73.8	75.2/76.3	27.4/25.8
PEGASUS	65.0/66.0	77.0/77.0	76.0/76.0	76.0/77.0	16.0/17.0
DAPT	61.6/61.8	74.0/75.3	74.0/75.8	-	24.7/24.6
Sardella2011	61.9/61.2	78.2/81.3	76.7/74.8	57.1/64.0	48.1/62.6
PRODIGY	70.0/68.0	75.0/78.0	71.0/72.0	62.0/66.0	12.0/15.0
Thukkani2015	64.3/64.3	98.5/98.5	97.1/97.8	-	34.8/33.3
ENDEAVOR	62.4/63.6	69.6/69.4	73.6/79.5	80.5/81.4	52.3/56.2
ITALIC	61.7/61.5	80.8/79.2	65.2/64.7	67.1/67.1	50.9/52.7

Abbreviations: *S* short term DAPT use, *L* prolonged DAPT use, *HT* hypertension, *Ds* dyslipidemia, *Cs* current smoking

Main analysis

Results of this analysis have been summarized in Table 4.

Table 4 Results of this analysis

Outcomes analyzed	OR with 95 % CI	*P* value	I^2 (%)
Primary endpoints	1.03 [0.65–1.64]	0.90	0
Net clinical outcomes	0.96 [0.69–1.34]	0.81	0
Mortality	0.87 [0.76–1.00]	0.05	0
MI	0.85 [0.70–1.04]	0.12	0
TVR	0.85 [0.58–1.24]	0.39	0
TLR	0.90 [0.57–1.41]	0.63	0
Stroke	0.94 [0.65–1.36]	0.75	0
ST (definite or probable)	0.56 [0.27–1.17]	0.12	0
Definite ST	0.63 [0.08–4.79]	0.65	0
TIMI major bleeding	0.91 [0.60–1.37]	0.65	0
TIMI minor bleeding	1.08 [0.62–1.91]	0.78	0
BARC defined bleeding	1.92 [1.58–2.34]	0.00001	0
BARC type 2	1.98 [1.50–2.61]	0.00001	0
BARC type 3	1.78 [1.34–2.37]	0.0001	0
BARC type 5	1.40 [0.59–3.30]	0.44	0

Abbreviations: *OR* odds ratios, *CI* confidence intervals, *MI* myocardial infarction, *TVR* target vessel revascularization, *TLR* target lesion revascularization, *ST* stent thrombosis, *TIMI* thrombolysis in myocardial infarction, *BARC* bleeding academic research consortium

This current analysis showed no significant differences in primary endpoints and net clinical outcomes in patients with DM whether with a short or prolonged treatment period with DAPT with OR: 1.03, 95 % CI: 0.65–1.64; *P* = 0.90 and OR: 0.96, 95 % CI: 0.69–1.34; *P* = 0.81 respectively. MI was also not significantly different with OR: 0.85, 95 % CI: 0.70–1.04; *P* = 0.12. However, even if mortality favored prolonged DAPT use, with OR: 0.87, 95 % CI: 0.76–1.00; *P* = 0.05, the result only approached statistical significance. These results have been illustrated in Fig. 2.

TVR and TLR were also similarly manifested between these 2 groups with OR: 0.85, 95 % CI: 0.58–1.24; *P* = 0.39 and OR: 0.90, 95 % CI: 0.57–1.41; *P* = 0.63 respectively. Stroke was also not significantly different with a short term or prolonged DAPT use with these patients with DM, with OR: 0.94, 95 % CI: 0.65–1.36; *P* = 0.75. However, even if stent thrombosis favored a prolonged DAPT use with OR: 0.56, 95 % CI: 0.27–1.17; *P* = 0.12, this result was not statistically significant. These results have been illustrated in Fig. 3.

Bleeding events were also analyzed in these patients with DM. Any bleeding was not significantly different between a short and a prolonged DAPT use with OR: 1.22, 95 % CI: 0.72–2.08; *P* = 0.46. TIMI defined major and minor bleeding were also not significantly different in these diabetic patients with OR: 0.91, 95 % CI: 0.60–1.37; *P* = 0.65 and OR: 1.08, 95 % CI: 0.62–1.91; *P* = 0.78 respectively. However, bleeding defined by the BARC classification was significantly higher with a prolonged

	long term DAPT		short term DAPT			Odds Ratio
Study or Subgroup	Events	Total	Events	Total	Weight	M-H, Fixed, 95% CI
1.1.1 Primary endpoints						
ARCTIC	7	198	10	222	1.3%	0.78 [0.29, 2.08]
ISAR-SAFE	8	484	7	495	0.9%	1.17 [0.42, 3.26]
ITALIC	5	344	5	331	0.7%	0.96 [0.28, 3.35]
RESET	12	305	12	316	1.6%	1.04 [0.46, 2.35]
Tarantini2016	5	223	3	206	0.4%	1.55 [0.37, 6.58]
Subtotal (95% CI)		**1554**		**1570**	**4.9%**	**1.03 [0.65, 1.64]**
Total events	37		37			
Heterogeneity: Chi² = 0.70, df = 4 (P = 0.95); I² = 0%						
Test for overall effect: Z = 0.12 (P = 0.90)						
1.1.2 Net clinical outcomes						
ARCTIC	9	198	10	222	1.2%	1.01 [0.40, 2.54]
ENDEAVOR	3	183	4	198	0.5%	0.81 [0.18, 3.66]
EXCELLENT	8	278	9	272	1.2%	0.87 [0.33, 2.28]
I-LOVE IT 2	13	203	15	211	1.9%	0.89 [0.41, 1.93]
ISAR-SAFE	7	484	6	495	0.8%	1.20 [0.40, 3.58]
OPTIMIZE	32	549	33	554	4.3%	0.98 [0.59, 1.61]
Subtotal (95% CI)		**1895**		**1952**	**9.9%**	**0.96 [0.69, 1.34]**
Total events	72		77			
Heterogeneity: Chi² = 0.30, df = 5 (P = 1.00); I² = 0%						
Test for overall effect: Z = 0.24 (P = 0.81)						
1.1.3 Mortality						
ARCTIC	2	198	3	222	0.4%	0.74 [0.12, 4.50]
Brar2008	78	371	104	378	11.2%	0.70 [0.50, 0.98]
ENDEAVOR	3	183	5	198	0.6%	0.64 [0.15, 2.73]
EXCELLENT	3	278	3	272	0.4%	0.98 [0.20, 4.89]
I-LOVE IT 2	3	203	3	211	0.4%	1.04 [0.21, 5.21]
ISAR-SAFE	3	484	2	495	0.3%	1.54 [0.26, 9.24]
ITALIC	3	344	3	331	0.4%	0.96 [0.19, 4.80]
OPTIMIZE	16	549	15	554	2.0%	1.08 [0.53, 2.20]
PEGASUS	72	1574	84	1950	9.8%	1.06 [0.77, 1.47]
PRODIGRY	1	36	4	35	0.5%	0.22 [0.02, 2.09]
RESET	2	305	1	316	0.1%	2.08 [0.19, 23.05]
Sardella2011	1	139	5	133	0.7%	0.19 [0.02, 1.61]
Tarantini2016	2	223	1	206	0.1%	1.86 [0.17, 20.61]
Thukkani2015	188	5949	238	6568	30.1%	0.87 [0.71, 1.05]
Subtotal (95% CI)		**10836**		**11869**	**57.2%**	**0.87 [0.76, 1.00]**
Total events	377		471			
Heterogeneity: Chi² = 8.38, df = 13 (P = 0.82); I² = 0%						
Test for overall effect: Z = 1.94 (P = 0.05)						
1.1.4 Myocardial infarction						
ARCTIC	3	198	3	222	0.4%	1.12 [0.22, 5.63]
Brar2008	7	371	17	378	2.3%	0.41 [0.17, 1.00]
ENDEAVOR	1	183	0	198	0.1%	3.26 [0.13, 80.61]
EXCELLENT	3	278	5	272	0.7%	0.58 [0.14, 2.46]
I-LOVE IT 2	8	203	10	211	1.3%	0.82 [0.32, 2.13]
ISAR-SAFE	3	484	3	495	0.4%	1.02 [0.21, 5.09]
ITALIC	2	344	2	331	0.3%	0.96 [0.13, 6.87]
OPTIMIZE	15	549	17	554	2.3%	0.89 [0.44, 1.79]
PEGASUS	61	1574	86	1950	10.2%	0.87 [0.63, 1.22]
PRODIGRY	1	36	3	35	0.4%	0.30 [0.03, 3.08]
RESET	1	305	1	316	0.1%	1.04 [0.06, 16.64]
Sardella2011	0	139	7	133	1.1%	0.06 [0.00, 1.07]
Tarantini2016	7	223	6	206	0.8%	1.08 [0.36, 3.27]
Thukkani2015	56	5949	60	6568	7.8%	1.03 [0.71, 1.49]
Subtotal (95% CI)		**10836**		**11869**	**28.0%**	**0.85 [0.70, 1.04]**
Total events	168		220			
Heterogeneity: Chi² = 9.02, df = 13 (P = 0.77); I² = 0%						
Test for overall effect: Z = 1.55 (P = 0.12)						
Total (95% CI)		**25121**		**27260**	**100.0%**	**0.88 [0.79, 0.98]**
Total events	654		805			
Heterogeneity: Chi² = 19.03, df = 38 (P = 1.00); I² = 0%						
Test for overall effect: Z = 2.33 (P = 0.02)						
Test for subgroup differences: Chi² = 0.84, df = 3 (P = 0.84), I² = 0%						

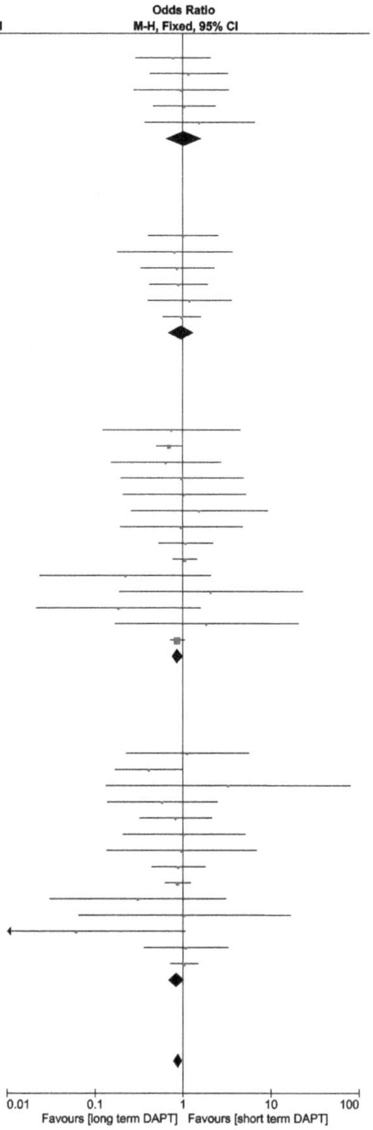

Fig. 2 Adverse clinical outcomes associated with a short versus prolonged DAPT use in patients with DM (part 1)

Study or Subgroup	long term DAPT Events	long term DAPT Total	short term DAPT Events	short term DAPT Total	Weight	Odds Ratio M-H, Fixed, 95% CI
1.1.1 Target vessel revascularization (TVR)						
EXCELLENT	8	278	8	272	4.4%	0.98 [0.36, 2.64]
I-LOVE IT 2	6	203	7	211	3.7%	0.89 [0.29, 2.69]
ITALIC	1	344	2	331	1.1%	0.48 [0.04, 5.31]
OPTIMIZE	20	549	25	554	13.3%	0.80 [0.44, 1.46]
PRODIGRY	6	36	5	35	2.3%	1.20 [0.33, 4.36]
RESET	8	305	9	315	4.8%	0.92 [0.35, 2.41]
Sardella2011	1	139	4	133	2.2%	0.23 [0.03, 2.12]
Tarantini2016	2	223	1	206	0.6%	1.86 [0.17, 20.61]
Subtotal (95% CI)		**2077**		**2057**	**32.4%**	**0.85 [0.58, 1.24]**
Total events	52		61			
Heterogeneity: Chi² = 2.36, df = 7 (P = 0.94); I² = 0%						
Test for overall effect: Z = 0.85 (P = 0.39)						
1.1.2 Target Lesion Revascularization (TLR)						
EXCELLENT	7	278	6	272	3.3%	1.15 [0.38, 3.45]
I-LOVE IT 2	5	203	6	211	3.2%	0.86 [0.26, 2.87]
OPTIMIZE	17	549	19	554	10.2%	0.90 [0.46, 1.75]
PRODIGRY	5	36	5	35	2.4%	0.97 [0.25, 3.69]
Sardella2011	1	139	4	133	2.2%	0.23 [0.03, 2.12]
Tarantini2016	2	223	1	206	0.6%	1.86 [0.17, 20.61]
Subtotal (95% CI)		**1428**		**1411**	**21.8%**	**0.90 [0.57, 1.41]**
Total events	37		41			
Heterogeneity: Chi² = 1.99, df = 5 (P = 0.85); I² = 0%						
Test for overall effect: Z = 0.48 (P = 0.63)						
1.1.3 Stent thrombosis (definite and probable)						
ARCTIC	0	198	1	222	0.8%	0.37 [0.02, 9.18]
ENDEAVOR	0	183	1	198	0.8%	0.36 [0.01, 8.86]
EXCELLENT	0	278	2	272	1.4%	0.19 [0.01, 4.06]
I-LOVE IT 2	2	203	3	211	1.6%	0.69 [0.11, 4.17]
ISAR-SAFE	1	484	1	495	0.5%	1.02 [0.06, 16.40]
ITALIC	0	344	1	331	0.8%	0.32 [0.01, 7.88]
OPTIMIZE	4	549	5	554	2.7%	0.81 [0.22, 3.02]
PRODIGRY	0	36	1	35	0.8%	0.32 [0.01, 8.00]
RESET	1	305	1	316	0.5%	1.04 [0.06, 16.64]
Tarantini2016	1	223	2	206	1.1%	0.46 [0.04, 5.11]
Subtotal (95% CI)		**2803**		**2840**	**11.2%**	**0.56 [0.27, 1.17]**
Total events	9		18			
Heterogeneity: Chi² = 1.58, df = 9 (P = 1.00); I² = 0%						
Test for overall effect: Z = 1.55 (P = 0.12)						
1.1.4 Definite stent thrombosis						
ENDEAVOR	0	183	1	198	0.8%	0.36 [0.01, 8.86]
I-LOVE IT 2	0	203	0	211		Not estimable
ISAR-SAFE	1	484	1	495	0.5%	1.02 [0.06, 16.40]
Subtotal (95% CI)		**870**		**904**	**1.3%**	**0.63 [0.08, 4.79]**
Total events	1		2			
Heterogeneity: Chi² = 0.24, df = 1 (P = 0.63); I² = 0%						
Test for overall effect: Z = 0.45 (P = 0.65)						
1.1.5 Stroke						
ENDEAVOR	1	183	1	198	0.5%	1.08 [0.07, 17.43]
EXCELLENT	2	278	1	272	0.6%	1.96 [0.18, 21.78]
I-LOVE IT 2	3	203	3	211	1.6%	1.04 [0.21, 5.21]
ISAR-SAFE	1	484	2	495	1.1%	0.51 [0.05, 5.65]
ITALIC	2	344	0	331	0.3%	4.84 [0.23, 101.18]
OPTIMIZE	2	549	2	554	1.1%	1.01 [0.14, 7.19]
PEGASUS	20	1574	33	1950	16.1%	0.75 [0.43, 1.31]
PRODIGRY	1	36	0	35	0.3%	3.00 [0.12, 76.16]
RESET	2	305	2	316	1.1%	1.04 [0.15, 7.40]
Sardella2011	0	133	0	139		Not estimable
Tarantini2016	2	223	1	206	0.6%	1.86 [0.17, 20.61]
Thukkani2015	17	5949	19	6568	10.0%	0.99 [0.51, 1.90]
Subtotal (95% CI)		**10261**		**11275**	**33.2%**	**0.94 [0.65, 1.36]**
Total events	53		64			
Heterogeneity: Chi² = 3.23, df = 10 (P = 0.98); I² = 0%						
Test for overall effect: Z = 0.32 (P = 0.75)						
Total (95% CI)		**17439**		**18487**	**100.0%**	**0.85 [0.69, 1.06]**
Total events	152		186			
Heterogeneity: Chi² = 10.66, df = 36 (P = 1.00); I² = 0%						
Test for overall effect: Z = 1.43 (P = 0.15)						
Test for subgroup differences: Chi² = 1.66, df = 4 (P = 0.80), I² = 0%						

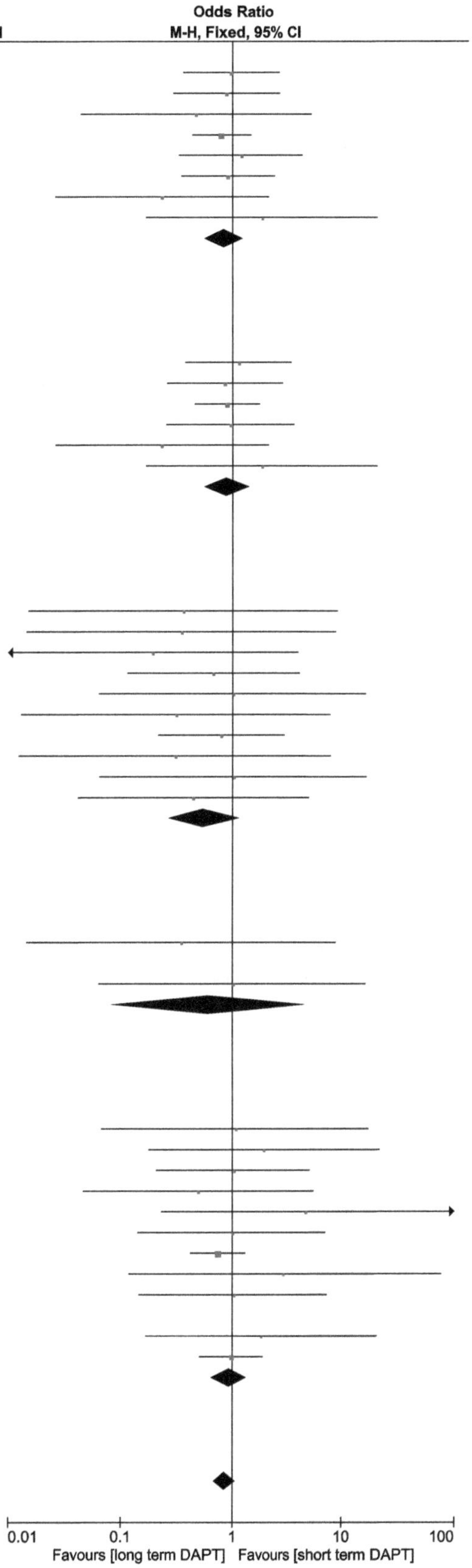

Fig. 3 Adverse clinical outcomes associated with a short versus prolonged DAPT use in patients with DM (part 2)

DAPT use in these diabetic patients with OR: 1.92, 95 % CI: 1.58–2.34; $P < 0.00001$. When bleeding defined by BARC classification was further subdivided, a significantly higher BARC bleeding types 2 and 3 were observed with a prolonged DAPT use with OR: 1.98, 95 % CI: 1.50–2.61; $P < 0.00001$ and OR: 1.78, 95 % CI: 1.34–2.37; $P < 0.0001$ respectively. But even if BARC type 5 also favored a short term DAPT use, with OR: 1.40, 95 % CI: 0.59–3.30; $P = 0.44$, the result was not statistically significant. Results analyzing bleeding events have been illustrated in Fig. 4.

Because the duration period of DAPT was not similar in all the studies included, that is, a few studies had a short term DAPT duration period of 3 months, 6 months and 12 months respectively, and a long term DAPT duration period of 12 months, 18 months or 24 months respectively, which might have influenced the results of this analysis, another subgroup analysis was conducted only with a short term DAPT duration of 6 months versus a long term duration of 12 months. However, this analysis also showed no significant difference in net clinical outcomes, mortality, MI, TVR, TLR, stent thrombosis and stroke with OR: 0.95, 95 % CI: 0.56–1.60; $P = 0.84$, OR: 1.14, 95 % CI: 0.44–2.97; $P = 0.79$, OR: 0.79, 95 % CI: 0.39–1.60; $P = 0.51$, OR: 0.94, 95 % CI: 0.45–1.96; $P = 0.86$, OR: 1.01, 95 % CI: 0.45–2.26; $P = 0.99$, OR: 0.55, 95 % CI: 0.15–2.01; $P = 0.36$ and OR: 1.02, 95 % CI: 0.33–3.18; $P = 0.97$ respectively. These results comparing 6 months versus 12 months DAPT use have been illustrated in Fig. 5.

Sensitivity analysis

For all of the above analyses, sensitivity analyses yielded consistent results. Based on a visual inspection of the funnel plots obtained, there has been very low evidence of publication bias for the included studies that assessed all clinical endpoints reported (including the adverse clinical outcomes and the bleeding events analyzed) in these patients with DM. The funnel plots have been illustrated in Figs. 6 and 7.

Discussion

This study aimed to compare the adverse clinical outcomes associated with a short and prolonged DAPT use in patients with DM following PCI. Results of this study showed that a prolonged duration of DAPT use was not associated with any significant difference in adverse clinical outcomes when compared to a short term duration of DAPT use in these patients with DM. The result for mortality which favored a prolonged DAPT use reached near significance but was not statistically significant in this analysis whereas even if stent thrombosis favored a prolonged DAPT use, the result was also not statistically significant. In addition, TIMI defined major and minor bleeding were also not significantly different. However, bleeding defined according to BARC classification was significantly higher with the prolonged DAPT use.

In part similar to the results of this current analysis, the systematic review and meta-analysis comparing the duration of DAPT following DES implantation showed short term DAPT use to be associated with a significantly lower rate of bleeding, and higher rates of stent thrombosis [29]. Note that their study involved more than 30 % of patients with DM. However, their meta-analysis showed all-cause mortality to be insignificantly higher in the long term duration group, which was not the case in our study. In addition, this current study only showed a significantly increased bleeding rate according to the BARC classification, without any significant difference for stent thrombosis. Another meta-analysis published by Navarese et al. showed that compared to a DAPT duration period of 12 months, a short term DAPT use was associated with a significantly lower rate of bleeding events, without any apparent increase in ischemic complications and therefore the authors concluded that a short term DAPT could be considered in most patients following PCI [5].

Furthermore, the meta-analysis published by Yang et al. showed no difference in efficacy outcomes associated with a short or prolonged duration of DAPT use after intracoronary DES implantation [30]. However, a longer duration of DAPT (≥12 months) was associated with increased risk of bleeding complications. The study by Udell et al. also concluded that DAPT use beyond one year was associated with increased bleeding events, without any increase in cardiovascular mortality [4]. In addition, the PRODIGY trial which involved more than 20 % of patients with DM, showed a 24 months of clopidogrel use not to be associated with any increase in adverse clinical outcomes compared to the use of clopidogrel during a short term period of 6 months [31]. This trial compared device specific outcomes relative to different duration of DAPT in 3 different types of DES (everolimus eluting stents, paclitaxel eluting stents, zotarolimus eluting stents) and bare metal stents, suggesting that the optimal duration of DAPT could also possibly be stent specific.

Moreover, patients with DM showed comparable adverse clinical outcomes to that of patients without DM whether during a 6-months treatment with DAPT or a prolonged duration of DAPT following PCI with implanted second generation DES [15].

Nevertheless, the study by Valgimigli et al. showed that along with an increased risk of bleeding associated with a prolonged duration of DAPT use, an increased risk of stroke was also observed [32]. However, our results which involved patients with DM, did not show any significant difference in stroke rate between these two

Study or Subgroup	long term DAPT Events	long term DAPT Total	short term DAPT Events	short term DAPT Total	Weight	Odds Ratio M-H, Fixed, 95% CI
1.2.1 All/Any bleeding						
EXCELLENT	4	278	2	272	0.5%	1.97 [0.36, 10.85]
I-LOVE IT 2	11	203	12	211	2.8%	0.95 [0.41, 2.20]
OPTIMIZE	16	549	12	554	2.9%	1.36 [0.64, 2.89]
Subtotal (95% CI)		**1030**		**1037**	**6.1%**	**1.22 [0.72, 2.08]**
Total events	31		26			
Heterogeneity: Chi² = 0.72, df = 2 (P = 0.70); I² = 0%						
Test for overall effect: Z = 0.74 (P = 0.46)						
1.2.2 TIMI major bleeding						
EXCELLENT	2	278	1	272	0.2%	1.96 [0.18, 21.78]
ISAR-SAFE	1	484	1	495	0.2%	1.02 [0.06, 16.40]
PEGASUS	38	1574	53	1950	11.5%	0.89 [0.58, 1.35]
PRODIGRY	0	36	0	35		Not estimable
Subtotal (95% CI)		**2372**		**2752**	**12.0%**	**0.91 [0.60, 1.37]**
Total events	41		55			
Heterogeneity: Chi² = 0.42, df = 2 (P = 0.81); I² = 0%						
Test for overall effect: Z = 0.45 (P = 0.65)						
1.2.3 TIMI minor bleeding						
ISAR-SAFE	2	483	1	495	0.2%	2.05 [0.19, 22.73]
PEGASUS	17	1574	21	1950	4.6%	1.00 [0.53, 1.91]
PRODIGRY	0	36	1	35	0.4%	0.32 [0.01, 8.00]
Sardella2011	4	139	2	133	0.5%	1.94 [0.35, 10.78]
Subtotal (95% CI)		**2232**		**2613**	**5.7%**	**1.08 [0.62, 1.91]**
Total events	23		25			
Heterogeneity: Chi² = 1.33, df = 3 (P = 0.72); I² = 0%						
Test for overall effect: Z = 0.28 (P = 0.78)						
1.2.4 BARC bleeding						
DAPT	274	4710	144	4649	33.9%	1.93 [1.57, 2.37]
ISAR-SAFE	18	484	8	495	1.9%	2.35 [1.01, 5.46]
PRODIGRY	8	36	7	35	1.4%	1.14 [0.36, 3.58]
Subtotal (95% CI)		**5230**		**5179**	**37.1%**	**1.92 [1.58, 2.34]**
Total events	300		159			
Heterogeneity: Chi² = 1.02, df = 2 (P = 0.60); I² = 0%						
Test for overall effect: Z = 6.52 (P < 0.00001)						
1.2.5 BARC 2						
DAPT	145	4710	72	4649	17.4%	2.02 [1.52, 2.69]
ISAR-SAFE	6	484	4	495	1.0%	1.54 [0.43, 5.49]
PRODIGRY	1	36	1	35	0.2%	0.97 [0.06, 16.16]
Subtotal (95% CI)		**5230**		**5179**	**18.6%**	**1.98 [1.50, 2.61]**
Total events	152		77			
Heterogeneity: Chi² = 0.41, df = 2 (P = 0.81); I² = 0%						
Test for overall effect: Z = 4.84 (P < 0.00001)						
1.2.6 BARC 3						
DAPT	122	4710	68	4649	16.5%	1.79 [1.33, 2.42]
ISAR-SAFE	5	484	1	495	0.2%	5.16 [0.60, 44.30]
PRODIGRY	3	36	3	35	0.7%	0.97 [0.18, 5.16]
Tarantini2016	4	223	3	206	0.8%	1.24 [0.27, 5.59]
Subtotal (95% CI)		**5453**		**5385**	**18.2%**	**1.78 [1.34, 2.37]**
Total events	134		75			
Heterogeneity: Chi² = 1.67, df = 3 (P = 0.64); I² = 0%						
Test for overall effect: Z = 3.97 (P < 0.0001)						
1.2.7 BARC 5						
DAPT	7	4710	4	4649	1.0%	1.73 [0.51, 5.91]
ISAR-SAFE	0	484	0	495		Not estimable
PRODIGRY	2	36	2	35	0.5%	0.97 [0.13, 7.30]
Tarantini2016	4	223	3	206	0.8%	1.24 [0.27, 5.59]
Subtotal (95% CI)		**5453**		**5385**	**2.2%**	**1.40 [0.59, 3.30]**
Total events	13		9			
Heterogeneity: Chi² = 0.27, df = 2 (P = 0.88); I² = 0%						
Test for overall effect: Z = 0.77 (P = 0.44)						
Total (95% CI)		**27000**		**27530**	**100.0%**	**1.69 [1.49, 1.91]**
Total events	694		426			
Heterogeneity: Chi² = 21.47, df = 22 (P = 0.49); I² = 0%						
Test for overall effect: Z = 8.33 (P < 0.00001)						
Test for subgroup differences: Chi² = 15.78, df = 6 (P = 0.01), I² = 62.0%						

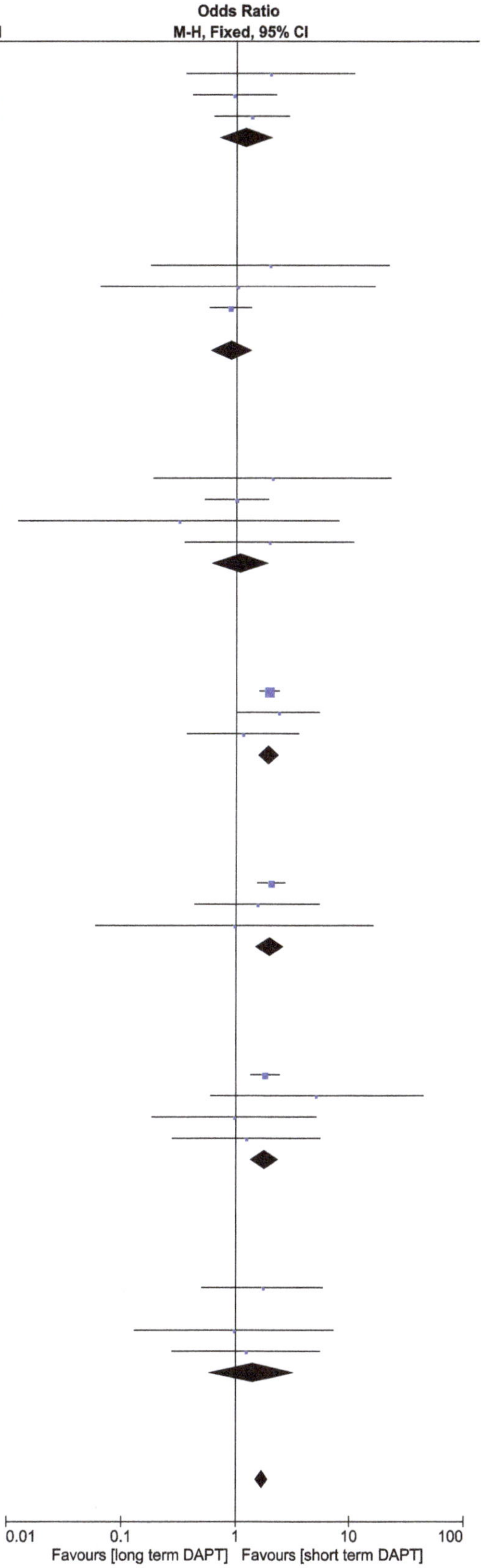

Fig. 4 Bleeding events associated with a short versus prolonged DAPT use in patients with DM

Study or Subgroup	long term DAPT Events	long term DAPT Total	short term DAPT Events	short term DAPT Total	Weight	Odds Ratio M-H, Fixed, 95% CI
1.1.1 Net clinical outcomes						
EXCELLENT	8	278	9	272	9.6%	0.87 [0.33, 2.28]
I-LOVE IT 2	13	203	15	211	14.9%	0.89 [0.41, 1.93]
ISAR-SAFE	7	484	6	495	6.3%	1.20 [0.40, 3.58]
Subtotal (95% CI)		**965**		**978**	**30.9%**	**0.95 [0.56, 1.60]**
Total events	28		30			
Heterogeneity: Chi² = 0.23, df = 2 (P = 0.89); I² = 0%						
Test for overall effect: Z = 0.20 (P = 0.84)						
1.1.2 Mortality						
EXCELLENT	3	278	3	272	3.3%	0.98 [0.20, 4.89]
I-LOVE IT 2	3	203	3	211	3.1%	1.04 [0.21, 5.21]
ISAR-SAFE	3	484	2	495	2.1%	1.54 [0.26, 9.24]
Subtotal (95% CI)		**965**		**978**	**8.5%**	**1.14 [0.44, 2.97]**
Total events	9		8			
Heterogeneity: Chi² = 0.15, df = 2 (P = 0.93); I² = 0%						
Test for overall effect: Z = 0.27 (P = 0.79)						
1.1.3 Myocardial infarction						
EXCELLENT	3	278	5	272	5.4%	0.58 [0.14, 2.46]
I-LOVE IT 2	8	203	10	211	10.2%	0.82 [0.32, 2.13]
ISAR-SAFE	3	484	3	495	3.2%	1.02 [0.21, 5.09]
Subtotal (95% CI)		**965**		**978**	**18.8%**	**0.79 [0.39, 1.60]**
Total events	14		18			
Heterogeneity: Chi² = 0.28, df = 2 (P = 0.87); I² = 0%						
Test for overall effect: Z = 0.66 (P = 0.51)						
1.1.4 Target vessel revascularization (TVR)						
EXCELLENT	8	278	8	272	8.5%	0.98 [0.36, 2.64]
I-LOVE IT 2	6	203	7	211	7.2%	0.89 [0.29, 2.69]
Subtotal (95% CI)		**481**		**483**	**15.8%**	**0.94 [0.45, 1.96]**
Total events	14		15			
Heterogeneity: Chi² = 0.02, df = 1 (P = 0.90); I² = 0%						
Test for overall effect: Z = 0.17 (P = 0.86)						
1.1.5 Target Lesion Revascularization (TLR)						
EXCELLENT	7	278	6	272	6.4%	1.15 [0.38, 3.45]
I-LOVE IT 2	5	203	6	211	6.2%	0.86 [0.26, 2.87]
Subtotal (95% CI)		**481**		**483**	**12.6%**	**1.01 [0.45, 2.26]**
Total events	12		12			
Heterogeneity: Chi² = 0.12, df = 1 (P = 0.73); I² = 0%						
Test for overall effect: Z = 0.01 (P = 0.99)						
1.1.6 Stent thrombosis (definite and probable)						
EXCELLENT	0	278	2	272	2.7%	0.19 [0.01, 4.06]
I-LOVE IT 2	2	203	3	211	3.2%	0.69 [0.11, 4.17]
ISAR-SAFE	1	484	1	495	1.1%	1.02 [0.06, 16.40]
Subtotal (95% CI)		**965**		**978**	**7.0%**	**0.55 [0.15, 2.01]**
Total events	3		6			
Heterogeneity: Chi² = 0.70, df = 2 (P = 0.70); I² = 0%						
Test for overall effect: Z = 0.91 (P = 0.36)						
1.1.7 Stroke						
EXCELLENT	2	278	1	272	1.1%	1.96 [0.18, 21.78]
I-LOVE IT 2	3	203	3	211	3.1%	1.04 [0.21, 5.21]
ISAR-SAFE	1	484	2	495	2.1%	0.51 [0.05, 5.65]
Subtotal (95% CI)		**965**		**978**	**6.4%**	**1.02 [0.33, 3.18]**
Total events	6		6			
Heterogeneity: Chi² = 0.60, df = 2 (P = 0.74); I² = 0%						
Test for overall effect: Z = 0.03 (P = 0.97)						
Total (95% CI)		**5787**		**5856**	**100.0%**	**0.92 [0.68, 1.23]**
Total events	86		95			
Heterogeneity: Chi² = 2.96, df = 18 (P = 1.00); I² = 0%						
Test for overall effect: Z = 0.58 (P = 0.56)						
Test for subgroup differences: Chi² = 1.08, df = 6 (P = 0.98), I² = 0%						

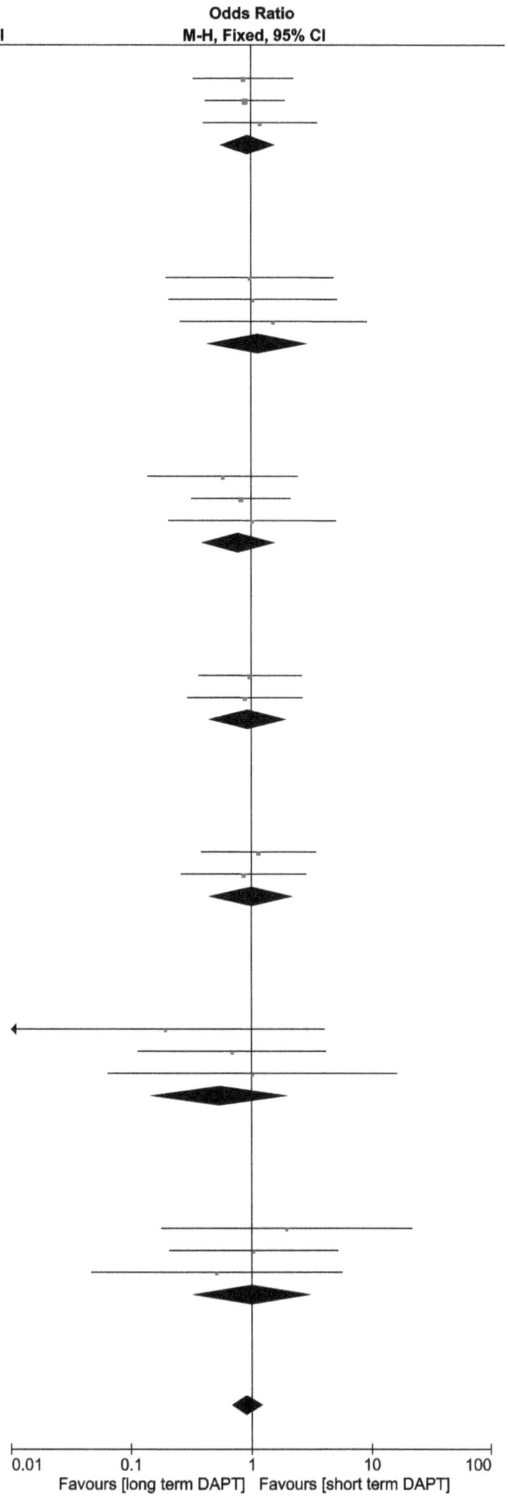

Fig. 5 Adverse clinical outcomes associated specifically with 6 versus 12 months DAPT use in patients with DM

groups. The ITALIC trial also showed no significantly different bleeding or thrombotic events when 6 months DAPT use was compared to 24 months DAPT use after PCI [25]. However, the ITALIC trial involved patients implanted with newer generation DES and also involved patients with good response to aspirin.

The study by Siddiqqi et al. which consisted of more than 50 % of patients with DM, showed a prolonged

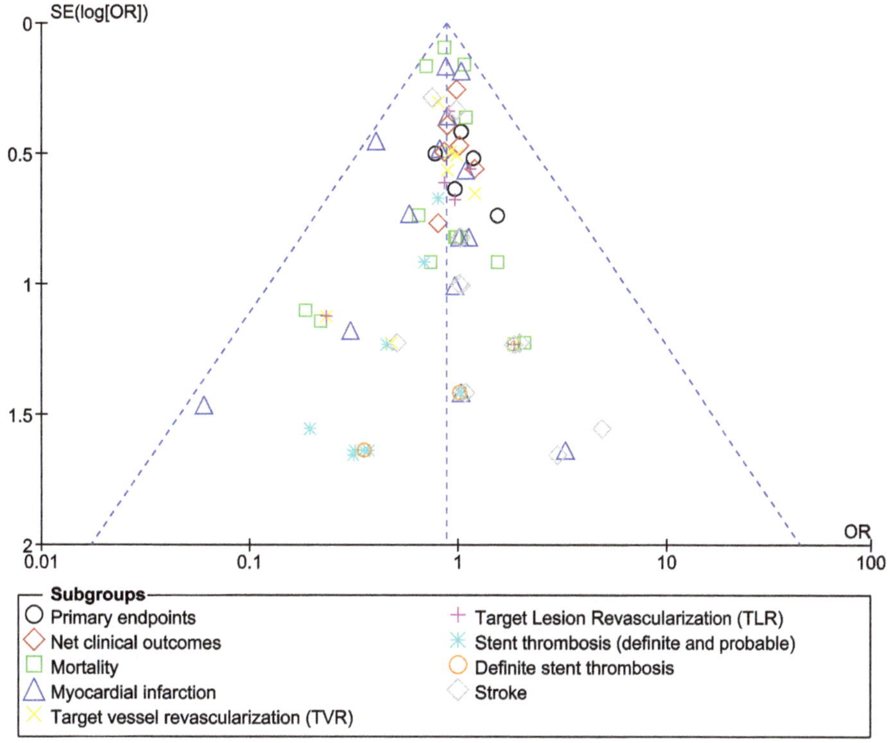

Fig. 6 Funnel plots representing sensitivity analyses

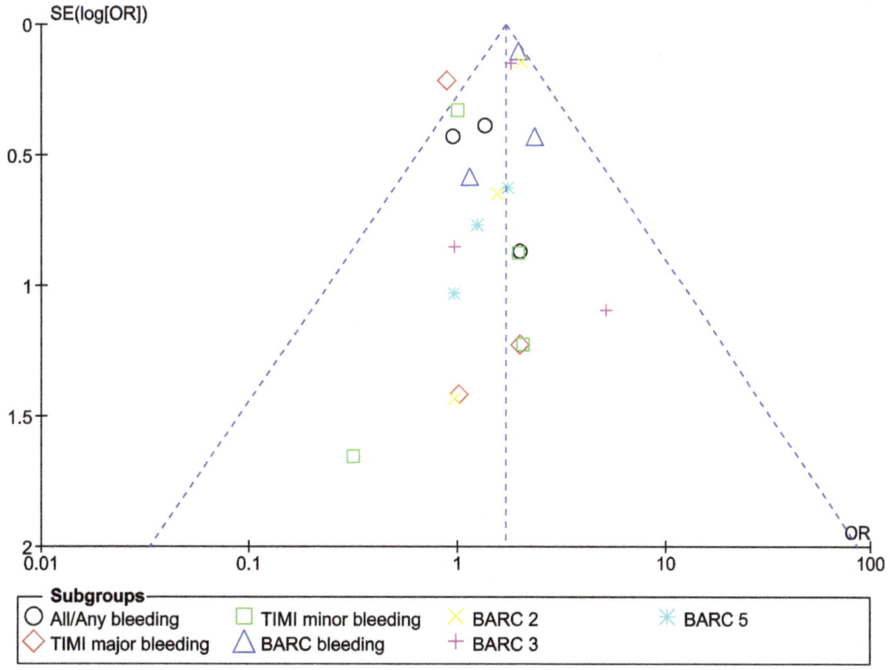

Fig. 7 Funnel plots representing sensitivity analyses

duration of DAPT not to be associated with any increased risk of bleeding. However, their study involved patients with chronic kidney disease and the exact type of bleeding assessed was not specified [33]. The study by Thukkani et al. also showed results that favored the prolonged use of clopidogrel to be associated with a lower risk of death and MI only in patients with DM implanted with DES [23]. However, that study did not show any benefit of prolonged clopidogrel use in patients without DM or in patients implanted with bare metal stents. Moreover, the DAPT trial also showed a lower rate of mortality to be associated with a prolonged use of clopidogrel after PCI [20]. However, result of this analysis which involved only patients with DM, did not reach statistical significance in the subgroup analyzing mortality.

Even if the subgroup analysis of the OPTIMIZE trial that assessed how short-term DAPT did not show any significantly increase risk for clinical events at 1 year in patients with DM undergoing PCI with a specific 2nd generation DES [34], other studies have shown second generation DES to be associated with higher adverse outcomes in patients with DM compared to the general population [35]. In addition, studies showed increasing adverse clinical outcomes to be associated with insulin-treated DM compared to non-insulin treated DM irrespective of the duration of DAPT [36, 37].

Furthermore, the observational study conducted by Eisenstein et al. examining consecutive patients receiving DES at Duke Heart Center between the year 2000 and 2005, concluded that the extended use of clopidogrel in patients implanted with DES might be associated with a lower risk of death and MI [2]. However, the authors concluded that only larger trials will be able to confirm their results, but unfortunately, even if this current analysis involved a pooling of data from several randomized trials (but only including patients with DM), the result analyzing mortality only nearly reached statistical significance, but was not statistically significant.

Even if the result for stent thrombosis was not significant in patients with DM, other studies have shown a prolonged use of DAPT to be associated with a lower risk of stent thrombosis compared to a shorter duration of DAPT use after PCI. To prove this point, the TYCOON registry showed an extended use of DAPT (2 years) to be associated with a lower rate of stent thrombosis following PCI with DES [38]. However, in contrast, other studies showed clopidogrel use beyond one year not to reduce the risk of stent thrombosis or other adverse clinical outcomes after PCI [39].

Previous studies have already compared the clinical outcomes associated with duration of DAPT in the subset of patients treated for in-stent restenosis [23]. This current analysis showed compared the adverse clinical outcomes between a short and prolonged DAPT use in patients with DM. To be noted, the duration of DAPT use might vary in other subgroups of patients. As it is said, one size shoe approach for DAPT duration is unlikely to fit all the patients, further investigations including other subgroups of patients such as patients with chronic obstructive pulmonary disease who underwent PCI [40, 41], should be conducted.

Novelty

This study is new in several ways. Even if many studies have compared the short and prolonged use of DAPT following PCI, this is among the first meta-analyses comparing the adverse clinical outcomes associated with the short and prolonged use of DAPT in patients with DM. Moreover, this analysis involved several newly published articles which were not included in other recently published meta-analyses representing another novelty.

Limitations

Similar to other studies, this study also has limitations. First of all, due to the small population of patients with DM, this study might not provide robust results. Secondly, different studies reported different duration of DAPT use, as well as different follow up periods. Even if we have tried to compare only 6 months versus 12 months DAPT use in these patients with DM in order to solve this particular issue, we might have only partly succeeded showing that this point should still be considered as a limitation in this study. Moreover, data analyzing several bleeding subgroups were limited, which might have influenced the results.

Conclusion

Following PCI, a prolonged DAPT use was associated with similar adverse clinical outcomes but with a significantly increased BARC defined bleeding compared to a short term DAPT use in these patients with DM. However, even if mortality and stent thrombosis favored a prolonged DAPT use, these outcomes only either reached statistical significance or were insignificant respectively, showing that a clear decision about recommending a prolonged duration of DAPT to patients with DM might not be possible at this moment, warranting further research in this particular subgroup.

Acknowledgement

This research was supported by Youth Science Foundation of Guangxi Medical University (No. GXMUYSF201308), Scientific Project of Guangxi Higher Education (No. KY2015ZD028) and National Natural Science Foundation of China (No. 81560046).

Funding

There was no external source of funding for this research.

Authors' contributions

PKB, CMY and FH were responsible for the conception and design, acquisition of data, analysis and interpretation of data, drafting the initial manuscript and revising it critically for important intellectual content. PKB wrote this manuscript. All authors read and approved the final manuscript.

Authors' information

Dr Pravesh Kumar Bundhun (M.D) is the first author. From the Department of Cardiovascular Diseases, the First Affiliated Hospital of Guangxi Medical University, Nanning, Guangxi, China.

Competing interests

The authors declare that they have no competing interests.

Author details

[1]Institute of Cardiovascular Diseases, the First Affiliated Hospital of Guangxi Medical University, Nanning, Guangxi 530021, People's Republic of China. [2]Department of Internal Medicine, EALING Hospital, University of Buckingham, Uxbridge road, Southall, UB1 3HW London, UK.

References

1. Task Force members, Windecker S, Kolh P, Alfonso F, et al. ESC/EACTS guidelines on myocardial revascularization: the Task Force on Myocardial Revascularization of the European Society of Cardiology (ESC) and the European Association for Cardio-Thoracic Surgery (EACTS) developed with the special contribution of the European Association of Percutaneous Cardiovascular Interventions (EAPCI). Eur Heart J. 2014;35:2541–619.
2. Eisenstein EL, Anstrom KJ, Kong DF, et al. Clopidogrel use and long-term clinical outcomes after drug-eluting stent implantation. JAMA. 2007;297(2):159–68.
3. Gwon HC, Hahn JY, Park KW, et al. Six-month versus 12-month dual antiplatelet therapy after implantation of drug-eluting stents: the Efficacy of Xience/Promus Versus Cypher to Reduce Late Loss After Stenting (EXCELLENT) randomized, multicenter study. Circulation. 2012;125(3):505–13.
4. Udell JA, Bonaca MP, Collet JP, et al. Long-term dual antiplatelet therapy for secondary prevention of cardiovascular events in the subgroup ofpatients with previous myocardial infarction: a collaborative meta-analysis of randomized trials. Eur Heart J. 2016;37(4):390–9.
5. Navarese EP, Andreotti F, Schulze V, et al. Optimal duration of dual antiplatelet therapy after percutaneous coronary intervention with drug eluting stents: meta-analysis of randomised controlled trials. BMJ. 2015;350:h1618.
6. Thygesen K, Alpert JS, White HD, et al. Universal definition of myocardial infarction. Circulation. 2007;116(22):2634–53.
7. Cutlip DE, Windecker S, Mehran R, Academic Research Consortium, et al. Clinical end points in coronary stent trials: a case for standardized definitions. Circulation. 2007;115(17):2344–51.
8. No authors. The Thrombolysis in Myocardial Infarction (TIMI) trial. Phase I findings. TIMI Study Group. N Engl J Med. 1985;312(14):932–6.
9. Mehran R, Rao SV, Bhatt DL, et al. Standardized bleeding definitions for cardiovascular clinical trials: a consensus report from the Bleeding Academic Research Consortium. Circulation. 2011;123(23):2736–47.
10. Higgins JP, Thompson SG, Deeks JJ, et al. Measuring inconsistency in meta-analyses. BMJ. 2003;327:557–60.
11. Liberati A, Altman DG, Tetzlaff J, et al. The PRISMA statement for reporting systematic reviews and meta-analyses of studies that evaluate healthcareinterventions: explanation and elaboration. BMJ. 2009;339:b2700.
12. Brar SS, Kim J, Brar SK, et al. Long-term outcomes by clopidogrel duration and stent type in a diabetic population with de novo coronary artery lesions. J Am Coll Cardiol. 2008;51(23):2220–7.
13. Han Y, Xu B, Xu K, et al. Six versus 12 months of dual antiplatelet therapy after implantation of biodegradable polymer sirolimus-ElutingStent: randomized substudy of the I-LOVE-IT 2 trial. Circ Cardiovasc Interv. 2016; 9(2):e003145.
14. Schulz-Schüpke S, Byrne RA, Ten Berg JM, et al. Intracoronary Stenting and Antithrombotic Regimen: Safety And EFficacy of 6 Months Dual Antiplatelet Therapy After Drug-Eluting Stenting (ISAR-SAFE) Trial Investigators. ISAR-SAFE: a randomized, double-blind, placebo-controlled trial of 6 vs. 12 months of clopidogrel therapy afterdrug-eluting stenting. Eur Heart J. 2015;36(20):1252–63.
15. Tarantini G, Nai Fovino L, Tellaroli P, et al. Optimal duration of dual antiplatelet therapy after second-generation drug-eluting stent implantation in patientswith diabetes: The SECURITY (Second-Generation Drug-Eluting Stent Implantation Followed By Six- VersusTwelve-Month Dual Antiplatelet Therapy)-diabetes substudy. Int J Cardiol. 2016;207:168–76.
16. Collet JP, Silvain J, Barthélémy O, ARCTIC investigators, et al. Dual-antiplatelet treatment beyond 1 year after drug-eluting stent implantation (ARCTIC-Interruption): a randomised trial. Lancet. 2014;384(9954):1577–85.
17. Feres F, Costa RA, Abizaid A, OPTIMIZE TrialInvestigators, et al. Three vs twelve months of dual antiplatelet therapy after zotarolimus-eluting stents: the OPTIMIZE randomized trial. JAMA. 2013;310(23):2510–22.
18. Kim BK, Hong MK, Shin DH, RESET Investigators, et al. A new strategy for discontinuation of dual antiplatelet therapy: the RESET Trial (REal Safety and Efficacy of 3-month dual antiplatelet Therapy following Endeavor zotarolimus-eluting stent implantation). J Am Coll Cardiol. 2012;60(15):1340–8.
19. Bonaca MP, Bhatt DL, Steg PG, Storey RF, Cohen M, Im K, Oude Ophuis T, Budaj A, Goto S, López-Sendón J, Diaz R, Dalby A, Van de Werf F, Ardissino D, Montalescot G, Aylward P, Magnani G, Jensen EC, Held P, Braunwald E, Sabatine MS. Ischaemic risk and efficacy of ticagrelor in relation to time from P2Y12 inhibitor withdrawal in patients withprior myocardial infarction: insights from PEGASUS-TIMI 54. Eur Heart J. 2016;37(14):1133–42.
20. Mauri L, Kereiakes DJ, Yeh RW, DAPT Study Investigators, et al. Twelve or 30 months of dual antiplatelet therapy after drug-eluting stents. N Engl J Med. 2014;371(23):2155–66.
21. Sardella G, Mancone M, Biondi-Zoccai G, et al. Beneficial impact of prolonged dual antiplatelet therapy after drug-eluting stent implantation. J Interv Cardiol. 2012;25(6):596–603.
22. Campo G, Tebaldi M, et al. Short- versus long-term duration of dual antiplatelet therapy in patients treated for in-stent restenosis: a PRODIGY trial substudy (Prolonging Dual Antiplatelet Treatment After Grading Stent-Induced Intimal Hyperplasia). J Am Coll Cardiol. 2014;63(6):506–12.
23. Thukkani AK, Agrawal K, Prince L, et al. Long-term outcomes in patients with diabetes mellitus related to prolonging clopidogrel more than 12 MonthsAfter coronary stenting. J Am Coll Cardiol. 2015;66(10):1091–101.
24. Kandzari DE, Barker CS, Leon MB, Mauri L, Wijns W, Fajadet J, Mehran R. Dual antiplatelet therapy duration and clinical outcomes following treatment with zotarolimus-eluting stents. JACC Cardiovasc Interv. 2011; 4(10):1119–28.
25. Gilard M, Barragan P, Noryani AA, et al. 6- versus 24-month dual antiplatelet therapy after implantation of drug-eluting stents in patients nonresistant toaspirin: the randomized, multicenter ITALIC trial. J Am Coll Cardiol. 2015; 65(8):777–86.
26. Colombo A, Chieffo A, Frasheri A, et al. Second-generation drug-eluting stent implantation followed by 6- versus 12-month dual antiplatelet therapy: the SECURITY randomized clinical trial. J Am Coll Cardiol. 2014; 64(20):2086–97.
27. Lee CW, Ahn JM, Park DW, et al. Optimal duration of dual antiplatelet therapy after drug-eluting stent implantation: a randomized, controlled trial. Circulation. 2014;129(3):304–12.
28. Park SJ, Park DW, Kim YH, et al. Duration of dual antiplatelet therapy after implantation of drug-eluting stents. N Engl J Med. 2010;362(15):1374–82.
29. Giustino G, Baber U, Sartori S, et al. Duration of dual antiplatelet therapy after drug-eluting stent implantation: a systematic review and meta-analysis of randomized controlled trials. J Am Coll Cardiol. 2015;65(13):1298–310.
30. Yang J, Fan ZX, Yang CJ, Wang HB. A meta-analysis of randomized clinical trials comparing shorter (less or equal than 6 months) and longer (more or equal than 12 months) dual anti-platelet therapy following drug-eluting coronary stents. Iran Red Crescent Med J. 2015;17(7):e26904.
31. Valgimigli M, Campo G, Monti M, Prolonging Dual Antiplatelet Treatment After Grading Stent-Induced Intimal Hyperplasia Study (PRODIGY) Investigators, et al. Short- versus long-term duration of dual-antiplatelet therapy after coronary stenting: a randomized multicenter trial. Circulation. 2012;125(16):2015–26.
32. Valgimigli M, Park SJ, Kim HS, et al. Benefits and risks of long-term duration of dual antiplatelet therapy after drug-eluting stenting: a meta-analysis of randomized trials. Int J Cardiol. 2013;168(3):2579–87.
33. Siddiqi OK, Smoot K, Dufour AB, et al. Outcomes with prolonged clopidogrel therapy after coronary stenting in patients with chronic kidney disease. Heart. 2015;101(19):1569–76.

34. Fausto F, Ricardo Costa D, et al. Impact pf short versus long term DAPT in patients with diabetes mellitus undergoing percutaneous intervention with endeavour zotarolimus eluting stents. A subanalysis of the large, prospective, randomized, multicenter OPTIMIZE trial. J Am Coll Cardiol. 2014;63(14):61862–3.
35. Silber S, Serruys PW, Leon MB, et al. Clinical outcome of patients with and without diabetes mellitus after percutaneous coronary intervention with the resolute zotarolimus-eluting stent: 2-year results from the prospectively pooled analysis of the international global RESOLUTE program. JACC Cardiovasc Interv. 2013;6(4):357–68.
36. Park KW, Lee JM, Kang SH, et al. Everolimus-eluting Xience v/Promus versus zotarolimus-eluting resolute stents in patients with diabetes mellitus. JACC Cardiovasc Interv. 2014;7(5):471–81.
37. Bundhun PK, Li N, Chen MH. Adverse cardiovascular outcomes between insulin-treated and non-insulin treated diabetic patients after percutaneous coronary intervention: a systematic review and meta-analysis. Cardiovasc Diabetol. 2015;14:135.
38. Tanzilli G, Greco C, Pelliccia F, et al. Effectiveness of two-year clopidogrel + aspirin in abolishing the risk of very late thrombosis after drug-eluting stent implantation (from the TYCOON [two-year ClOpidOgrel need] study). Am J Cardiol. 2009;104(10):1357–61.
39. Park DW, Yun SC, Lee SW, et al. Stent thrombosis, clinical events, and influence of prolonged clopidogrel use after placement of drug-elutingstent data from an observational cohort study of drug-eluting versus bare-metal stents. JACC Cardiovasc Interv. 2008;1(5):494–503.
40. Campo G, Guastaroba P, Marzocchi A, Santarelli A, Varani E, Vignali L, Sangiorgio P, Tondi S, Serenelli C, De Palma R, Saia F. Impact of COPD on long-term outcome after ST-segment elevation myocardial infarction receiving primary percutaneous coronary intervention. Chest. 2013;144(3):750–7.
41. Campo G, Pavasini R, Malagù M, Mascetti S, Biscaglia S, Ceconi C, Papi A, Contoli M. Chronic obstructive pulmonary disease and ischemic heart disease comorbidity: overview of mechanisms and clinical management. Cardiovasc Drugs Ther. 2015;29(2):147–57.

6

Recurrent acute coronary syndrome and restenosis after percutaneous coronary intervention in a patient with idiopathic thrombocytopenic purpura

Ge Li-Sha[1], Chen Peng[2] and Li Yue-Chun[2*]

Abstract

Background: Platelets play a pivotal role in the pathogenesis of acute coronary syndrome (ACS) and acute and chronic complications following percutaneous coronary intervention (PCI). Platelet inhibition is a cornerstone in the management of these patients. Idiopathic thrombocytopenic purpura (ITP) is a bleeding disorder characterized by premature platelet destruction mediated by autoantibodies. The safety of antiplatelet therapy and PCI in patients who have ACS and ITP is unknown. The aim of the present study is to discuss the management strategies for patients who have ACS and ITP and to review limited data available in the literature.

Case presentation: We report the case of a patient with ITP who underwent three separate coronary interventions. The first PCI with stenting was performed in the left anterior descending artery 5 years ago while the patient suffered an anterior acute myocardial infarction, and the platelet count at admission was 90×10^9/L. The patient presented with recurrent ACS and severe in-stent restenosis 5 years after the first PCI, and the platelet count at admission was 18×10^9/L, and elevated to 87×10^9/L after platelets transfusion. He was treated successfully with cutting balloon angioplasty under anticoagulation with unfractionated heparin and antiagregation with acetylsalicylic acid and clopidogrel. Four months later after cutting balloon angioplasty, the patient received an intracoronary stent when he once again presented with recurrent ACS in the setting of restenosis. The patient has been observed for 1.5 years without restenosis after the third PCI.

Conclusion: We reviewed all the cases in the literature involving PCI and discussed the management strategies in patients with ITP and ACS. Available data suggest that PCI can be safe and feasible, and the risk–benefit equation of PCI procedures and antiplatelet therapies should be carefully evaluated, and the treatment should be individualized.

Keywords: Acute coronary syndrome, Idiopathic thrombocytopenic purpura, Percutaneous coronary intervention, Antiplatelet therapy

* Correspondence: liyuechun1980@sina.com
[2]Department of Cardiology, Second Affiliated Hospital of Wenzhou Medical University, 109 Xueyuan Road, Wenzhou, Zhejiang, China
Full list of author information is available at the end of the article

Background

Platelets play a pivotal role in the pathogenesis of acute coronary syndrome (ACS) [1]. Treatment for ACS usually involves antiplatelet, anticoagulant, and antithrombotic therapy, and the performance of percutaneous coronary intervention (PCI) [1, 2]. In addition, platelet aggregation also plays a crucial role in the pathogenesis of acute and chronic complications following PCI [1–3]. The combination of acetylsalicylic acid and thienopyridine derivatives is a mainstay in the management of patients undergoing PCI [1–3]. All of these medications are associated with bleeding sequelae and are generally contraindicated in patients with thrombocytopenia.

Idiopathic thrombocytopenic purpura (ITP) is an autoimmune syndrome involving antibody and cell-mediated destruction of platelets and suppression of platelet production that may predispose to bleeding [4]. Spontaneous mucocutaneous bleeding is common and death from hemorrhage occurs in approximately 5 % of the ITP patients [4]. The decision to treat ITP is based on the platelet count, the degree of bleeding, and the patient's lifestyle. Many patients with ITP require no therapy and only careful monitoring. Treatment is indicated when platelets are $<30 \times 10^9$/L, and is generally based on steroids and splenectomy [4]. Since the incidence of ITP is around 100 cases in 1 million persons per year, ACS patients with ITP are seen very rare. The safety of antiplatelet therapy and PCI in patients who have ACS and ITP is unknown, and to our knowledge, there are no guidelines or randomized studies to suggest treatment approaches in such patients.

We present here a case of a patient with ITP who experienced recurrent ACS and restenosis after PCI and we discuss the management strategies, including antiplatelet therapy.

Case presentation

A 75-year-old Chinese man was admitted to our hospital with increasing chest pain and dyspnea upon exertion. The chest pain developed 4 weeks previously when he was climbing stairs, and this was relieved by several minutes rest. He also reported that 2 day preceding hospitalization, the pain was triggered by minimum exertion, appearing even at rest. His chest pain was characterized by a squeezing pattern and this was located in the substernal area and it radiated to his left arm. He had no history of hypertension, hypercholesterolemia, diabetes mellitus, smoking and drinking, and there was no history of ischemic heart disease in his family.

Eight years ago he was diagnosed of chronic ITP, but didn't take any treatment. His platelet counts through the years had always been above 60×10^9/L. This earlier diagnosis of ITP was based on the observation of moderate thrombocytopenia and antiplatelet antibodies, with bone marrow findings consistent with the diagnosis. Five years ago primary PCI was performed in the proximal left anterior descending coronary artery using a drug-eluting stent (DES) because of acute anterior ST-segment elevation myocardial infarction at other hospital. At the time of the first PCI, his platelet count had been around 90×10^9/L. He received 300 mg of clopidogrel and 300 mg of aspirin along with 5000 units of heparin bolus before PCI. He was discharged on aspirin 100 mg and clopidogrel 75 mg orally daily for 1 year, and he never had bleeding before.

On physical examination, his blood pressure was 135/70 mmHg. His heart rate was regular at 76 beats/min. The chest was clear to auscultation and percussion bilaterally. There was no heart murmur. Findings of abdominal and neurological examinations were unremarkable, and lower extremities were without edema. A 12-lead ECG recorded on admission in the patient showed normal sinus rhythm and biphasic or inverted T waves in leads V_{1-3} (Fig. 1a). Blood examination revealed a platelet count of 18×10^9/L, mean platelet volume 13.6 fl (normal range: 6.5–11.0), troponin I level of 0.55 ng/mL (reference, <0.1), creatine kinase of 105 IU/L (normal range: 38–171), total cholesterol of 4.47 mmol/l, low density lipoprotein-cholesterol of 1.88 mmol/l, high density lipoprotein-cholesterol of 1.40 mmol/l, triglyceride of 1.29 mmol/l and fasting blood-glucose of 5.2 mmol/l. Blood coagulation tests showed a prothrombin time of 12.4 s (normal range: 12–15), an international normalized ratio of 0.97 (normal range: 0.85–1.15) and an activated partial thromboplastin time of 35.0 s (normal: 30–45 s). Brain natriuretic peptide and chest X-ray were normal. A transthoracic echocardiography demonstrated a normal left ventricular end-diastolic internal diameter of 50 mm with a slightly decreased left ventricular ejection fraction of 0.50. Diagnosis of ACS (acute non-ST-segment elevation myocardial infarction) was made. The GRACE (Global Registry of Acute Coronary Events) risk score of the patient was 143. The patient was administered high doses of intravenous nitroglycerin and oral metrolol and atorvastatin. Ten units of platelets were transfused after the patient was assessed by a hematologist, and the platelet count elevated to 87×10^9/L in the second day, and the patient was given 300 mg of aspirin and 300 mg of clopidogrel, prepared for a coronary artery angiography. Bolus injection of 3000 units unfractionated heparin was done at the beginning of the coronary angiography, and the activated clotting time (ACT) was monitored for the dose of heparin required, and then additional 3000 units were added during the PCI procedure, but GP IIb/IIIa inhibitors were not used. Coronary angiography was carried out via the radial artery, and revealed a 95 % in-stent restenosis in the middle part of left anterior descending artery (LAD; Fig. 2a, b). No other lesions were detected. The lesion in

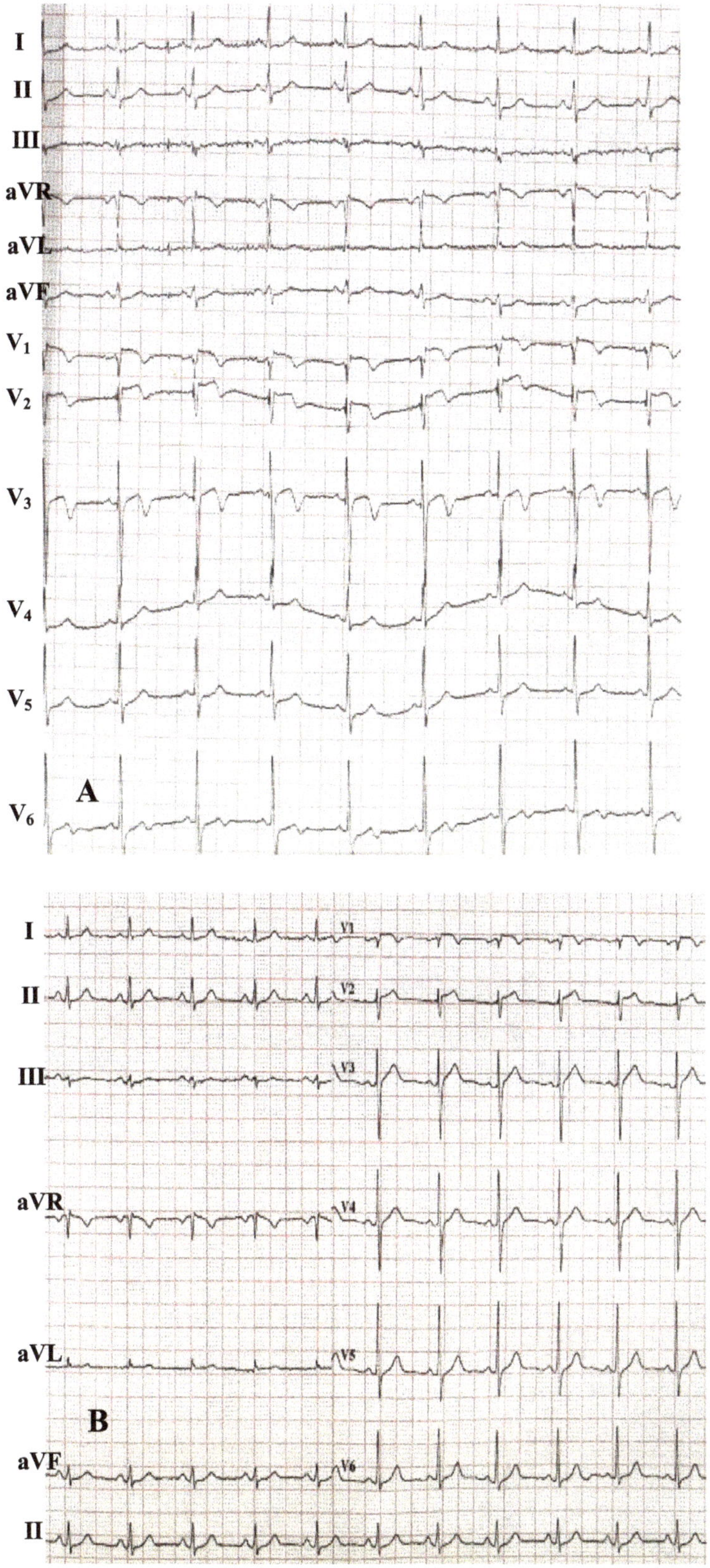

Fig. 1 Electrocardiography on admission and after PCI. **a** Electrocardiography performed on admission showing biphasic or inverted T waves in leads V_{1-3}. **b** Electrocardiography performed after PCI showing a resolution of the T wave abnormalities in V_{1-3}

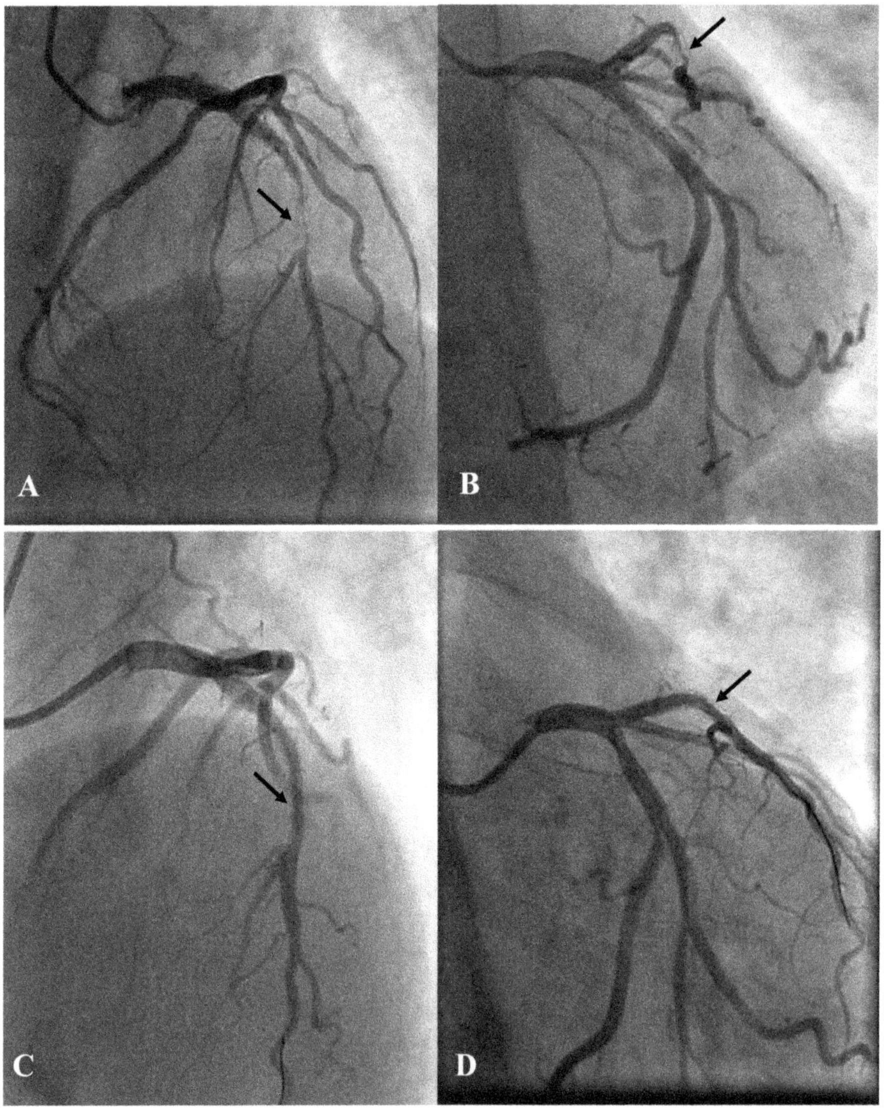

Fig. 2 Coronary angiography in a CRA projection (**a**) and an RAO + CAU projection (**b**) showing a severe in-stent restenosis of approximately 95 % in the middle part of left anterior descending artery (arrow). Repeat left coronary angiography following successful cutting balloon angioplasty (arrow) in a CRA projection (**c**) and an RAO + CAU projection (**d**)

the left anterior descending artery was treated using a cutting balloon (Boston Scientific) with no complications (Fig. 2c, d). Heparin was not administered any more after the PCI, but combined anti-platelet therapy (aspirin 100 mg and clopidogrel 75 mg daily) was performed as usual. The ECG showed the T wave abnormalities in $V_{1\text{-}3}$ were resolved after PCI (Fig. 1b). The patient was discharged asymptomatically at 3 days after PCI. Neither bleeding nor ischemic events were noted during hospitalization.

A week after discharge the platelet count was declined to 27×10^9/L, and aspirin and clopidogrel were stopped in outpatient clinic. Oral methylprednisolone was begun at 1 mg/kg per day and tapered over the subsequent 6 weeks. The platelet count gradually recovered to 200×10^9/L after receiving 1 week of methylprednisolone. He continued the treatment with aspirin 100 mg/day, and clopidogrel 75 mg/day for one month without any further problems.

Four months later, the patient was readmitted due to exertional chest pain he had felt for 1 month, even though he took all the medications (aspirin, clopidogrel, metrolol, atorvastatin and oral methylprednisolone) prescribed every day. On admission, the platelet count was 124×10^9/L, ECG showed normal sinus rhythm and ST segment depression in leads V_{2-5}, and troponin I was mildly elevated (0.26 ng/ml; reference, <0.1). Diagnosis of unstable angina was made. Coronary angiography showed a 99 % restenosis at the site of the previous

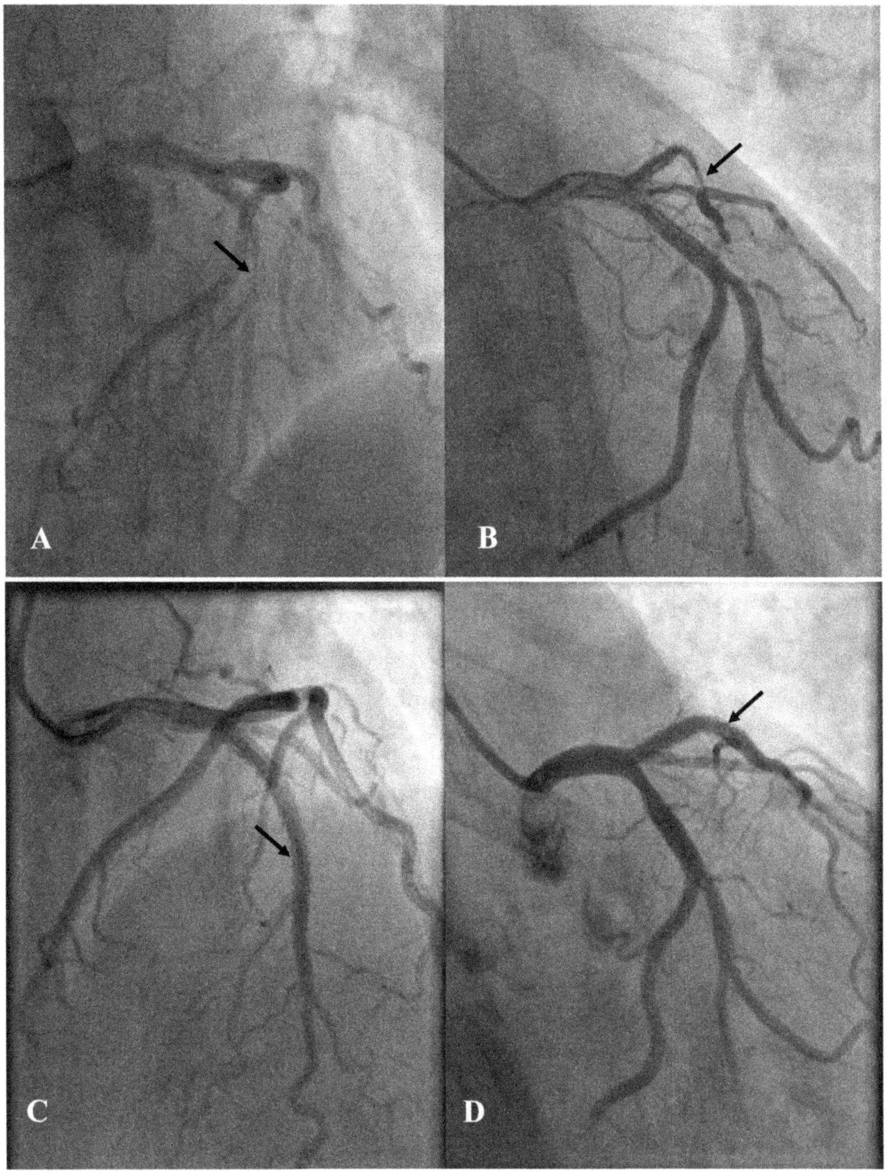

Fig. 3 Coronary angiography in a CRA projection (**a**) and an RAO + CAU projection (**b**) showing a severe in-stent restenosis of approximately 99 % in the left anterior descending artery (arrow) 4 months after cutting balloon angioplasty. Repeat left coronary angiography after successful stenting without residual stenosis (arrow) in a CRA projection (**c**) and an RAO + CAU projection (**d**)

lesion and a 40 % stenosis in the proximal left circumflex artery (LCX; Fig. 3a, b). We used unfractionated heparin, a dose of 100 U/kg, aspirin 300mg and clopidogrel 600 mg were administrated. An activated clotting time of 358 s was achieved. A 3.5*28 mm sirolimus eluted stent was deployed in the LAD with optimal angiographic result and Thrombolysis in Myocardial Infarction (TIMI) flow 3 in the LAD (Fig. 3c, d). There were no bleedings during or after the procedure, and at discharge the platelet count was 203×10^9/L.

He was then discharged on aspirin, clopidogrel, atorvastatin and oral methylprednisolone. Clopidogrel was discontinued 1 year after the procedure. During 18-month follow-up, the patient remained clinically free of symptoms without any ischemia events or bleeding complications. Coronary angiography showed stent patency at 11 months' follow-up (Fig. 4a, b). The platelet count remained stable.

Results in previous case reports

Previous reports focusing on ITP patients who underwent PCI were identified by searching PubMed and Google Scholar. Key words used included "ITP", "coronary artery disease", "ACS", "myocardial infarction", "angioplasty",

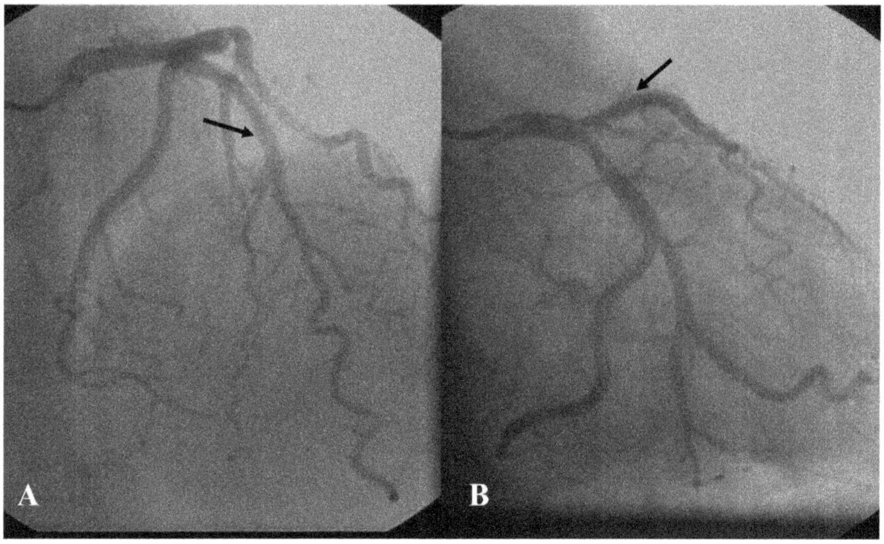

Fig. 4 Coronary angiography in a CRA projection (**a**) and an RAO + CAU projection (**b**) showing stent patency 11 months after stenting performed in in-stent restenotic lesion (arrow)

"PCI" and "stent". From 1999 to January 2013, 17 studies involving 18 patients affected by ITP who underwent PCI were reported in the literature (Table 1) [5–21]. The mean age of the patients was 59.7 ± 15.1 years (range 23–80 years). Eleven patients were male, and 7 patients were female. Two patients were affected by stable angina, 4 patients by unstable angina, 6 patients by acute non-ST elevation myocardial infarction, and 6 patients by acute ST elevation myocardial infarction. Thirteen patients (72 %) had single vessel coronary artery disease (10 patients for LAD disease, 1 patient for LCX disease, 1 patient for right coronary artery (RCA) disease, 1 patient for obtuse marginal branch disease), 4 patients (22 %) had two-vessel disease, the remaining 1 patient (6 %) had three-vessel disease. The 18 patients underwent 22 PCI procedures. A total of 29 vessels [15 LAD (51.7 %), 8 LCX (27.6 %), 4 RCA (13.8 %), 1 left main coronary artery (LM; 3.4 %), 1 obtuse marginal branch of LCX (3.4 %)] were treated in the 22 PCI procedures. Re-PCI was underwent in 4 patients (22 %), 1 patient because of acute coronary thrombosis [6], 2 patients because of restenosis [10, 15], 1 patient because of staged procedure [17]. Transfemoral and transradial approaches were used for PCI in 12 and 3 patients, respectively, and approach of PCI was not specifed in remaining 3 patients. Only PTCA without subsequent stent placement were underwent in 5 of 22 procedures (22.7 %), PCI with bare metal stent placement in 13 of 22 procedures (59.1 %), and PCI with drug-eluting stent placement in 4 of 22 procedures (18.2 %). PCI was performed with extremely different platelet counts, ranging from 3×10^9/L to 322×10^9/L (mean $78.5 \pm 81.5 \times 10^9$/L). Glycoprotein IIb/IIIa inhibitors were administrated during PCI in 4 PCI procedures, clopidogrel was administrated before and during PCI in 9 PCI procedures, ticlopidine in 1 PCI procedure, acetylsalicylic acid in 9 PCI procedures, and no any antiplatelet agents were administrated before and during PCI in 5 PCI procedures. Twelve patients (66.7 %) received steroid therapy, 10 patients (55.6 %) received intravenous immunoglobulin (IVIG) therapy, and platelet transfusions were completed in 4 patients (22.2 %). One instance (5.6 %) of major bleeding (large hematom around the puncture site of the right femoral artery) [6] and 6 of minor bleeding (ecchymoses in 4 patients, small hematoma in 1 patient, diffuse petechiae in 1 patient) were observed. Ten patients (55.6 %) were discharged on double antiplatelet therapy of acetylsalicylic acid and clopidogrel, and 3 patients only on aspirin or ticlopidine, and 3 patients did not receive any antiplatelet agent at discharge. In 2 reports, antiplatelet therapy at discharge was not specifed.

Discussion

Platelets play an important role in the atherosclerotic process and are intrinsically involved in the pathogenesis of ACS [1–3]. Thrombocytosis has been correlated with high incidence of ischemic heart disease, such as acute myocardial infarction [22]. Since platelets play a major role in thrombotic events, the association of ITP and ACS is rare. Nevertheless, acute myocardial infarction has been reported in even severely thrombocytopenic patients [5]. This implies that some factor other than platelet numbers alone is involved.

Table 1 Case reports on percutaneous coronary intervention in patients with idiopathic thrombocytopenic purpura

Study	Pt age (Y) and sex	CAD	Pre-PCIPLT count ($\times 10^9$/L)	Antiplatelet agent before and during PCI	Treated vessels	PCI and approach	Treatment of ITP	Bleeding	Restenosis	Discharge therapy
Fuchi et al., 1999 [20] (twice)	72, F	NSTEMI	59	None	LAD	PTCA, Femoral	STER	Large hematoma	NA	None
		STEMI	23	None	LAD	PTCA, Femoral	STERIVIGPLTT	No	NA	
Caputo et al., 2000 [6]	62, M	Unstable angina	3	NA	LAD	BMS stenting, Radial	STER	No	NA	ASA Clop
Segal et al., 2001 [21]	49, M	NSTEMI	41	ASAClopAbciximab	RCA, LCX	BMS stenting, Femoral	STER	No	NA	ASA Clop
Kikuchi et al., 2002 [22]	68, F	STEMI	22	Ticlopidine	LAD	BMS stenting, Femoral	NA	No	No	Ticlopidine
Méndez et al., 2004 [23]	70, M	NSTEMI	170	ASAClopAbciximab	RCA, LCX	BMS stenting, Radial	IVIGPLTT	ECC	NA	NA
Stouffer et al., 2004 [24] (twice)	77, M	Unstable angina	64	ASA	LCX	PTCA	None	No	yes	ASA
		NSTEMI	78	ASA Eptifibatide	LCX	BMS stenting	STER	Petechiae	No	ASA Clop
Amit et al., 2005 [25]	46, M	NSTEMI	38	ASA	LAD	PTCA	IVIG	No	NA	ASA
Marques et al., 2005 [26]	54, M	Unstable angina	15	None	LAD, LCX	BMS stenting, Brachial	STERIVIGPLTT	No	NA	None
Kim et al., 2006 [27]	47, F	STEMI	21	Clop	RCA	BMS stenting, Femoral	IVIG	ECC	NA	ASA Clop
Fong et al., 2006 [28]	71, F	NSTEMI	119	ASA	LAD	DES stenting, Radial	STERIVIG	No	No	ASA Clop
Park et al., 2007 [29] 3 times	61, F	Stable angina	4	None	None	CAG, Femoral	STER	Hematoma	No	None
			34	None	LAD, LCX	BMS stenting, Femoral	STERIVIGPLTT	No	yes	None
			20	None	LAD, LCX	PTCA, Femoral	STER	No	NA	None
Gracia et al., 2008 [30]	37, M	STEMI	39	ASA Clop	LAD	BMS stenting, Femoral	None	No	NA	ASA Clop
Moretti et al., 2008 [31] (twice)	66, M	Unstable angina	110	NA	RCA, LCX	BMS stenting	STERIVIG	No	NA	ASA Clop
			200	NA	LM, LAD	DES stenting, Femoral	STER	No	NA	ASA Clop
Can et al., 2009 [32]	76, M	Stable angina	100	Clop	LAD	BMS stenting, Femoral	Danazol	No	NA	NA
Yildiz et al., 2010 [33]	23, F	STEMI	35	Clop	LAD	BMS stenting, Femoral	STER	ECC	NA	ASA Clop

Table 1 Case reports on percutaneous coronary intervention in patients with idiopathic thrombocytopenic purpura *(Continued)*

Neskovic et al., 2010 [34]	80, M	STEMI	5	ASA Clop	LAD	BMS stenting, Femoral	STER Danazol	No	NA	ASA Clop
Torbey et al., 2013 [35] 2 cases	61, F	STEMI	322	ASA Clop Abciximab	LAD	DES stenting, Femoral	SPLSTERIVIG	ECC	NA	ASA Clop
	55, M	NSTEMI	208	Clop	Obtusemarginal branch	DES stenting, Femoral	STERIVIG	No	yes	ASA Clop

Pt patient, *Y* years, *F* femal, *M* male, *CAD* coronary artery disease, *NSTEMI* non-ST elevation myocardial infarction, *STEMI* ST elevation myocardial infarction, *PCI* percutaneous coronary intervention, *PLT* Platelet, *NA* data not available, *ASA* acetylsalicylic acid, *Clop* clopidogrel, *LAD* left anterior descending artery, *RCA* right coronary artery, *LCX* left circumflex artery, *LM* left main artery, *PTCA* Percutaneous transluminal coronary angioplasty, *BMS* bare metal stent, *DES* drug-eluting stent, *ITP* idiopathic thrombocytopenic purpura, *STER* steroids, *IVIG* intravenous immunoglobulin, *PLTT* Platelets transfusion, *SPL* Splenectomy, *ECC* Ecchymoses

If a patient with chronic thrombocytopenia has coronary artery disease, the concomitance of known coronary risk factors, such as hypertension, diabetes, dyslipidemia, cigarette smoking or a family history for cardiovascular disease, should be considered. Sometimes, in patients without these coronary risk factors like the present case, it could be related with some other causes. First, platelets in patients with ITP was larger, younger, and more adhesive to the vascular surface [23]. In acute myocardial infarction or stroke patients, mean platelet volume is significantly increased despite a concomitant decrease in platelet count [24–26]. In the present case, the mean platelet volume of the patient was significantly increased. Previous studies have demonstrated that large platelets have a higher thrombotic potential [24–26]. Osuna et al [27] analysed the relationship between mean platelet volume and recurrent myocardial infarction, and found that increased mean platelet volume and platelet size contributed to reinfarction and death. Karpatkin [28] reported that the platelet aggregation velocity was directly in proportion to the platelet volume and correlated best with the megathrombocyte index. Second, elevated platelet microparticles in the ITP patients with ACS were observed [29, 30]. Microparticles are membrane vesicles released from many different cell types, including platelets. They have a potent pro-inflammatory effect, promote coagulation and affect vascular function [29, 30]. Circulating platelet microparticles and the risk of thromboembolic complications have repeatedly been demonstrated [29–31]. Therefore, platelet microparticles may be associated with coronary thrombosis in patients with ITP. Third, antigenic mimicry between platelets and endothelial cells may lead to damage of the platelets and the endothelium, caused by autoantibodies directed against platelet surface antigens, notably IIb/IIIa receptors [32, 33]. Finally, a rise of the platelet count with administration of steroids, intravenous immunoglobulin, or platelet transfusion in ITP might be "procoagulant" and might aggravate the potentially adverse effect of increased plasma viscosity leading to increased susceptibility to fatal thrombotic events, such as myocardial infarction or stroke [23, 34, 35].

The combination of ITP and coronary artery disease poses serious management problems in which a good balance between the prevention of thrombosis and hemorrhagic risk must be achieved. Indeed, ITP increases risks of bleeding in general and medications to inhibit platelet function are generally not recommended. However, antiplatelet agents should be used in patients with coronary artery disease unless contraindication exists, especially after stent implantation. This dilemma leads to difficulty in managing concomitant ITP and coronary artery disease. Performance of PCI in a patient with ITP presents a unique situation in which platelet function needs to be inhibited sufficiently to perform PCI safely but not to the extent that bleeding complications result. Our initial strategy was to treat the patient with drugs, but our patient had refractory symptoms and ischemic ECG changes and elevated troponin I despite therapy with nitrates, β-blockers and statins, and revascularization was, therefore, indicated. Since our patient was categorized as having high risk for major bleeding and had only a single coronary lesion, PCI was a better choice than bypass surgery. We decided to administer antiplatelet agents after platelets transfusion, and then proceed using cutting balloon angioplasty without stent implantation because of the risk of subacute stent thrombosis in a patient in whom it was unknown whether he would be tolerant of combination therapy of acetylsalicylic acid and clopidogrel after stent implantation. The patient was given steroids following cutting balloon angioplasty, and the platelet count increased and remained normal level. The patient did receive an intracoronary stent 4 months later when he once again presented with recurrent ACS in the setting of restenosis. Coronary angiography showed stent patency 11 months after stent implantation.

Based on the results of the previous case reports [5–21, 31, 36] and present report, we concluded that PCI can be a useful strategy in patients with ITP and severe coronary artery disease even when the patient has severe thrombocytopenia, and major bleeding was rare. Both transfemoral and transradial approaches were successfully used for PCI. Implanting a bare metal stent (BMS) appears to be reasonable choice during PCI, since dual antiplatelet therapy with acetylsalicylic acid and clopidogrel could be administered for a shorter period of time to allow stent endothelialization. DES implantation was also reported in 4 patients, and 5 cases of PCI without subsequent stent placement were also reported. Perioperative ITP treatment certainly minimized the complication rate in the PCI population as well. Steroids should be first choice to increase the platelet count, but if a rapid platelet count elevation were required, platelet transfusions and IVIG supplementation could be administered. A safe cutoff platelet count above which invasive procedures can be performed has not been yet established. Russo et al. [36] have suggested that when the platelet counts $>50 \times 10^9$/L intervention either percutaneously or surgically can be safely performed. The combined therapy of acetylsalicylic acid and clopidogrel after PCI was well tolerated in most of patients. In addtion, most of patients had single vessel coronary artery disease and LAD artery was the most commonly occluded of the coronary arteries in patient with ITP, which was the same with the general population. Among 7 cases who underwent reexamined coronary angiography, 3 patients had coronary restenosis. The restenosis developed after percutaneous transluminal coronary angioplasty without stent placement in 1 patient, after BMS implant in 1 patient, and after DES implant in 1 patient. The present case also occurred repeatedly in-stent restenosis. Repeat revascularization was successfully done in all 4 patients. Many factors may be involved in the pathophysiology of restenosis. Norgaz et al [37] found that mean platele volume before PCI is correlated with subsequent development of in-stent restenosis, and if preprocedural mean platele volume is greater than 8.4 fl, restenosis is more probable to occur. Generally, The mean platelet volume in patients with ITP was significantly increased. Therefore, platelet size may play a role in the development of restenosis after PCI in a patient with ITP.

Conclusions

Available data suggest that PCI can be safe and feasible, and the risk–benefit equation of PCI procedures and antiplatelet therapies should be carefully evaluated, and the treatment should be individualized.

Consent statement

Written informed consent was obtained from the patient for publication of this case report and any accompanying images.

Abbreviations

ACS: Acute coronary syndrome; ACT: Activated clotting time; BMS: Bare metal stent; DES: Drug-eluting stent; GRACE: Global Registry of Acute Coronary Events; ITP: Idiopathic thrombocytopenic purpura; IVIG: Intravenous immunoglobulin; LAD: Left anterior descending artery; LCX: Left circumflex artery; PCI: Percutaneous coronary intervention; RCA: Right coronary artery; TIMI: Thrombolysis in Myocardial Infarction.

Competing interests

The authors declare that they have no competing interests.

Authors' contributions

LYC and CP performed the PCI and helped writing the paper. GLS wrote the paper. All authors read and approved the final manuscript.

Author details

[1]Department of Pediatric, Second Affiliated Hospital of Wenzhou Medical University, Wenzhou 325000, China. [2]Department of Cardiology, Second Affiliated Hospital of Wenzhou Medical University, 109 Xueyuan Road, Wenzhou, Zhejiang, China.

References

1. Ault KA, Cannon CP, Mitchell J, McCahan J, Tracy RP, Novotny WF, et al. Platelet activation in patients after an acute coronary syndrome: results from the TIMI-12 trial. Thrombolysis in Myocardial Infarction. J Am Coll Cardiol. 1999;33:634–9.
2. Giugliano RP, Braunwald E. The year in acute coronary syndrome. J Am Coll Cardiol. 2014;63:201–14.
3. Varenhorst C, Jensevik K, Jernberg T, Sundström A, Hasvold P, Held C, et al. Duration of dual antiplatelet treatment with clopidogrel and aspirin in patients with acute coronary syndrome. Eur Heart J. 2014;35:969–78.
4. Cines DB, Blanchette VS. Immune thrombocytopenic purpura. N Engl J Med. 2002;346:995–1008.
5. Caputo RP, Abraham S, Churchill D. Transradial coronary stent placement in a patient with severe idiopathic autoimmune thrombocytopenic purpura. J Invasive Cardiol. 2000;12:365–8.
6. Fuchi T, Kondo T, Sase K, Takahashi M. Primary percutaneous transluminal coronary angioplasty performed for acute myocardial infarction in a patient with idiopathic thrombocytopenic purpura. Jpn Circ J. 1999;63:133–6.
7. Segal OR, Baker CS, Banim S. Percutaneous coronary intervention with adjunctive abciximab and clopidogrel in a patient with chronic idiopathic thrombocytopaenic purpura. Int J Cardiovasc Intervent. 2001;4:35–8.
8. Kikuchi S, Hayashi Y, Fujioka S, Kukita H, Ochi N. A case of intracoronary stent implanted for acute myocardial infarction in an elderly patient with idiopathic thrombocytopenic purpura. Nippon Ronen Igakkai Zasshi. 2002;39:88–93.
9. Méndez TC, Díaz Ó, Enríquez L, Baz JA, Fernández F, Goicolea J. Severe thrombocytopenia refractory to platelet transfusion secondary to abciximab readministration in a patient previously diagnosed with idiopathic thrombocytopenic purpura A possible etiopathogenic link. Rev Esp Cardiol. 2004;57:789–91.
10. Stouffer GA, Hirmerova J, Moll S, Rubery B, Napoli M, Ohman EM, et al. Percutaneous coronary intervention in a patient with immune thrombocytopenia purpura. Catheter Cardiovasc Interv. 2004;61:364–7.
11. Amit G, Yermiyahu T, Gilutz H, Ilia R, Zahger D. Thrombocytopenia, immunoglobulin treatment, and acute myocardial infarction–a case report. Angiology. 2005;56:229–31.
12. Marques LG, Furukawa MK, Leitão TP, Quiñones JL, Queiroz FC, Tiossi RF, et al. Percutaneous transluminal coronary angioplasty in a patient with idiopathic thrombocytopenic purpura. Arq Bras Cardiol. 2005;84:337–9.
13. Kim JH, Park KU, Chum WJ, Kim SH, Nah DY. Primary percutaneous coronary intervention for acute myocardial infarction with idiopathic thrombocytopenic purpura: a case report. J Korean Med Sci. 2006;21:355–7.
14. Fong MC, Chen KC, Leu HB, Chen LC. Coronary revascularization in a patient with immune thrombocytopenic purpura. J Chin Med Assoc. 2006;69:436–8.
15. Park HJ, Seung KB, Kim PJ, Kang HH, Park CS, Kil UH, et al. Intracoronary stent deployment without antiplatelet agents in a patient with idiopathic thrombocytopenic purpura. Korean Circ J. 2007;37:87–90.
16. Gracia MC, Cebollero IC, Lezcano JS, Osuna GG, Miguel JA, Peralta LP. Invasive treatment performed for acute myocardial infarction in a patient with immune thrombocytopenic purpura. Int J Cardiol. 2008;127:183–5.
17. Moretti C, Teresa Lucciola M, Morena L, Biondi-Zoccai G, Laudito A, Anselmino M, et al. Idiopathic thrombocytopenic purpura and percutaneous coronary stenting: a dangerous duo? Int J Cardiol. 2008;130:e96–7.
18. Can MM, Tanboga IH, Boztosun B, Kaymaz C. Antiplatelet treatment after percutaneous coronary intervention in a patient with idiopathic thrombocytopenic purpura. Arch Turk Soc Cardiol. 2009;37:575–7.
19. Yildiz A, Coskun U, Batukan OE, Keskin K. Primary percutaneous coronary intervention for acute myocardial infarction in a young female with idiopathic thrombocytopenic purpura: a case report and review. Case Rep Med. 2010;2010:854682.
20. Neskovic A, Stankovic I, Milicevic P, Aleksic A, Vlahovic-Stipac A, Calija B, et al. Primary PCI for acute myocardial infarction in a patient with idiopathic thrombocytopenic purpura. Herz. 2010;35:43–9.
21. Torbey E, Yacoub H, McCord D, Lafferty J. Two cases and review of the literature: primary percutaneous angiography and antiplatelet management in patients with immune thrombocytopenic purpura. ISRN Hematol. 2013;2013:174659.
22. Nanavati A, Patel N, Burke J. Thrombocytosis and coronary occlusion. JACC Cardiovasc Interv. 2012;5:e18–9.
23. Rand ML, Dean JA. Platelet function in autoimmune (idiopathic) thrombocytopenic purpura. Acta Paediatr Suppl. 1998;424:57–60.
24. Martin JF, Bath PM, Burr ML. Influence of platelet size on outcome after myocardial infarction. Lancet. 1991;338:1409–11.
25. Endler G, Klimesch A, Sunder-Plassmann H, Schillinger M, Exner M, Mannhalter C, et al. Mean platelet volume is an independent risk factor for myocardial infarction but not for coronary artery disease. Br J Haematol. 2002;117:399–404.
26. Furiozzi F. Mean platelet volume and acute ischemic stroke. Stroke. 1996;27:1010–1.
27. Pabón Osuna P, Nieto Ballesteros F, Moríñigo Muñoz JL, Sánchez Fernández PL, Arribas Jiménez A, Diego Domínguez M, et al. The effect

of the mean platelet volume on the short-term prognosis of acute myocardial infarct. Rev Esp Cardiol. 1998;51:816–22.
28. Karpatkin S. Heterogeneity of human platelets. VI. Correlation of platelet function with platelet volume. Blood. 1978;51:307–16.
29. VanWijk MJ, VanBavel E, Sturk A, Nieuwland R. Microparticles in cardiovascular diseases. Cardiovasc Res. 2003;59:277–87.
30. Puddu P, Puddu GM, Cravero E, Muscari S, Muscari A. The involvement of circulating microparticles in inflammation, coagulation and cardiovascular diseases. Can J Cardiol. 2010;26:140–5.
31. Yusuf SW, Iliescu C, Bathina JD, Daher IN, Durand JB. Antiplatelet therapy and percutaneous coronary intervention in patients with acute coronary syndrome and thrombocytopenia. Tex Heart Inst J. 2010;37:336–3340.
32. Thiagarajan P, Shapiro SS, Levine E, DeMarco L, Yalcin A. A monoclonal antibody to human platelet glycoprotein IIIa detects a related protein in cultured human endothelial cells. J Clin Invest. 1985;75:896–901.
33. Leeksma OC, Zandbergen-Spaargaren J, Giltay JC, van Mourik JA. Cultured human endothelial cells synthesize a plasma membrane protein complex immunologically related to the platelet glycoprotein IIb/IIIa complex. Blood. 1986;67:1176–80.
34. Woodruff RK, Grigg AP, Firkin FC, Smith IL. Fatal thrombotic events during treatment of autoimmune thrombocytopenia with intravenous immunoglobulin in elderly patients. Lancet. 1986;2:217–8.
35. Paolini R, Zamboni S, Ramazzina E, Zampieri P, Cella G. Idiopathic thrombocytopenic purpura treated with steroid therapy does not prevent acute myocardial infarction: a case report. Blood Coagul Fibrinolysis. 1999;10:439–42.
36. Russo A, Cannizzo M, Ghetti G, Barbaresi E, Filippini E, Specchia S, et al. Idiopathic thrombocytopenic purpura and coronary artery disease: comparison between coronary artery bypass grafting and percutaneous coronary intervention. Interact Cardiovasc Thorac Surg. 2011;13:153–7.
37. Norgaz T, Hobikoglu G, Aksu H, Bolca O, Uyarel H, Eren M, et al. The relationship between preprocedural platelet size and subsequent in-stent restenosis. Acta Cardiol. 2004;59:391–5.

7

Is the concomitant use of clopidogrel and Proton Pump Inhibitors still associated with increased adverse cardiovascular outcomes following coronary angioplasty?

Pravesh Kumar Bundhun[1], Abhishek Rishikesh Teeluck[2], Akash Bhurtu[2] and Wei-Qiang Huang[1*]

Abstract

Background: Controversies were previously observed with the concomitant use of clopidogrel and Proton Pump Inhibitors (PPIs), especially omeprazole, following coronary angioplasty. Even though several studies showed no interaction between clopidogrel and PPIs, questions have been raised about the decrease in antiplatelet effects of clopidogrel with PPIs. A previously published meta-analysis showed concomitant use of clopidogrel and PPIs to be associated with higher adverse cardiovascular outcomes. However, data which were used were extracted from studies published before the year 2012. Whether these controversies still exist in this new era is not clear. Therefore, we aim to show if the concomitant use of clopidogrel and PPIs is still associated with higher adverse outcomes following Percutaneous Coronary Intervention (PCI) using data obtained from recently published studies (2012 to 2016).

Methods: Electronic databases were searched for recent publications (2012–2016) comparing (clopidogrel plus PPIs) versus clopidogrel alone following PCI. Adverse cardiovascular outcomes were considered as the clinical endpoints. Odds Ratios (OR) with 95% Confidence Intervals (CI) were used as the statistical parameters and the pooled analyses were performed with RevMan 5.3 software.

Results: Eleven studies with a total number of 84,729 patients (29,235 patients from the PPIs group versus 55,494 patients from the non-PPIs group) were included. Results of this analysis showed that short term mortality and Target Vessel Revascularization (TVR) significantly favored the non-PPIs group with OR: 1.55; 95% CI: 1.43–1.68, $P < 0.00001$ and OR: 1.26; 95% CI: 1.06–1.49, $P = 0.009$ respectively. Long-term Major Adverse Cardiac Events (MACEs), Myocardial Infarction (MI), Stent Thrombosis (ST) and TVR significantly favored patients who did not use PPIs with OR: 1.37; 95% CI: 1.23–1.53, $P < 0.00001$, OR: 1.41; 95% CI: 1.26–1.57, $P < 0.00001$ and OR: 1.38; 95% CI: 1.13–1.70, $P = 0.002$ and OR: 1.28; 95% CI: 1.01–1.61, $P = 0.04$ respectively. However, the result for long term mortality was not statistically significant.

Conclusion: The combined use of clopidogrel with PPIs is still associated with significantly higher adverse cardiovascular events such as MACEs, ST and MI following PCI supporting results of the previously published meta-analysis. However, long-term mortality is not statistically significant warranting further analysis with randomized patients.

Keywords: Proton pump inhibitors, Clopidogrel, Percutaneous coronary intervention, Major adverse cardiac events

* Correspondence: huangwq1029@126.com
[1]Institute of Cardiovascular Diseases, the First Affiliated Hospital of Guangxi Medical University, Nanning, Guangxi 530021, People's Republic of China
Full list of author information is available at the end of the article

Background

Controversies still exist with the concomitant use of clopidogrel, one of the components of the Dual Anti-Platelet Therapy (DAPT) with Proton Pump Inhibitors (PPIs), especially omeprazole following Percutaneous Coronary Intervention (PCI). Even if the American College of Cardiology/Gastroenterology and the American Heart Association recommend prophylactic treatment with a PPI in those patients who require DAPT and those patients who are at high risk of gastrointestinal injury [1], recent studies have shown clopidogrel and PPIs to be metabolized by the same cytochrome P450 2C19 (CYP2C19) pathway [2].

Several studies showed no interaction between clopidogrel and PPIs. For example, Rassen et al. showed a slight increase in the rate of Myocardial Infarction (MI) and mortality in older patients discharged on clopidogrel and PPIs, but the authors were not able to conclude any interaction between PPIs and clopidogrel in terms of major clinical relevance [3]. Zairis et al. also showed no impact of omeprazole on the clinical efficacy of clopidogrel during the first year following PCI [4].

However, decrease in antiplatelet effects of clopidogrel with the concomitant use of PPIs has been observed. Patients had a higher level of platelet reactivity which resulted in an increased risk of adverse clinical outcomes [5]. For example, Gupta et al. concluded that the concomitant use of clopidogrel with PPIs following coronary stents implantation was associated with a significantly higher risk of major adverse cardiac events (MACEs) [6].

In 2012, Huang et al. conducted a meta-analysis based on the current idea, using old data (2009–2011) [7]. Results from their meta-analysis showed significantly increased risk of MACEs in patients with the concomitant use of clopidogrel and PPIs. Unfortunately, the high level of heterogeneity observed among the different subgroups analyzed was their major limitation.

Recently, many new studies were published based on the cardiovascular outcomes observed in patients treated with clopidogrel plus PPIs and clopidogrel alone following PCI. However, whether these controversies still exist in this new era is not clear. Therefore, we aim to show if the concomitant use of clopidogrel and PPIs is still associated with higher adverse outcomes following PCI using data obtained from recently published studies (2012 to 2016).

Methods

Data sources and search strategy

Three reviewers (P.K.B, A.R.T and A.B) carefully searched EMBASE, PubMed/Medline databases, and the Cochrane library for Randomized Controlled Trials (RCTs) and observational studies comparing the concomitant use clopidogrel with PPI and clopidogrel alone following PCI. The terms 'proton pump inhibitor and clopidogrel', 'proton pump inhibitor and percutaneous coronary intervention' and 'proton pump inhibitor and dual antiplatelet therapy' were searched carefully. In addition, abbreviations such as PPI, PCI and DAPT were also used. In order to widen the search process, individual PPIs namely 'omeprazole, pantoprazole, lansoprazole, esomeprazole, and rabeprazole' were also used in this search strategy. Because this current meta-analysis was based on recently published English articles, and since the previously published meta-analysis already included old data published before or in the year 2011, only studies published after the year 2011 (2012 to 2016) were considered relevant. Unpublished data were not included.

Inclusion and exclusion criteria

RCTs and observational studies were included if:

(a) They compared patients treated with (clopidogrel and PPIs) and patients treated with clopidogrel but without PPIs following coronary stenting.
(b) Adverse cardiovascular outcomes were reported as their clinical endpoints.
(c) They were published after the year 2011.

RCTs and observational studies were excluded if:

(a) They did not compare patients (clopidogrel and PPIs) with clopidogrel alone following coronary stenting.
(b) Adverse cardiovascular outcomes were not reported as their clinical endpoints.
(c) They were published before or in the year 2011.
(d) They were duplicates.

Outcomes and follow up periods

Reported outcomes which have been listed in Table 1 included:

(a) All-cause mortality
(b) MI
(c) Target vessel revascularization (TVR)
(d) Stent thrombosis (ST)
(e) MACEs which consisted of death, MI and repeated revascularization.

Follow up period was divided into a short term follow up period (<1 year) and a long term follow up period (≥ 1 year).

Data extraction and quality assessment

Three authors (P.K.B, A.R.T and A.B) independently reviewed the data extracted from the studies included in this meta-analysis. Information regarding the type of study, the total number of patients in the study group and the control group respectively, data regarding the baseline characteristics of the patients involved,

Table 1 Reported outcomes and their follow up periods

Study	Reported outcomes	Follow up periods	Type of follow up
Bhurke 2012 [17]	MI and revascularization	9 months	Short term
Burkard 2012 [18]	Death, MI, ST, MACE, TVR	3 years	Long term
Chitose 2012 [19]	Death, MI	18 months	Long term
Douglas 2012 [20]	Death, MI	10 months	Short term
Dunn 2013 [21]	Death, MI, TVR	1 month	Short term
Goodman 2012 [22]	Death, MI, ST	1 year	Long term
Hsieh 2015 [23]	MI, revascularization	1 year	Long term
Macaione 2012 [24]	Death, MI, TVR	3 years	Long term
Weisz 2015 [25]	Death, MACEs, MI, ST, TVR	In hospital, 2 years	Short and long term
Zou 2014 [26]	Death, MACEs, MI, ST, TVR	1 year	Long term
Gargiolo 2016 [16]	Death, MACEs, MI, ST	2 years	Long term

Abbreviations: *MI* Myocardial infarction, *ST* Stent thrombosis, *MACEs* Major adverse cardiac events, *TVR* Target vessel revascularization

information regarding the cardiovascular outcomes reported as well as the follow up periods associated with each eligible study were systematically extracted. At a certain point, when the authors disagreed about including certain studies, disagreements were resolved and a final decision was made by the fourth author (W.Q.H). Since only two trials were included in this meta-analysis whereas the other studies were observational cohorts, the risk of bias was not assessed [8].

Methodological quality and statistical analysis

Recommendations from the Preferred Reporting Items for Systematic Reviews and Meta-Analyses guideline were followed [9]. Heterogeneity was assessed using the following:

(a) Cochrane Q-statistic test based on a *P* value with a cut-off point of 0.05 whereby a value less or equal to 0.05 was considered statistically significant.
(b) I^2-statistic test whereby an increasing value denoted an increasing heterogeneity.

A fixed effects model ($I^2 < 50\%$) or a random effects model ($I^2 > 50\%$) was used based on the value of I^2 obtained.

Odds Ratios (OR) with 95% Confidence Intervals (CIs) were calculated. The pooled analyses were performed with RevMan 5.3 software.

Publication bias was assessed by observing funnel plots. The reason for using funnel plots was the fact that studies with a smaller volume were used. For studies of smaller volumes, due to the higher degree of random changes, they have a wider distribution of results compared to studies of greater volumes. This might cause asymmetry in the funnels whereby publication bias could therefore be visually estimated.

Ethical approval was not necessary for such types of research articles.

Results

Study selection

A total number of 1153 articles were obtained from the searched databases. One thousand and ninety-six articles were rejected since they were either not related to this current topic or they were duplicates. Fifty-seven full text articles were assessed for eligibility. A further six articles were eliminated since they were case studies and meta-analyses. Three more articles were eliminated because their data could not be used (outcomes were reported in terms of Hazard Ratio which was not appropriate to be used in meta-analysis). In addition, 37 more articles were eliminated since they were published before the year 2012. Finally, 11 articles were included in this analysis (Fig. 1).

Baseline characteristics

A total number of 84,729 patients were included in this analysis (29,235 patients treated with clopidogrel plus PPIs and 55,494 patients treated with clopidogrel alone). The general features of the studies have been summarized in Table 2.

Study Douglas 2012, which was conducted in United Kingdom, consisted of the highest number of patients, followed by the studies Bhurke 2012, Dunn 2013 and Goodman 2012 respectively.

The baseline features of the patients have been listed in Tables 3 and 4 lists the different types of PPIs used by the patients.

According to the baseline features, there was no significant difference among the patients who were treated with (clopidogrel plus PPIs) and clopidogrel alone.

Main results of this meta-analysis

Results of this analysis (summarized in Table 5) showed that during a short term follow up period, using a fixed effects model, mortality and TVR significantly favored

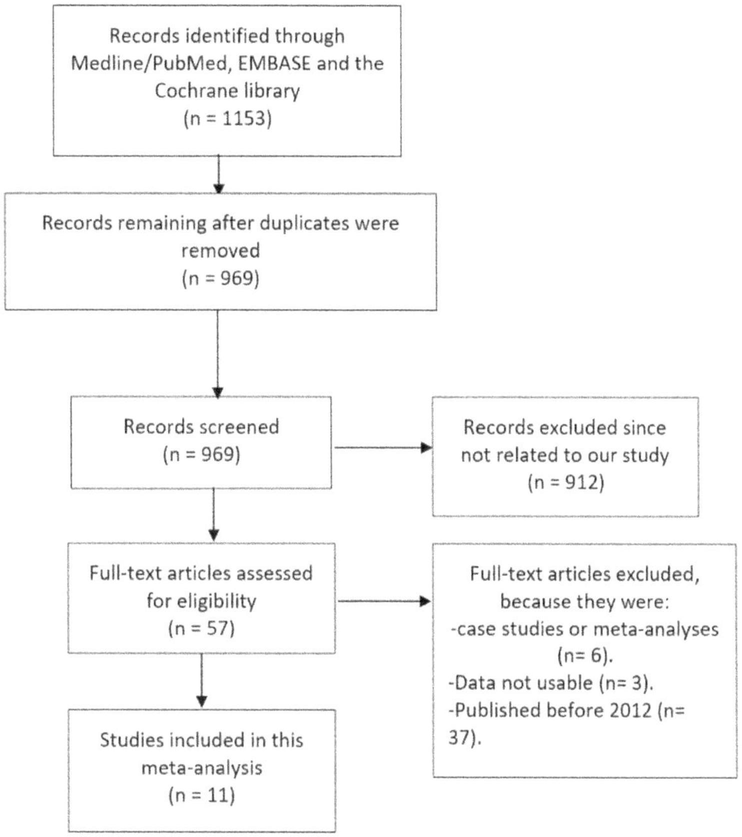

Fig. 1 Flow diagram for the study selection

clopidogrel alone with OR: 1.55; 95% CI: 1.43–1.68, $P <$ 0.00001 and OR: 1.26; 95% CI: 1.06–1.49, $P = 0.009$ respectively. This result has been represented in Fig. 2. However, result for the short-term MI which was analyzed using a random effects model, was not statistically significant with OR: 1.17; 95% CI: 0.86–1.58, $P = 0.32$ (Fig. 3).

During the long-term follow up period, MACEs, MI and ST significantly favored clopidogrel alone with OR: 1.37; 95% CI: 1.23–1.53, $P < 0.00001$, OR: 1.41; 95% CI:

Table 2 General features of the studies included

Studies	No of patients using clopidogrel + PPIs (*n*)	No of patients using clopidogrel alone (*n*)	Type of study	Region
Bhurke 2012	2958	7143	Retrospective	United states
Burkard 2012	109	692	Retrospective	United states
Chitose 2012	187	443	Observational	Japan
Douglas 2012	12439	16900	Observational	United Kingdom
Dunn 2013	408	9191	Retrospective	Charlottesville
Goodman 2012	3255	6021	RCT	Canada
Hsieh 2015	670	5933	Observational	Taiwan
Macaione 2012	121	55	Retrospective	Italy
Weisz 2015	2162	6419	Observational	Israel
Zou 2014	6188	1465	Observational	China
Gargiolo 2016	738	1232	RCT	Italy
Total no of patients (*n*)	29,235	55,494		

Abbreviations: *PPIs* Proton pump inhibitor, *RCT* Randomized controlled trial

Table 3 Baseline characteristics of the patients

Study	Age (year)	Males (%)	HT (%)	Ds (%)	DM (%)	CS (%)
	C + PPI/C alone	C + PPI/C alone	C + PPI/C alone	C + PPI/C alone	C + PPI/C alone	C + PPI/C alone
Bhurke 2012	61.5/59.6	68.7/76.3	-	-	28.9/26.4	-
Burkard 2012	66.5/63.3	68.8/79.9	72.5/65.0	73.4/75.9	29.6/17.2	24.8/29.8
Chitose 2012	70.3/68.9	71.6/72.2	77.9/79.0	61.9/61.7	35.3/33.7	23.9/26.2
Douglas 2012	71.0/68.0	58.0/65.0	-	-	34.0/29.0	16.0/18.0
Dunn 2013	63.9/62.5	69.3/72.3	49.5/51.5	39.4/41.2	16.5/20.3	23.9/29.6
Goodman 2012	63.0/62.0	72.4/71.2	65.6/65.4	49.8/45.0	25.8/24.7	36.2/35.7
Hsieh 2015	68.4/66.5	63.6/66.4	-	-	-	-
Macaione 2012	63.7/65.8	80.2/87.3	70.2/81.8	53.7/58.2	41.3/49.1	37.2/27.3
Weisz 2015	64.4/63.2	70.1/75.9	83.7/77.8	76.9/73.2	34.8/31.4	22.7/22.6
Zou 2014	66.2/65.7	73.5/73.9	71.3/70.4	60.2/62.3	25.8/23.6	32.2/31.0
Gargiolo 2016	71.2/68.1	72.5/79.2	72.5/71.3	53.8/55.3	23.3/24.8	22.6/24.4

Abbreviations: *C* Clopidogrel, *PPI* Proton pump inhibitor, *HT* Hypertension, *Ds* Dyslipidemia, *DM* Diabetes mellitus, *CS* Current smoker

1.26–1.57, $P < 0.00001$ and OR: 1.38; 95% CI: 1.13–1.70, $P = 0.002$ respectively (Fig. 4).

However, since a high level of heterogeneity was observed when analyzing the long-term mortality and TVR, a random effects model was used. Long term TVR also significantly favored the non-PPI group with OR: 1.28; 95% CI: 1.01–1.61, $P = 0.04$ whereas the result for the long-term mortality was not statistically significant with OR: 1.26; 95% CI: 0.99–1.60, $P = 0.06$ (Fig. 5).

Based on a visual inspection of the funnel plot, there has been a low evidence of publication bias among the studies that assessed several subgroups of adverse cardiovascular endpoints. These funnel plots have been illustrated in Fig. 6a and b.

Discussion

Controversies still exist with the concomitant use of clopidogrel and PPIs following coronary stenting, which remain to be solved in this new era. In this analysis, we aimed to compare the adverse clinical outcomes associated with the concomitant use of clopidogrel and PPIs versus clopidogrel alone following PCI using data obtained from recently published articles (2012–2016).

This current analysis showed that during a short term follow up period, mortality and revascularization were significantly lower in those patients who did not require treatment with PPIs. Moreover, during the long term follow up period, adverse cardiovascular outcomes such as MACEs, ST, MI and TVR significantly favored patients in the non-PPI group. However, result for the long-term mortality was similar manifested in both groups.

The previously published meta-analysis [7] which included 32 studies with publication date before the year 2012 (29 studies published in English and 3 studies published in Chinese), showed the concomitant use of PPI and clopidogrel to be associated with higher MACEs with OR: 1.27, 95% CI: 1.13–1.42 when a combination of data obtained from randomized trials and observational

Table 4 Types of Proton Pump Inhibitors used by the patients

Studies	Omeprazole	Esomeprazole	Lansoprazole	Pantoprazole	Rabeprazole
Bhurke 2012	27.1	23.1	17.6	25.8	6.30
Burkard 2012	17.0	51.0	7.00	25.0	-
Chitose 2012	-	-	-	-	-
Douglas 2012	-	-	-	-	-
Dunn 2013	14.0	-	18.1	3.03	1.60
Goodman 2012	48.9	11.7	7.80	30.1	1.48
Hsieh 2015	-	-	-	-	-
Macaione 2012	43.0	11.6	10.7	34.7	-
Weisz 2015	-	-	-	-	-
Zou 2014	-	-	-	-	-
Gargiolo 2016	0.5	0.5	90.9	7.60	0.5

Percentage (%) has been used to represent these data

Table 5 Results of the main analysis

Outcomes analyzed	OR with 95% CI	*P* value	I^2 (%)
Short term follow up			
Mortality	1.55 [1.43–1.68]	0.00001	0
TVR	1.26 [1.06–1.49]	0.009	22
MI	1.17 [0.86–1.58]	0.32	91
Long term follow up			
MACEs	1.37 [1.23–1.53]	0.00001	0
MI	1.41 [1.26–1.57]	0.00001	29
ST	1.38 [1.13–1.70]	0.002	0
Mortality	1.26 [0.99–1.60]	0.06	61
TVR	1.28 [1.01–1.61]	0.04	72

Abbreviations: *OR* Odds ratio, *CI* Confidence interval, *TVR* Target vessel revascularization, *MI* Myocardial infarction, *MACEs* Major adverse cardiac events, *ST* Stent thrombosis

studies was used. However, pooling data only from randomized trials did not show any increase risk of MACEs with OR: 0.92, 95% CI: 0.53–1.58; $P = 0.72$, $I^2 = 0\%$. When mortality was analyzed using a random effects model, a significant increase was observed with HR: 1.30, 95% CI: 0.91–1.86. But when a fixed effects model was used to analyze mortality, no significant increase was observed with clopidogrel plus PPI with OR: 0.92, 95% CI: 0.82–1.04.

Several reasons have been suggested for such a result. First of all, PPIs involve the same metabolic pathway (mainly CYP2C19 isoenzyme) with that of clopidogrel [10]. In other words, by occupying the same metabolic pathway as clopidogrel, PPIs are expected to reduce the antiplatelet effects of clopidogrel. Because PPIs can act as both, inhibitors and substrates of CYP2C19, patients treated with clopidogrel and PPIs are vulnerable to a reduced effectiveness of clopidogrel. This could in turn result in a higher platelet activity following PCI finally causing an increase in adverse clinical outcomes. Gilard et al. were the first ones to show the interaction of clopidogrel and PPIs [11]. Moreover, PPIs not only showed a high platelet reactivity but also showed an increased inflammatory state due to the rise in the level of interleukins-6 which in turn could increase the occurrence of ischemic events [12]. However, whether PPIs really have an effect on clopidogrel's antiplatelet effect is still being debated.

Similar to the results of this current analysis, many other previously published studies showed that adverse clinical outcomes were significantly increased in the PPIs group. Gupta et al. concluded that the concomitant use of clopidogrel with PPIs was associated with an increased risk of MACEs following PCI [6]. In addition, Ho et al. showed increased risk of adverse outcomes with clopidogrel plus PPIs [13].

However, even if many studies supported these current results, several other studies showed results which were completely different. For example, Rassen et al. showed that although a slight increase in hospitalization due to MI and death was observed in older patients who were prescribed PPIs and clopidogrel together, there was not enough evidence to conclude any major interaction between these 2 drugs [3]. In the analysis from the Guthrie Health Off-Label Stent (GHOST) Investigators, the

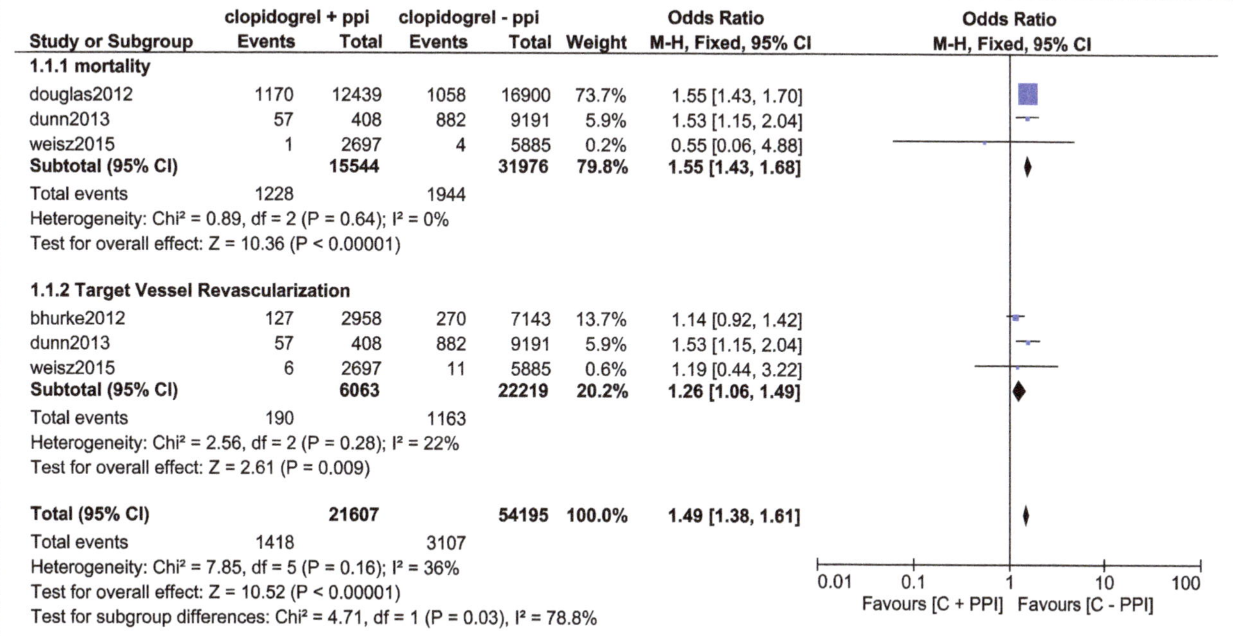

clopidogrel + ppi
clopidogrel - ppi
Odds Ratio
Odds Ratio
Study or Subgroup Events Total Events Total Weight M-H, Fixed, 95% CI
M-H, Fixed, 95% CI
1.1.1 mortality
douglas2012 1170 12439 1058 16900 73.7% 1.55 [1.43, 1.70]
dunn2013 57 408 882 9191 5.9% 1.53 [1.15, 2.04]
weisz2015 1 2697 4 5885 0.2% 0.55 [0.06, 4.88]
Subtotal (95% CI) 15544 31976 79.8% 1.55 [1.43, 1.68]
Total events 1228 1944
Heterogeneity: Chi² = 0.89, df = 2 (P = 0.64); I² = 0%
Test for overall effect: Z = 10.36 (P < 0.00001)
1.1.2 Target Vessel Revascularization
bhurke2012 127 2958 270 7143 13.7% 1.14 [0.92, 1.42]
dunn2013 57 408 882 9191 5.9% 1.53 [1.15, 2.04]
weisz2015 6 2697 11 5885 0.6% 1.19 [0.44, 3.22]
Subtotal (95% CI) 6063 22219 20.2% 1.26 [1.06, 1.49]
Total events 190 1163
Heterogeneity: Chi² = 2.56, df = 2 (P = 0.28); I² = 22%
Test for overall effect: Z = 2.61 (P = 0.009)
Total (95% CI) 21607 54195 100.0% 1.49 [1.38, 1.61]
Total events 1418 3107
Heterogeneity: Chi² = 7.85, df = 5 (P = 0.16); I² = 36%
Test for overall effect: Z = 10.52 (P < 0.00001)
Test for subgroup differences: Chi² = 4.71, df = 1 (P = 0.03), I² = 78.8%
0.01 0.1 1 10 100
Favours [C + PPI] Favours [C - PPI]

Fig. 2 Short term adverse clinical outcomes associated with the concomitant use of clopidogrel and PPIs

Study or Subgroup	clopidogrel + ppi Events	clopidogrel + ppi Total	clopidogrel - ppi Events	clopidogrel - ppi Total	Weight	Odds Ratio M-H, Random, 95% CI
1.1.1 Myocardial Infarction						
bhurke2012	1232	2958	3210	7143	28.8%	0.87 [0.80, 0.95]
douglas2012	365	12345	369	16680	27.6%	1.35 [1.16, 1.56]
dunn2013	57	408	882	9191	23.3%	1.53 [1.15, 2.04]
weisz2015	41	2697	85	5885	20.3%	1.05 [0.72, 1.53]
Subtotal (95% CI)		**18408**		**38899**	**100.0%**	**1.17 [0.86, 1.58]**
Total events	1695		4546			
Heterogeneity: Tau² = 0.08; Chi² = 33.42, df = 3 (P < 0.00001); I² = 91%						
Test for overall effect: Z = 0.99 (P = 0.32)						
Total (95% CI)		**18408**		**38899**	**100.0%**	**1.17 [0.86, 1.58]**
Total events	1695		4546			
Heterogeneity: Tau² = 0.08; Chi² = 33.42, df = 3 (P < 0.00001); I² = 91%						
Test for overall effect: Z = 0.99 (P = 0.32)						
Test for subgroup differences: Not applicable						

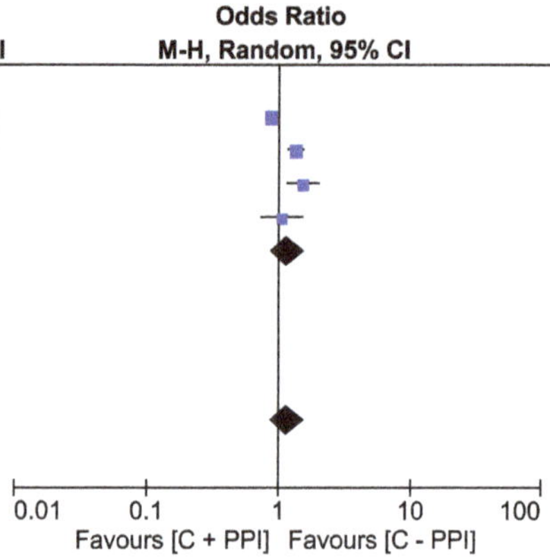

Fig. 3 Short term Myocardial Infarction associated with the concomitant use of clopidogrel and PPIs

Study or Subgroup	C + PPI Events	C + PPI Total	C - PPI Events	C - PPI Total	Weight	Odds Ratio M-H, Fixed, 95% CI
2.1.1 Myocardial Infarction						
burkard2012	16	109	51	692	1.0%	2.16 [1.18, 3.95]
chitose2012	1	187	3	443	0.1%	0.79 [0.08, 7.63]
Gargiulo2016	32	738	48	1232	2.8%	1.12 [0.71, 1.77]
goodman2012	245	3255	354	6021	18.6%	1.30 [1.10, 1.54]
hsieh2015	133	949	827	8856	11.2%	1.58 [1.30, 1.93]
macaione2012	38	121	7	55	0.5%	3.14 [1.30, 7.58]
weisz2015	79	2162	190	6419	7.5%	1.24 [0.95, 1.62]
zou2014	69	6188	9	1465	1.2%	1.82 [0.91, 3.66]
Subtotal (95% CI)		**13709**		**25183**	**42.9%**	**1.41 [1.26, 1.57]**
Total events	613		1489			
Heterogeneity: Chi² = 9.89, df = 7 (P = 0.20); I² = 29%						
Test for overall effect: Z = 6.22 (P < 0.00001)						
2.1.2 Major Adverse Cardiac Events						
burkard2012	33	109	144	692	2.2%	1.65 [1.06, 2.59]
Gargiulo2016	85	738	113	1232	6.1%	1.29 [0.96, 1.74]
weisz2015	238	2162	531	6419	19.3%	1.37 [1.17, 1.61]
zou2014	860	6188	155	1465	17.5%	1.36 [1.14, 1.64]
Subtotal (95% CI)		**9197**		**9808**	**45.1%**	**1.37 [1.23, 1.53]**
Total events	1216		943			
Heterogeneity: Chi² = 0.84, df = 3 (P = 0.84); I² = 0%						
Test for overall effect: Z = 5.70 (P < 0.00001)						
2.1.3 Stent Thrombosis						
burkard2012	12	109	56	692	1.1%	1.41 [0.73, 2.72]
Gargiulo2016	9	738	19	1232	1.1%	0.79 [0.35, 1.75]
goodman2012	89	3238	121	5978	6.7%	1.37 [1.04, 1.80]
weisz2015	26	2162	58	6419	2.3%	1.33 [0.84, 2.13]
zou2014	63	6188	6	1465	0.8%	2.50 [1.08, 5.79]
Subtotal (95% CI)		**12435**		**15786**	**12.1%**	**1.38 [1.13, 1.70]**
Total events	199		260			
Heterogeneity: Chi² = 3.85, df = 4 (P = 0.43); I² = 0%						
Test for overall effect: Z = 3.08 (P = 0.002)						
Total (95% CI)		**35341**		**50777**	**100.0%**	**1.39 [1.29, 1.49]**
Total events	2028		2692			
Heterogeneity: Chi² = 14.70, df = 16 (P = 0.55); I² = 0%						
Test for overall effect: Z = 8.96 (P < 0.00001)						
Test for subgroup differences: Chi² = 0.12, df = 2 (P = 0.94), I² = 0%						

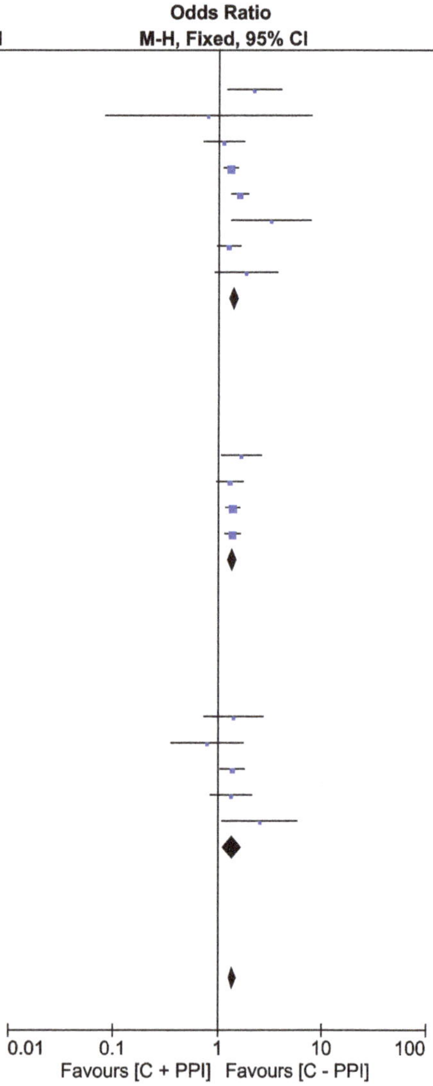

Fig. 4 Long term adverse clinical outcomes associated with the concomitant use of clopidogrel and PPIs

Study or Subgroup	C + PPI Events	C + PPI Total	C - PPI Events	C - PPI Total	Weight	Odds Ratio M-H, Random, 95% CI
2.1.1 Mortality						
burkard2012	9	109	51	692	3.5%	1.13 [0.54, 2.37]
chitose2012	4	187	5	443	1.3%	1.91 [0.51, 7.21]
Gargiulo2016	53	738	77	1232	8.9%	1.16 [0.81, 1.67]
goodman2012	213	3255	286	6021	14.0%	1.40 [1.17, 1.69]
macaione2012	2	121	0	55	0.3%	2.32 [0.11, 49.18]
weisz2015	111	2162	200	6419	12.3%	1.68 [1.33, 2.13]
zou2014	223	6188	63	1465	10.9%	0.83 [0.63, 1.11]
Subtotal (95% CI)		**12760**		**16327**	**51.2%**	**1.26 [0.99, 1.60]**
Total events	615		682			
Heterogeneity: $Tau^2 = 0.05$; $Chi^2 = 15.57$, df = 6 (P = 0.02); $I^2 = 61\%$						
Test for overall effect: Z = 1.88 (P = 0.06)						
2.1.2 Target Vessel revascularization						
burkard2012	22	109	106	692	6.0%	1.40 [0.84, 2.33]
hsieh2015	185	949	1753	8856	14.4%	0.98 [0.83, 1.16]
macaione2012	25	121	3	55	1.4%	4.51 [1.30, 15.66]
weisz2015	266	2162	580	6419	14.8%	1.41 [1.21, 1.65]
zou2014	427	6188	82	1465	12.2%	1.25 [0.98, 1.59]
Subtotal (95% CI)		**9529**		**17487**	**48.8%**	**1.28 [1.01, 1.61]**
Total events	925		2524			
Heterogeneity: $Tau^2 = 0.04$; $Chi^2 = 14.42$, df = 4 (P = 0.006); $I^2 = 72\%$						
Test for overall effect: Z = 2.05 (P = 0.04)						
Total (95% CI)		**22289**		**33814**	**100.0%**	**1.27 [1.08, 1.48]**
Total events	1540		3206			
Heterogeneity: $Tau^2 = 0.04$; $Chi^2 = 30.73$, df = 11 (P = 0.001); $I^2 = 64\%$						
Test for overall effect: Z = 2.98 (P = 0.003)						
Test for subgroup differences: $Chi^2 = 0.01$, df = 1 (P = 0.94), $I^2 = 0\%$						

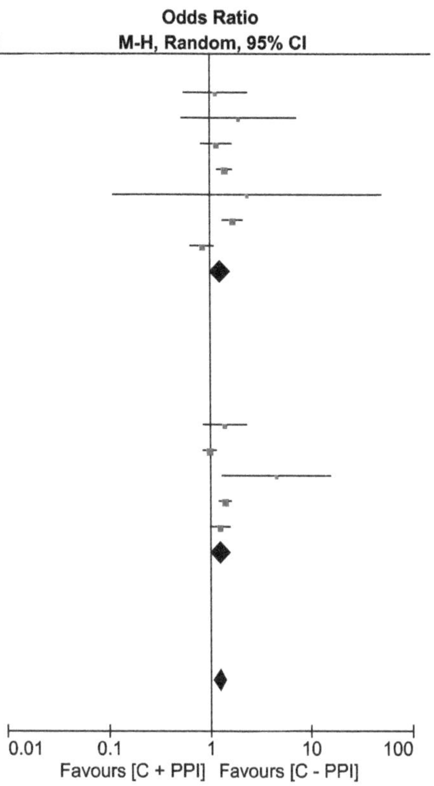

Fig. 5 Long term mortality and TVR associated with the concomitant use of clopidogrel and PPIs

authors also concluded that the use of PPIs with DAPT was not associated with any increase in MACEs following PCI [14]. However, their study had a follow up period of only 6 months. Zairis et al. also showed no impact of omeprazole on the clinical efficacy of clopidogrel during the first year following successful PCI [4]. However, the authors concluded that further highly powered studies should be conducted to confirm whether or not, omeprazole has any effect on the antiplatelet mechanism of clopidogrel. In addition, the COGENT study also did not observe any apparent interaction between clopidogrel and omeprazole, but however, the authors strictly mentioned that their results did not rule out clinically meaningful differences in adverse cardiovascular outcomes due to the use of PPIs [15].

Nevertheless, among all the PPIs, omeprazole is considered to have a higher effect on the mechanism of clopidogrel. Other studies did not show any notable inter-reaction among non-omeprazole PPIs and clopidogrel. For example, when pantoprazole was used along with clopidogrel, no increase in adverse events was observed and therefore pantoprazole has been recommended compared to omeprazole in patients treated with clopidogrel. In addition, in a sub-analysis of the randomized PRODIGY trial, it was reported that the concomitant use of PPIs, when clinically indicated, in patients receiving clopidogrel, was not associated with adverse clinical outcomes. However, it should also be noted that only less than 1.5% of the patients used omeprazole while more than 90% of the patients in that particular trial used lansoprazole, suggesting that this type of PPIs might be safer to use with clopidogrel [16].

Since the adverse clinical events associated with non-omeprazole PPIs and clopidogrel have still not clearly been studied, further research is recommended with these individual PPIs (esomeprazole, rabeprazole, lansoprazole, and pantoprazole). In addition, bleeding events especially gastrointestinal bleeding associated with the concomitant use of clopidogrel with these individual PPIs should also be carefully studied.

A moderate level of heterogeneity was observed among certain subgroups analyzing the cardiovascular outcomes. Only English publications were considered, and articles written in other languages were ignored, therefore, a language bias might most probably be present. Moreover, data obtained from conference abstracts and other unpublished studies were not included. However, since most of the data used in this analysis were obtained from observational studies, it could be one of the reasons contributing to the moderate risk of bias observed. In addition, a high level of heterogeneity could also have been due to the fact

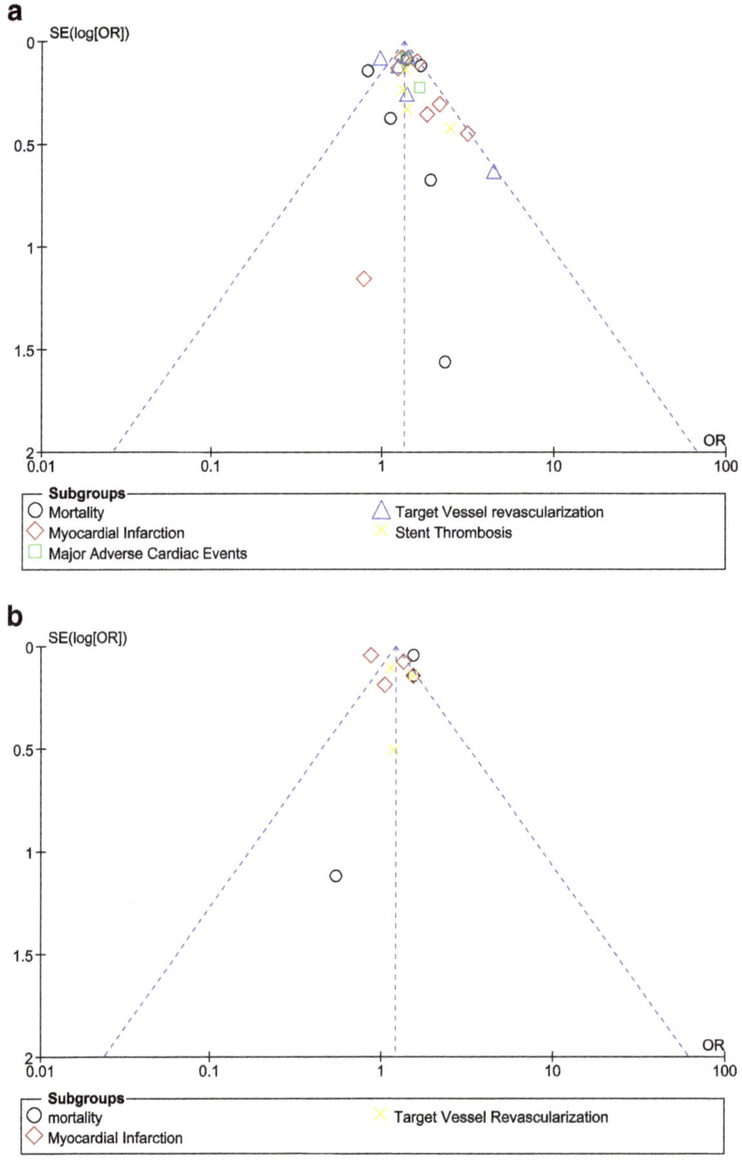

Fig. 6 a and **b** Funnel plots showing publication bias

that different types of patients were included (chronic stable angina, STEMI, NSTEMI) and the type of stent following PCI was also not taken into consideration; patients implanted with DES and BMS were combined and analyzed.

Novelty in this study is the fact that a lower level of heterogeneity was present among several subgroups compared to the previously published meta-analysis. Moreover, different from other studies which mainly report either short term, mid-term or long term outcomes, this analysis has compared the long term and short term adverse clinical outcomes in patients with and without the concomitant use of clopidogrel and PPIs. In addition, this analysis included data obtained from newly published research articles.

Limitations

Several limitations are present. Due to a limited number of patients, the result of this analysis might be affected. Moreover, this analysis involved mainly data obtained from observational studies which might be another limitation, and because of this reason, the bias risk of the studies included in this analysis was not assessed using recommendations from the Cochrane Collaboration. In addition, one study reported death, MI and revascularization together. Since data for each outcome could not be separated, we have included the same data for this particular study in the different subgroups analyzing mortality, MI and TVR. Also, adverse bleeding events (GI bleeding) were not analyzed because only a few studies reported bleeding outcomes, which were also different in each of the study, making it difficult to compare.

Conclusion

The combined use of clopidogrel with PPIs is still associated with significantly higher adverse cardiovascular events such as MACEs, ST and MI following PCI supporting results of the previously published meta-analysis. However, long-term mortality is not statistically significant warranting further analysis with randomized patients.

Abbreviations

DAPT: Dual antiplatelet therapy; MACEs: Major adverse cardiac events; PCI: Percutaneous coronary intervention; PPI: Proton pump inhibitor; ST: Stent thrombosis

Acknowledgements

Not applicable.

Funding

This research was supported by the Promotional Project of Guangxi Medical and Health Appropriate Technology (No. S201518).

Authors' contributions

PKB, ART, AB and WQH were responsible for the conception and design, acquisition of data, analysis and interpretation of data, drafting the initial manuscript and revising it critically for important intellectual content. PKB wrote this manuscript. All authors read and approved the final manuscript.

Competing interests

The authors declare that they have no competing interests.

Author details

[1]Institute of Cardiovascular Diseases, the First Affiliated Hospital of Guangxi Medical University, Nanning, Guangxi 530021, People's Republic of China. [2]Guangxi Medical University, Nanning, Guangxi 530027, People's Republic of China.

References

1. Abraham NS, Hlatky MA, Antman EM, et al. ACCF/ACG/AHA. ACCF/ACG/AHA 2010 expert consensus document on the concomitant use of proton pump inhibitors and thienopyridines: a focused update of the ACCF/ACG/AHA 2008 expert consensus document on reducing thegastrointestinal risks of antiplatelet therapy and NSAID use. A Report of the American College of CardiologyFoundation Task Force on Expert Consensus Documents. J Am Coll Cardiol. 2010;56(24):2051–66.
2. Shah BS, Parmar SA, Mahajan S, Mehta AA. An insight into the interaction between clopidogrel and proton pump inhibitors. Curr Drug Metab. 2012; 13(2):225–35.
3. Rassen JA, Choudhry NK, Avorn J, Schneeweiss S. Cardiovascular outcomes and mortality in patients using clopidogrel with proton pump inhibitors after percutaneous coronary intervention or acute coronary syndrome. Circulation. 2009;120(23):2322–9. doi:10.1161/CIRCULATIONAHA.109.873497.
4. Zairis MN, Tsiaousis GZ, Patsourakos NG, et al. The impact of treatment with omeprazole on the effectiveness of clopidogrel drug therapy during the first yearafter successful coronary stenting. Can J Cardiol. 2010;26(2):e54–7.
5. Gaglia Jr MA, Torguson R, Hanna N, et al. Relation of proton pump inhibitor use after percutaneous coronary intervention with drug-eluting stents to outcomes. Am J Cardiol. 2010;105(6):833–8.
6. Gupta E, Bansal D, Sotos J, Olden K. Risk of adverse clinical outcomes with concomitant use of clopidogrel and proton pump inhibitors followingpercutaneous coronary intervention. Dig Dis Sci. 2010;55(7):1964–8.
7. Huang B, Huang Y, Li Y, et al. Adverse cardiovascular effects of concomitant use of proton pump inhibitors and clopidogrel in patients with coronary artery disease: a systematic review and meta-analysis. Arch Med Res. 2012;43(3):212–24.
8. Higgins JPT, Altman DG. Assessing risk of bias in included studies. In: Higgins JPT, Green S, eds. Cochrane handbook for systematic reviews of interventions. Wiley, 2008:187–241.
9. Liberati A, Altman DG, Tetzlaff J, et al. The PRISMA statement for reporting systematic reviews and meta-analyses of studies that evaluate healthcareinterventions: explanation and elaboration. BMJ. 2009;339:b2700.
10. Lettino M. Inhibition of the antithrombotic effects of clopidogrel by proton pump inhibitors: facts or fancies? Eur J Intern Med. 2010;21(6):484–9.
11. Gilard M, Arnaud B, Cornily JC, et al. Influence of omeprazole on the antiplatelet action of clopidogrel associated with aspirin: the randomized, double-blind OCLA (Omeprazole CLopidogrel Aspirin) study. J Am Coll Cardiol. 2008;51(3):256–60.
12. Jakubowski A, Chlopicki S, Olszanecki R, et al. Endothelial action of thienopyridines and thienopyrimidinones in the isolated guinea pig heart. Prostaglandins Leukot Essent Fatty Acids. 2005;72(2):139–45.
13. Ho PM, Maddox TM, Wang L, et al. Risk of adverse outcomes associated with concomitant use of clopidogrel and proton pump inhibitors followingacute coronary syndrome. JAMA. 2009;301(9):937–44.
14. Harjai KJ, Shenoy C, Orshaw P, Usmani S, Boura J, Mehta RH. Clinical outcomes in patients with the concomitant use of clopidogrel and proton pump inhibitors after percutaneous coronary intervention: an analysis from the Guthrie Health Off-Label Stent (GHOST) investigators. Circ Cardiovasc Interv. 2011;4(2):162–70.
15. Bhatt DL, Cryer BL, Contant CF, et al. COGENT Investigators. Clopidogrel with or without omeprazole in coronary artery disease. N Engl J Med. 2010; 363(20):1909–17.
16. Gargiulo G, Costa F, Ariotti S, et al. Impact of proton pump inhibitors on clinical outcomes in patients treated with a 6- or 24-month dual-antiplatelet therapy duration: Insights from the PROlonging Dual-antiplatelet treatment after Gradingstent-induced Intimal hyperplasia studY trial. Am Heart J. 2016;174:95–102.
17. Bhurke SM, Martin BC, Li C, Franks AM, Bursac Z, Said Q. Effect of the clopidogrel-proton pump inhibitor drug interaction on adverse cardiovascular events in patients with acute coronary syndrome. Pharmacotherapy. 2012;32(9):809–18.
18. Burkard T, Kaiser CA, Brunner-La Rocca H, Osswald S, Pfisterer ME, Jeger RV. BASKET Investigators. Combined clopidogrel and proton pump inhibitor therapy is associated with higher cardiovascular event ratesafter percutaneous coronary intervention,: a report from the BASKET trial. J Intern Med. 2012;271(3):257–63.
19. Chitose T, Hokimoto S, Oshima S, et al. Kumamoto Intervention Conference Study (KICS) Investigators. Clinical outcomes following coronary stenting in Japanese patients treated with and without proton pump inhibitor. Circ J. 2012;76(1):71–8.
20. Douglas IJ, Evans SJ, Hingorani AD, et al. Clopidogrel and interaction with proton pump inhibitors: comparison between cohort and within person study designs. BMJ. 2012;345:e4388.
21. Dunn SP, Steinhubl SR, Bauer D, Charnigo RJ, Berger PB, Topol EJ. Impact of proton pump inhibitor therapy on the efficacy of clopidogrel in the CAPRIE and CREDO trials. J Am Heart Assoc. 2013;2(1):e004564.
22. Goodman SG, Clare R, Pieper KS, et al. Platelet Inhibition and Patient Outcomes Trial Investigators. Association of proton pump inhibitor use on cardiovascular outcomes with clopidogrel and ticagrelor: insightsfrom the platelet inhibition and patient outcomes trial. Circulation. 2012;125(8):978–86.

8

Instructive percutaneous coronary intervention to avoid the risk of side branch occlusion at a lesion with a lotus root appearance

Tetsuya Nomura*, Taku Kato, Hiroshi Kubota, Daisuke Miyawaki, Ryota Urata, Takeshi Sugimoto, Yusuke Higuchi, Natsuya Keira and Tetsuya Tatsumi

Abstract

Background: A lotus root appearance is a rare entity, and there is little opportunity to perform coronary intervention for this kind of lesion. Because of its peculiar anatomical characteristics, one of the problems regarding percutaneous coronary intervention (PCI) for these lesions is related to the involvement of branch vessels.

Case presentation: We encountered a case of PCI for a stenotic lesion with a lotus root appearance in the mid-portion of the right coronary artery (RCA). To avoid the risk of right ventricular (RV) branch occlusion due to stent deployment in the main RCA, we re-crossed the third guidewire into the main RCA via the nearest point to the RV branch ostium through the communicating vascular lumen. Thereafter, we deployed a drug-eluting stent in the main RCA crossing over the RV branch, and the ostium of the RV branch remained intact, as we expected.

Conclusions: This case is the first report in the world describing the details of how to maintain the patency of the side branch bifurcating from a lesion with a lotus root appearance under optical coherence tomography guidance.

Keywords: Case report, Lotus root appearance, Optical coherence tomography, Dual lumen microcatheter, Bifurcation, Side branch

Background

A lotus root appearance is a rare entity that can be detected by intravenous ultrasound sonography (IVUS) or optical coherence tomography (OCT) during the daily practice of coronary catheterization. Lesions with a lotus root appearance are characterized by multiple vascular channels separated by wall partitions, communicating with each other and converging into a single lumen at proximal and distal sites. The detailed origin of the lotus root appearance is still unknown. Although there is little opportunity to perform coronary intervention for this kind of lesion, we always have to be aware of how to maintain the patency of a side branch (SB) bifurcating from a lesion with a lotus root appearance.

* Correspondence: t2-ya@nike.eonet.ne.jp
Department of Cardiovascular Medicine, Nantan General Hospital, 25, Yagi-Ueno, Yagi-cho, Nantan City, Japan

Case presentation

A 70-year-old male was admitted to our hospital complaining of exertional chest pain on effort. His coronary risk factor was only hypertension. A twelve-lead electrocardiogram at rest demonstrated a normal sinus rhythm and no significant ST-segment change. Ultrasound echocardiography showed slight motion abnormality in the inferior wall. Coronary computed tomography angiography revealed an image which resembled coronary dissection in the mid-portion of the right coronary artery (RCA). Therefore, we performed cardiac catheterization with a left trans-radial approach, and a moderate stenotic lesion with some linear opacity was observed there (Fig. 1a). Also, the right ventricular (RV) branch bifurcated from the stenotic lesion (Fig. 1a,b). Considering his clinical background and the findings of the examinations, we decided to perform percutaneous coronary intervention (PCI) for this lesion in the mid RCA.

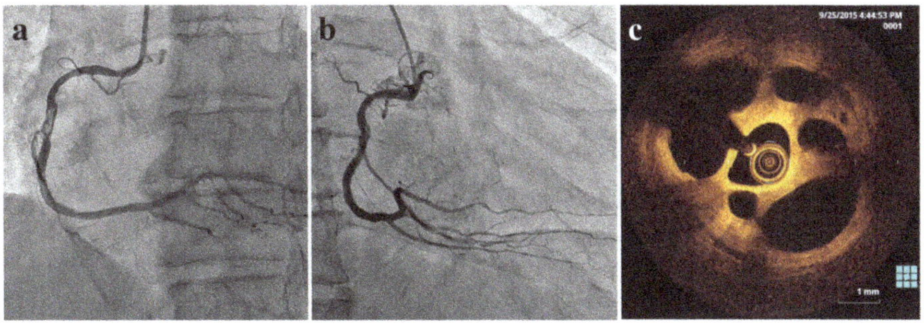

Fig. 1 **a** A control image demonstrates a moderate stenotic lesion with some linear opacity in the mid-portion of the RCA. **b** The RV branch bifurcates from the stenotic lesion. **c** A typical image of a lotus root appearance is observed for the full length of the stenotic lesion

A 6Fr Sherpa NX ACTIVE JR4 guiding catheter (Medtronic Inc., MN, USA) was engaged in the RCA ostium, and a Sion blue guidewire (Asahi Intecc Co., Ltd., Aichi, Japan) was advanced along the side of the greater curvature of the RCA toward the distal RV branch. Then, we tried to introduce the Sion guidewire (Asahi Intecc) along the side of the lesser curvature of the RCA toward the distal RCA (Fig. 2a-c). We performed OCT scanning with a Dragonfly imaging catheter (St. Jude Medical, Inc., MN, USA) around the lesion, and typical pictures of a lotus root appearance were observed along the full length of the stenotic lesion (Fig. 1c). The OCT findings also clearly showed that the Sion blue guidewire branched off toward the RV branch from a point (Fig. 2c,e *Red arrows*) more proximal than the true bifurcation point (Fig. 2c, *Arrowheads*) and some partition walls existed between the two guidewires (Fig. 2d,e). Therefore, we tried to re-cross the new third guidewire into the main RCA

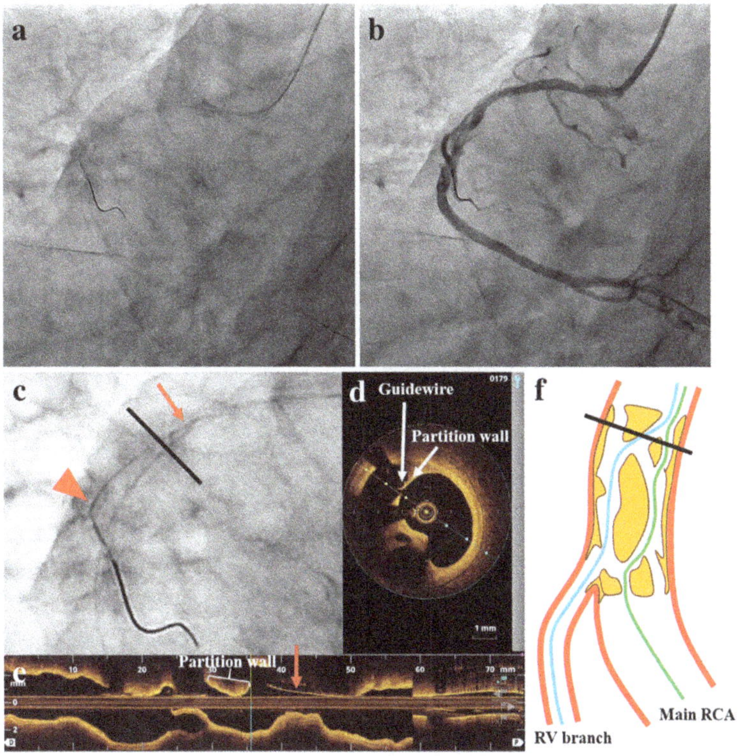

Fig. 2 **a**, **b** Two guidewires initially pass through both the main RCA and RV branch. **c** The magnified image around the lesion shows the difference between the positions of the two guidewires in the RCA. The *red arrow* indicates the point where the guidewire branches off toward the RV branch. The *red arrowhead* indicates the true bifurcation point. **d**, **e** The OCT findings clearly show that the guidewire branches off toward the RV branch from a point more proximal than the true bifurcation point. **d** is a cross-sectional image at the distance indicated with the *black bar* in **c**, **f**. **f** The outlook of the lesion with the lotus root appearance after initial guidewire passage. *Blue* and *green lines* indicate the guidewires passing into the RV branch and main RCA, respectively

before deploying the stent. For that purpose, we used the Crusade catheter (KANEKA Corp., Osaka, Japan), a dual lumen microcatheter, mounted on the Sion blue guidewire in the RV branch, and re-crossed the third guidewire Fielder FC guidewire (Asahi Intecc) through the over-the-wire lumen of the Crusade catheter toward the main RCA via the nearer point to the RV branch ostium as close as possible (Fig. 3a). After re-crossing the third guidewire to the distal RCA, we checked the OCT mounted on this third guidewire (Fig. 3b-e). It was verified that the third guidewire crossed from the nearest point of the RV branch ostium to the distal RCA through the communicating vascular lumen (Fig. 3d-f).

We inflated the scoring balloon NSE ALPHA (GOODMAN Co., Ltd., Aichi, Japan) with a 2.5-mm diameter and then deployed a Resolute Integrity drug-eluting stent (Medtronic) of 3.5/22 mm in the main RCA crossing over the RV branch (Fig. 4a). After re-wiring with the Sion guidewire through the stent strut to the RV branch with the Crusade catheter, we completed the procedure with kissing balloon inflation using a TREK balloon catheter (Abbott Laboratories, IL, USA) with a 3.5-mm diameter in the main RCA and Kamui balloon catheter (Asahi Intecc) with a 2.0-mm diameter in the RV branch (Fig. 4b). We inflated both balloon catheters to a pressure of 10 atmospheres. Finally, we performed proximal optimization therapy using a Hiryu balloon catheter (Terumo Corp., Tokyo, Japan) with a 4.0-mm diameter at the proximal lesion in the stent. The final angiogram demonstrated favorable dilation of the lesion in the mid RCA with good patency of the RV branch (Fig. 4c,d).

His chest symptom fully resolved after this intervention and no adverse events have been observed since then. We performed follow-up coronary angiography (CAG) at 8-month after PCI. Favorable blood flow was observed in both the main RCA and the RV branch, and OCT findings showed better strut apposition and coverage with neointimal formation.

Discussion

We encountered a patient who required coronary intervention for the mid-portion of the RCA with a lotus root appearance detected during a survey with OCT. A lotus root appearance was firstly reported as a lesion composed of multiple channels observed by IVUS in a young

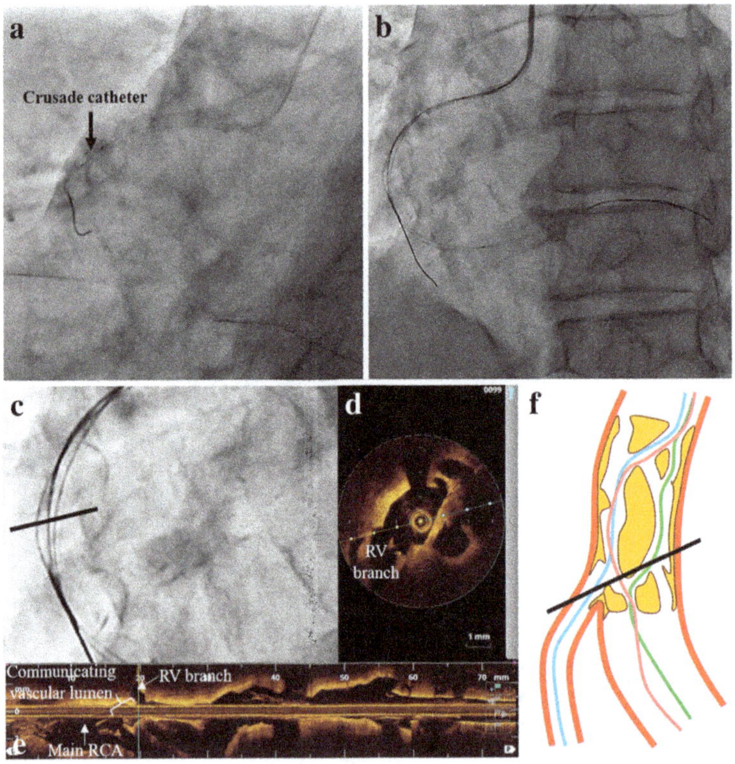

Fig. 3 **a**, **b** An attempt is made to pass the Fielder FC guidewire toward the main RCA via the true bifurcation point using the Crusade catheter. **c** The magnified image around the re-crossing point of the third guidewire shows the three different courses of the guidewire-passing routes. **d**, **e** The OCT findings clearly show the third guidewire crossing from the nearest point of the RV branch ostium to the distal RCA through the communicating vascular lumen. **d** is a cross sectional image at the distance indicated with the *black bar* in **c**, **f**. **f** The outlook of the lesion with the lotus root appearance after the third guidewire re-crossing. *Blue* and *green lines* indicate the initial guidewires passing into the RV branch and main RCA, respectively. The pink line indicates the third guidewire

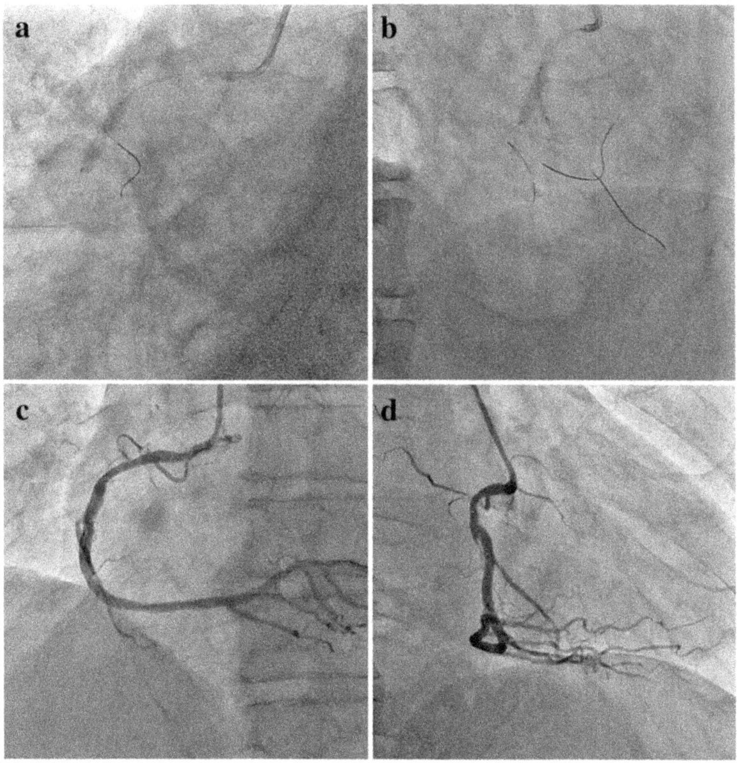

Fig. 4 **a** A Resolute Integrity drug-eluting stent is deployed in the main RCA crossing over the RV branch. **b** Kissing balloon inflation using two semi-compliant balloons is performed. **c**, **d** The final angiogram demonstrates favorable dilation of the lesion in the mid RCA with good patency of the RV branch

patient who had a history of suspected Kawasaki disease in 2002 [1]. Although the detailed origin of the lotus root appearance is still unknown, "arteries within the artery" was first described as spontaneous recanalization after coronary thrombotic events in a patient with Kawasaki disease [2], and it is believed to be identical to a lotus root appearance.

A lesion with a lotus root appearance is characterized by multiple vascular channels separated by wall partitions, communicating with each other and converging into a single lumen at proximal and distal sites. As the OCT has become widely used, more and more cases with this kind of lesion have been reported not only in coronary arteries [3, 4] but also in carotid arteries [5]. However, not so many cases have received PCI for this kind of lesion. Several cases verified the validity of performing PCI for these lesions based on a significant decrease of the fractional flow reserve value [6, 7]. Functionally significant ischemic findings are often demonstrated at a lesion with a lotus root appearance, whereas the stenosis rate at that lesion angiographically shows a moderate degree. The reason for the "visual -functional mismatch" is suggested from the OCT images in which the dead end of the majority of multiple intraluminal channels except a skinny channel can cause markedly limited coronary flow.

It is considered that one of the problems regarding PCI for these lesions is related to the involvement of the branch vessels. A previous case report described a strategy to prevent occlusion of the SB which bifurcated from a lesion with a lotus root appearance [8]. In this case report, the operator confirmed the route through which the guidewire passed from the main vessel (MV) to the SB using IVUS. However, the authors did not describe the details about the methods to cross the guidewire into the SB through the optimal branch ostium at the lesion with the lotus root appearance. Similarly in our case, we were concerned about the risk of SB occlusion after stenting in the MV. To avoid this problem, we considered it important to deposit the guidewire using the optimal route. From the findings of OCT, the point at that the vascular lumen most distally branching from the MV was thought to be the true bifurcation point. The Sion blue guidewire branched off toward the RV branch from a point more proximal than the true bifurcation point, and some partition walls existed between the two guidewires (Fig. 2f). Therefore, to avoid SB occlusion due to deploying a stent in the MV, we had to re-cross the guidewire using the optimal route in the main RCA via the nearest point to the RV branch ostium.

Regarding the guidewire re-cross, there were two choices which direction we should take either from the main RCA to the RV branch or its opposite direction. Because the vascular lumens are intricately connected with each other around the bifurcation point in the main RCA and the lumen size at just distal site of the bifurcation in the RV branch was smaller than that in the main RCA, we thought it was more difficult to re-cross a guidewire from the main RCA to the RV branch. Therefore, we adopted a strategy to manipulate the third guidewire with the Crusade dual lumen microcatheter mounted on the guidewire passing into the RV branch (Fig. 3f). If we deploy a stent in the main RCA without re-crossing the guidewire, the RV branch may be occluded with a high probability due to compression of the partition walls toward the ostium of the RV branch. On the other hand, in the case of third guidewire re-crossing from the side of the RV branch to the MV, the partition walls are compressed to the opposite side of the vascular wall from the RV branch ostium by deploying a stent in the MV (Fig. 5). Actually the ostium of the RV branch was intact after deploying a stent, as we expected.

We performed all PCI procedures with the guidance of OCT. The high resolution of OCT remarkably helped us to clearly detect the guidewire position in the lesion with a lotus root appearance. Moreover, OCT is also very useful for characterization of stent healing and vascular responses in the chronic phase as well as accurate procedures in PCI. As shown in recent systemic review, we confirmed better strut apposition and coverage with neointimal formation after zotarolimus-eluting stent implantation in the follow-up CAG [9].

In this case, we took advantage of the Crusade dual lumen microcatheter when introducing the third guidewire along the optimal route. The dual lumen microcatheter allows the operator to deliver the second guidewire through the over-the-wire lumen into the same vascular lumen where the first guidewire exists. Because the vascular lumens are intricately connected with each other around the lesion with a lotus root appearance, we think the dual lumen microcatheter is optimal for this kind of lesion. The dual lumen microcatheter is a very useful device for multipurpose use in practical PCI. It can help us to perform complex PCI procedures more safely, speedily, and steadily.

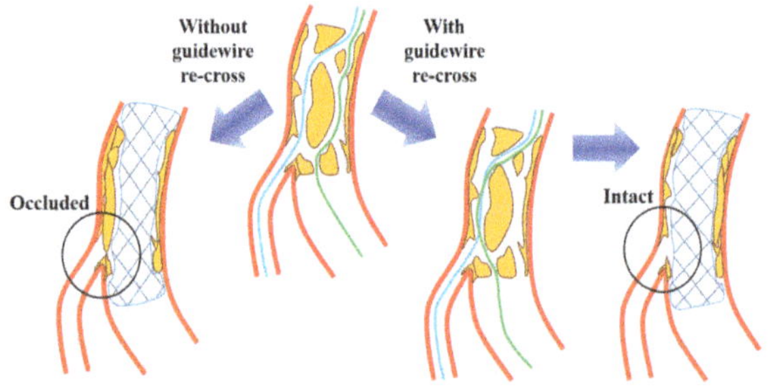

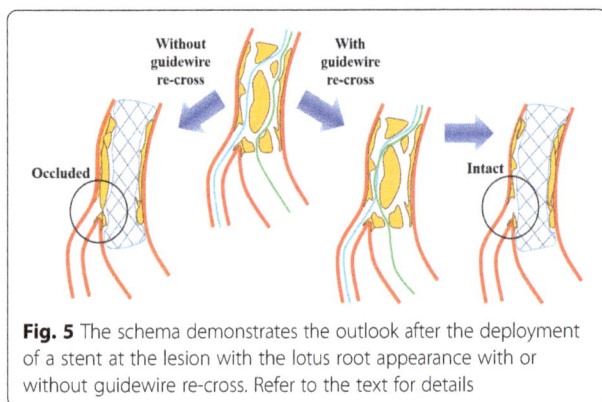

Fig. 5 The schema demonstrates the outlook after the deployment of a stent at the lesion with the lotus root appearance with or without guidewire re-cross. Refer to the text for details

Conclusions

A lotus root appearance is a rare entity detected by IVUS or OCT during the daily practice of coronary catheterization. Although there is little opportunity to perform coronary intervention for a lesion with a lotus root appearance, we always have to pay attention to how to maintain the patency of the SB bifurcating from a lesion with a lotus root appearance.

Abbreviations

CAG, coronary angiography; IVUS, intravenous ultrasound sonography; MV, main vessel; OCT, optical coherence tomography; PCI, percutaneous coronary intervention; RCA, right coronary artery; RV, right ventricular; SB, side branch

Acknowledgements

None.

Funding

None.

Authors' contributions

TN is the primary author of this paper. TK, HK, DM, RU, TS, YH, NK and TT made substantial editorial revisions to the manuscript. TK made major contributions to the conception and design. All authors read and approved the final manuscript.

Competing interests

The authors declare that they have no conflicting interests.

References

1. Terashima M, Awano K, Honda Y, Yoshino N, Mori T, Fujita H, et al. Images in cardiovascular medicine. "Arteries within the artery" after kawasaki disease: A lotus root appearance by intravascular ultrasound. Circulation. 2002;106:887.
2. Takahashi K, Hirota H, Naoe S, Tsukada T, Masuda H, Tanaka N. A morphological study of intimal thickening in sequelae of coronary arterial lesions of Kawasaki disease. J Jpn Coll Angiol. 1991;31:17–25.
3. Kato M, Dote K, Sasaki S. Recanalized image of thrombotic occlusion with coronary plaque rupture: A lotus root-like appearance by optical coherence tomography. Can J Cardiol. 2011;27:871 e1–2.
4. Sakurai S, Takashima H, Waseda K, Ando H, Kurita A, Amano T. Multiple recanalized images of thrombotic occlusion 19 years after percutaneous coronary intervention: Insights from optical coherence tomography and intravascular ultrasound. Int J Cardiol. 2014;172:480–1.
5. Chang H, Yoon HJ, Hong JH, Kim CH, Sohn SI, Lee CY. A lotus root-like appearance in carotid stenosis on optical coherence tomography. J Neurointerv Surg. doi:10.1136/neurintsurg-2015-011685.rep.

6. Kadowaki H, Taguchi E, Kotono Y, Suzuyama H, Yoshida M, Miyamoto S, et al. A lotus root-like appearance in both the left anterior descending and right coronary arteries. Heart Vessels. 2016;31:124–8.
7. Suzuki M, Seki A, Nishikawa K, Takamisawa I, Tobaru T, Sumiyoshi T. Novel physiological insight into a lotus root appearance in stable coronary artery diseases; report of two cases. Cardiovasc Interv Ther. doi:10.1007/s12928-015-0325-5.
8. Nakanishi T, Kawata M, Matsuura T, Kuroda M, Mori K, Hirayama Y, et al. A case of coronary lesion with lotus root appearance treated by percutaneous coronary intervention with intravascular ultrasound guidance. Cardiovasc Interv Ther. 2010;25:131–4.
9. Iannaccone M, D'Ascenzo F, Templin C, Omede P, Montefusco A, Guagliumi G, et al. Optical coherence tomography evaluation of intermediate-term healing of different stent types: systemic review and meta-analysis. Eur Heart J Cardiovasc Imaging. 2016. [Epub ahead of print].

Association of serum transaminases with short- and long-term outcomes in patients with ST-elevation myocardial infarction undergoing primary percutaneous coronary intervention

Ming Gao[1], Yi Cheng[1,2,3], Yang Zheng[1], Weihua Zhang[1], Lin Wang[1] and Ling Qin[1*]

Abstract

Background: Alanine transaminase (ALT) and aspartate aminotransferase (AST) are referred to as liver transaminases. Although used routinely in clinical practice for decades, their role as predictors of mortality has not been examined until recently. We studied the predictive value of these serum transaminases in patients with ST-segment elevation myocardial infarction (STEMI) treated with primary percutaneous coronary intervention (PCI).

Methods: We analyzed records of 2417 consecutive STEMI patients with no preexisting liver disease who were treated with primary PCI at the Cardiovascular Center in the First Hospital of Jilin University. The outcomes measured were all-cause mortality at the first month and at 2 years. The relationship between the baseline serum transaminase levels and primary outcome was determined.

Results: We found a significant correlation between elevated liver transaminases and the Killip classification ($P < 0.001$ for ALT; $P < 0.001$ for AST), cardiac troponin I ($P = 0.002$ for ALT; $P < 0.001$ for AST), infarct-related coronary artery ($P = 0.036$ for ALT; $P = 0.011$ for AST), and pre-thrombolysis-in-myocardial-infarction (pre-TIMI) flow ($P < 0.001$ for ALT and AST). The serum level of ALT and AST were high along with the increasing of the grade of Killip classification. The primary infarct-related coronary artery in patients with ALT ≥95th percentage was left anterior descending artery (56%), followed by right coronary artery (36%). The OR for all-cause mortality at 2 years for participants with ALT ≥95th percentage was 5.370 (95% CI: 2.899–9.948), 7.034 (95% CI: 3.718–13.307) after adjustment for age and gender and 1.051 (95% CI: 0.302–3.652) after adjustment for all covariables. The OR for all-cause mortality at 2 years for participants with AST ≥95th percentage was 5.370 (95% CI 2.899–9.948) and 5.699 (95% CI 3.030–10.718) after adjustment for age and gender and 1.796 (95% CI: 0.588–5.481) after adjustment for all covariables. ALT (HR 1.004, 95% CI 1.001–1.006, $P = 0.010$) and AST (HR 0.999, 95% CI 0.998–1.000, $P = 0.030$) were associated with early all-cause mortality in patients with STEMI treated with PCI but not at 2 years post-procedure, unless for AST and ALT levels ≥95th percentage. Moreover, short- and long-term outcomes were significantly worse when both AST and ALT levels ≥95th percentage ($P < 0.001$).

Conclusions: Serum transaminases ≥95th percentage were associated with a significantly increased incidence of short- and long-term all-cause mortality.

Keywords: ST-elevation myocardial infarction, Serum transaminase, Primary percutaneous coronary intervention

* Correspondence: 1071927028@qq.com
[1]The Cardiovascular Center, the First Hospital of Jilin University, 71 Xinmin Street, Changchun 130021, China
Full list of author information is available at the end of the article

Background

Alanine transaminase (ALT) and aspartate aminotransferase (AST) are referred to as liver transaminases. Although their levels have been tested routinely in clinical practice for decades, their role as predictors of mortality has not been examined until recently. ALT is found predominantly in hepatocytes and is a widely used specific serum marker of liver disease. AST is mainly derived from the liver; although, a significant portion is derived from other tissues, such as heart, red blood cells, and muscle, which makes it an imperfect marker of liver function. Recent studies have demonstrated an increasing interest in investigating the role of liver transaminases in independently predicting cardiac-related morbidity and mortality [1–3].

Several prospective epidemiological studies have suggested that hepatic dysfunction is common in cardiac disease [4, 5]. If no other causes of liver injury are identified, the elevations of liver aminotransferases are associated with a higher incidence of cardiac-related mortality [6]. However, the results from these studies have been inconsistent and have revealed geographical variations in the association between ALT and all-cause mortality [7–11]. Little is known about the association between hepatic dysfunction and mortality in patients with ST-segment elevation myocardial infarction (STEMI) treated with stents or angioplasty for coronary artery stenosis. The goal of this study was to evaluate the association between elevated liver transaminases and all-cause mortality in patients with STEMI undergoing primary percutaneous coronary intervention (PCI) at 1-month and 2-years post-procedure.

Methods

Study population

In this study, we examined digital data from the First Hospital of Jilin University, Cardiovascular Department, which is located in an agricultural province of Northeast China, populated by members of the Chinese Han ethnic group. This prospective observational cohort study aimed to investigate the association between ALT and AST levels and the incidence of all-cause mortality at 1 month and 2 years following treatment. From January 1, 2013 to December 31, 2014, 6017 patients were hospitalized with a diagnosis of acute myocardial infarction. Among those patients, 3692 had ST-segment elevation myocardial infarction. From those patients, 1056 were excluded who did not undergo angiography. Finally we included in this study all 2636 (71.3%) consecutive STEMI patients who underwent PCI without thrombolysis or conservative therapy. From this group, we excluded 219 patients for the following reasons: insufficient AST or ALT data ($n = 126$), cirrhosis ($n = 1$), fatty liver ($n = 64$), and hepatitis ($n = 8$). In addition, we excluded 14 patients of another ethnic group. Finally, we excluded 16 patients because there was missing follow-up information. The final number of patients enrolled in this study was 2417. Their baseline demographic data, medical history, laboratory data, and clinical data during hospitalization were retrieved from the department's heart disease electronic database (Table 1). The mean time to follow up was 2 years (30–1165 days) in the included patients. Angiographic features, angiographic results, and treatment characteristics are provided in Table 2. The study protocol was approved by the ethics review board of the First Hospital of Jilin University (No.2016-263).

Laboratory data

Peripheral blood samples were obtained at the time of admission and the following were tested: creatinine, cardiac troponin I (Tn I), creatine kinase MB (CKMB), K^+, Na^+, and N-terminal pro-brain natriuretic peptide (NT-proBNP). Total cholesterol (TC), triglyceride (TG), high-density lipoprotein cholesterol (HDL-C), glucose, ALT, AST, alkaline phosphatase (ALP), -glutamyl transpeptidase (GGT), and low-density lipoprotein cholesterol (LDL-C) were measured after 12-hours fasting following admission. All blood samples obtained at the time of admission were analyzed in the certified laboratory department of First Hospital of Jilin University. ALT and AST were determined using ultraviolet-lactate dehydrogenase method and ultraviolet-malic acid dehydrogenase method according to the manufacturers' instructions (Kehua Bio-Engineering, China). According to local recommended guidelines, an abnormal ALT level was defined as a serum concentration >50 U/L for men and >40 U/L for women; an abnormal AST level was defined as a serum concentration >40 U/L for men and >35 U/L for women.

Protocol and definition

STEMI was diagnosed in accordance with the European Society of Cardiology/American College of Cardiology consensus document, using at least two separate measurements for the following parameters: a past history of chest pain, diagnostic electrocardiographic changes, and serial elevation of serum cardiac biomarkers [12]. The Killip classification is a system used in individuals with an acute myocardial infarction, taking physical examination and the development of heart failure to predict and stratify their risk [13]. It was determined as follows: Killip class I, no clinical signs of heart failure; Killip class II, rales or crackles in the lungs, an S_3, and elevated jugular venous pressure; Killip class III, frank acute pulmonary edema; and Killip class IV, cardiogenic shock or hypotension and evidence of peripheral vasoconstriction [13].

All patients enrolled were pre-medicated with either 1) 300 mg aspirin or 2) 600 mg clopidogrel orally and unfractionated heparin (1000 IU/L intravenous injection).

Table 1 Baseline characteristics of participants ($n = 2417$)

Characteristic	N (%) or mean ± SD
Demographic data	
Age (year)	59.5 ± 11.1
Male, n (%)	1748 (72)
Living in the city	11,148 (48)
Hospital days	7.2 ± 3.8
Medical history (n)	
Dyslipidemia	931 (38)
Diabetes mellitus	545 (23)
Hypertension	1088 (45)
Myocardial disease	160 (7)
Previous myocardial infarction	24 (1)
Arrhythmias	492 (20)
Previous stroke	75 (3)
Malignancies	6 (0.2)
Peripheral vascular disease	24 (1)
COPD	30 (1)
Infarct location by ECG	
Inferior	1189 (49)
Anterior	1172 (48)
Lateral	56 (2)
Killip classification	
Cardiogenic shock	101 (4)
Noncardiogenic shock	2316 (96)
Laboratory data	
K^+ (mmol/L)	3.9 ± 0.5
Creatinine (mmol/L)	75.3 ± 29.8
Na^+ (mmol/L)	139.4 ± 4.1
Total cholesterol (mmol/L)	4.5 ± 1.0
HDL-C (mmol/L)	1.1 ± 0.3
LDL-C (mmol/L)	2.8 ± 0.9
Triglycerides (mmol/L)	1.7 ± 1.2
Glucose (mmol/L)	7.1 ± 3.1
ALT (unit/L)	55.5 ± 108.3
AST (unit/L)	165.3 ± 283.1
ALP (unit/L)	72.4 ± 24.4
GGT (unit/L)	47.4 ± 69.4
Cardiac troponin I (ng/mL)	20.9 ± 60.9
Creatine kinase MB (ng/ml)	38.3 ± 75.9
NT-proBNP (pg/mL)	1829.9 ± 6019.6

SD standard deviation, *COPD* chronic obstructive pulmonary disease, *ECG* electrocardiographic, *HDL-C* high-density lipoprotein cholesterol, *LDL-C* low-density lipoprotein cholesterol, *ALT* alanine aminotransferase, *AST* aspartate aminotransferase, *ALP* Alkaline phosphatase, *GGT* ɣ-glutamyl transpeptidase, *NT-proBNP* N-terminal pro-brain natriuretic peptide

Table 2 Angiographic features, angioplasty results, and mortality of participants ($n = 2417$)

Characteristic/Outcome	N (%)
Infarct related artery	
RCA	1044 (43)
LAD	1,172 (48)
LCX	201 (8)
Pre-TMI flow	
TIMI-0 flow	475 (20)
≥TIMI −1 flow	1,942 (80)
Multivessel disease (≥2 vessels)	1145 (47)
Method of reperfusion, n (%)	
Balloon	282 (12)
Stent implantation	2135 (88)
All-cause mortality	
1-month death	59 (2)
24-month death	128 (5)

RCA right coronary artery, *LAD* left anterior descending, *LCX* left circumflex coronary artery, *TIMI* thrombolysis in myocardial infarction

Coronary angiography was performed through the femoral or radial artery using standard techniques to evaluate coronary artery lesions. Multivessel coronary artery disease was defined as significant stenosis of two or more major coronary arteries, stenosis of ≥50% of the diameter in the left main or proximal segment of the left anterior descending artery (LAD), and stenosis of ≥70% of the diameter in two of these three vessels: left coronary artery, right coronary artery (RCA), and left circumflex coronary artery (LCX). An artery was considered infarct-related if one of the following criteria was present: definite or suspected thrombus, a ruptured or ulcerated plaque, the presence of thrombolysis-in-myocardial-infarction (TIMI) flow grade ≤2, or stenosis ≥70% of the diameter. The coronary artery flow was assessed using TIMI flow grades [14]. The strategy for multivessel arteries disease in our center was infarct-related artery only according to current guideline recommendations which encourage culprit-only PCI in patients with STEMI and multivessel disease (excluding cardiogenic shock) [15, 16].

Follow-up

To monitor for all-cause mortality following discharge, the clinical course of the patients was monitored by telephone until death or April 1, 2016, whichever occurred first. In the case of patients who were lost to follow-up, we reviewed all medical records and contacted the patients' families. The endpoint of the present study was defined in separate analyses of all-cause mortality at 1-month and at 2-years post-procedure. Two independent observers performed statistical analysis.

Statistical analysis

After testing for normality by the Kolmogorov-Smirnov test, the data were presented as mean ± standard deviation (SD) or median [interquartile range]. Separate analyses were conducted for ALT and AST. Serum ALT and AST levels were categorized into percentiles separately (<25th, 25th to <50th, 50th to <75th, 75th to <95th, and ≥95th percentages). Liver enzyme levels <25th percentage were used as a reference. Logistic regression was performed to evaluate the power of percentiles for each liver enzyme with all-cause mortality. AUC curves were constructed to further illuminate the best cut-off values for ALT and AST for predicting the all-cause mortality. Multiple linear regression was used in order to test the association of the liver enzymes and other previously identified prognostic factors in STEMI with the measured outcomes. Survival curves were generated by the Kaplan–Meier method, and survival among groups was compared using the Log Rank test. To evaluate the independent contribution of the baseline clinical characteristics, medical history, and laboratory data on the occurrence of major events, two consecutive models of Cox multiple regression analysis were performed with forward stepwise selection to determine predictors for all-cause mortality at 1 month and 2 years separately. In the first model, the baseline clinical characteristics and laboratory data were included. Only those clinical and laboratory variables found to be independent in the first model were included in the second model. For all analyses, a two-sided $P < 0.05$ was considered statistically significant. All analyses were conducted using Stata software, version 12 (Stata Corp., College Station, TX).

Results

Baseline characteristics

The baseline data of the participants included demographic characteristics, medical history, laboratory data, culprit vessel, and PCI procedure. The median age of the 2417 patients was 60 years [interquartile range: 52–67] with 72% male patients. Using the definitions of abnormal liver enzyme levels defined previously, 38.9% of the study population had elevated ALT and 71.9% of the study population had elevated AST (Table 1). During the median 2 years (ranging from 30 to 1165 days, median 775 days) of follow up, the cumulative data for all-cause mortality was 2% (59 deaths) at the first month and 5% (122 deaths) at 2 years (Table 2).

Risk factors and elevated liver enzymes

We found some differences in the associations between known risk factors and elevated liver enzymes between ALT and AST. Variables found to be independent in the first regression model and further analyzed included age, gender, living in rural regions, hospital days, medical history, Killip classification, infarct-related coronary artery, Tn I, pre-TIMI, and multivessel disease. In multivariate regression analysis, elevated ALT and AST were both related to Killip classification ($P < 0.001$ for ALT; $P < 0.001$ for AST), Tn I ($P = 0.002$ for ALT; $P < 0.001$ for AST), infarct-related coronary artery ($P = 0.036$ for ALT; $P = 0.011$ for AST), and pre-TIMI flow ($P < 0.001$ for ALT and AST). ALT was also related to age ($P = 0.002$) and dyslipidemia ($P = 0.048$) (Table 3). The serum level of ALT and AST were high along with the increasing of the grade of Killip classification (Fig. 1). The primary infarct-related coronary artery in patients with ALT ≥95th percentage was LAD (56%), followed by RCA (36%).

At cox proportional hazards regression, ALT (hazard ratio [HR] 1.004, 95% confidence interval [CI] 1.001–1.007, $P = 0.010$) and AST (HR 0.999, 95% CI 0.098–1.000, $P = 0.030$) were associated with of all-cause mortality at 1 month but not at 2 years after adjustment for potential confounders (Additional file 1: Table S1 and Table S2).

Transaminases stratification and clinical outcome

Values for the percentages of ALT and AST in males and females in the study population are shown (Additional file 1: Table S3). The odds ratio (OR) for all-cause mortality at 2 years for participants with ALT ≥95th percentage was 5.370 (95% CI: 2.899–9.948), 7.034 (95% CI: 3.718–13.307) after adjustment for age and gender and 1.051 (95% CI: 0.302–3.652) after adjustment for all covariables. The OR for all-cause mortality at 2 years for participants with AST ≥95th percentage was 5.370 (95% CI 2.899–9.948), 5.699 (95% CI 3.030–10.718) after adjustment for age and gender and 1.796 (95% CI: 0.588–5.481) after adjustment for all covariables (Table 4). For predicting outcomes, we constructed the receiver operating characteristic area under the curve (ROC-AUC) to value the best cut-off of ALT and AST. Using a cut-off level of 63.65 IU/L, ALT predicted 1 month mortality with a sensitivity of 75.19% and specificity of 50.85% (ROC-AUC: 0.635, 95% CI: 0.552 to 0.719, $P < 0.001$) and 2 year mortality with a sensitivity of 75.56% and specificity of 44.26% (ROC-AUC: 0.604, 95% CI: 0.546 to 0.662, $P < 0.001$). Using a cut-off level of 310.5 IU/L, AST predicted 1 month mortality with a sensitivity of 84.56% and specificity of 42.37% (ROC-AUC: 0.665, 95% CI: 0.587 to 0.743, $P < 0.001$) and 2 year mortality with a sensitivity of 84.75% and specificity of 31.97% (ROC-AUC: 0.577, 95% CI: 0.520 to 0.634, $P = 0.004$).

The 2 year all-cause mortality was significantly high along with an increasing level of ALT and AST (Table 4). Kaplan-Meier curves were constructed to explore the additive prognostic value of combinations of ALT and AST levels. We divided the study patients into four groups by ≥95th percentage of ALT and AST or not.

Table 3 Association between liver enzymes and covariables in univariate analyses

Variable	CC for ALT (SE)	*P* value	CC for AST (SE)	*P* value
Age (year)	30.456 (3.275)	0.002	−0.467 (0.546)	0.392
Male, n (%)	4.316 (5.199)	0.407	14.206 (13.344)	0.287
Living in the city	−5.163 (4.548)	0.256	−17.423 (11.674)	0.136
Hospital days	0.164 (0.602)	0.785	−2.807 (1.545)	0..069
Dyslipidemia (n)	−9.094 (4.604)	0.048	−20.057 (11.818)	0.090
Diabetes mellitus (n)	−3.187 (5.399)	0.555	−11.918 (13.859)	0.390
Hypertension (n)	1.631 (4.536)	0.719	3.295 (11.642)	0.777
Myocardial disease (n)	−17.047 (9.239)	0.065	−38.681 (23.715)	0.103
Killip classification	30.456 (3.275)	<0.001	83.942 (8.406)	<0.001
Infarct-related coronary artery	8.766 (4.176)	0.036	27.303 (10.718)	0.011
cardiac troponin I (ng/mL)	0.116 (0.037)	0.002	0.809 (0.094)	<0.001
Pre-TMI flow	−29.730 (5.587)	<0.001	−69.304 (14.339)	<0.001
Multivessel disease (≥2 vessels)	7.055 (4.539)	0.120	17.559 (11.650)	0.132

CC correlation coefficient, *ALT* alanine aminotransferase, *SE* standard error, *AST* aspartate aminotransferase, *NT-proBNP* N-terminal pro-brain natriuretic peptide

The all-cause mortality at 1 month and 2 years were significantly increased in patients with both AST and ALT levels ≥95th percentage ($P < 0.001$) (Fig. 2).

Discussion

Liver function tests usually comprise ALT, AST, ALP, GGT, other nonenzymatic proteins (e.g., albumin), and heme metabolites, such as bilirubin. Among these markers, AST and ALT are often elevated in patients with STEMI [17]. Serum ALT is predominantly found in the liver. AST is mainly derived from liver and, hence, also considered as a marker of liver function; however, a significant portion of AST is derived from the heart and other tissues. Nevertheless, it remains unclear whether ALT or AST provide any long- or short-term independent prognostic value in STEMI patients who underwent PCI and whether ALT and AST levels are associated with any other risk factors.

To our knowledge, this is the first prospective study evaluating the association between ALT and AST and short- and long-term all-cause mortality in STEMI patients who underwent PCI. We demonstrated in the Chinese Han ethnic group that AST and ALT levels on admission were significant correlated with Killip classification, pre-TIMI flow, infarct-related coronary artery, and cardiac troponin I. Serum transaminases ≥95th percentage were associated with a significantly increased incidence of short- and long-term all-cause mortality.

Recent studies investigating the relationship between ALT and AST with mortality have yielded conflicting results. A large national population-based cohort study conducted in the United States showed a lack of association between overall or cardiovascular-disease (CVD) mortality with ALT [18]. However, a similar study of a population-based cohort of Caucasian persons aged 55 years or older found AST and ALT are associated with all-cause mortality [19]. Furthermore, a recent meta-analysis study with aggregate data on over 9.24 million participants and 242,953 instances of all-cause mortality found a comparatively moderate association of AST with all-cause mortality and geographical variations in the association of ALT with all-cause mortality risk in

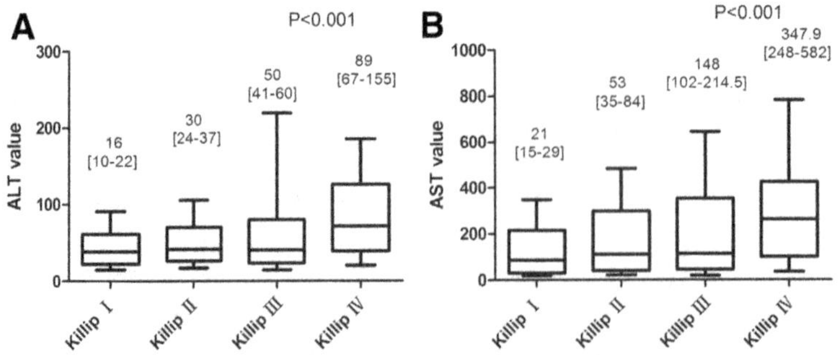

Fig. 1 ALT (**a**) and AST (**b**) values stratified according to Killip classification. The *horizontal line* shows the median value. The box showed the interquartile range. The *vertical line* shows the 10th–90th percentage

Table 4 Association of liver enzymes with long-term all-cause mortality

	Association of ALT with all-cause mortality									
Category	ALT (unit/L)	Crude univariate model			Adjusted for age and sex			Adjusted for all covariables		
		OR	95% CI	*P*-value	OR	95% CI	P-value	OR	95% CI	*P*-value
ALT (1)[a]	≤23	1 (ref)		<0.001	1 (ref)		<0.001	1 (ref)		<0.001
ALT (2)	>23 to ≤39	0.957	0.534–1.714		1.126	0.624–2.030		1.358	0.650–2.834	
ALT (3)	>39 to ≤64	0.914	0.506–1.648		1.124	0.618–2.041		1.413	0.658–3.036	
ALT (4)	>64 to ≤125	1.654	0.957–2.858		2.144	1.226–3.751		1.650	0.732–3.719	
ALT (5)	≥125	5.370	2.899–9.948		7.034	3.718–13.307		1.051	0.302–3.652	
	Association of AST with all-cause mortality									
Category	AST (unit/L)	Crude univariate model			Adjusted for age and sex			Adjusted for all covariables		
		OR	95% CI	*P*-value	OR	95% CI	*P*-value	OR	95% CI	*P*-value
AST (1)[a]	≤32	1 (ref)		<0.001	1 (ref)		<0.001	1 (ref)		<0.001
AST (2)	>32 to ≤93	1.442	0.844–2.462		1.432	0.834–2.459		1.379	0.700–2.717	
AST (3)	>93 to ≤233	0.785	0.425–1.448		0.744	0.401–1.382		0.786	0.361–1.715	
AST (4)	>233 to ≤492	1.206	0.672–2.164		1.152	0.639–2.080		0.989	0.439–2.225	
AST (5)	≥492	5.370	2.899–9.948		5.699	3.030–10.718		1.796	0.588–5.481	

HR hazard ratio, *CI* confidence interval, *ALT* alanine aminotransferase, *AST* aspartate aminotransferase
[a]Percentiles are shown in categories: (1) ≤25th percentage; (2) 25th - < 50th percentage; (3) 50th- < 75th percentage; (4) 75th- < 95th percentage; (5) ≥95th percentage

general populations [7]. Interestingly, other studies have found elevation of common markers, including ALT and AST, in patients with heart failure and CVD with liver injury resulting from ischemia or congestion [20–23]. These results further confirm the association between ALT/AST and mortality risk. Considering that liver enzymes are routine parameters of liver function assessed in STEMI patients before PCI, we investigated the association between ALT/AST and all-cause mortality in the Chinese Han ethnic group.

Notably, increased ALT levels are found in STEMI patients with acute liver injury [24–26]. Cardiac disorders

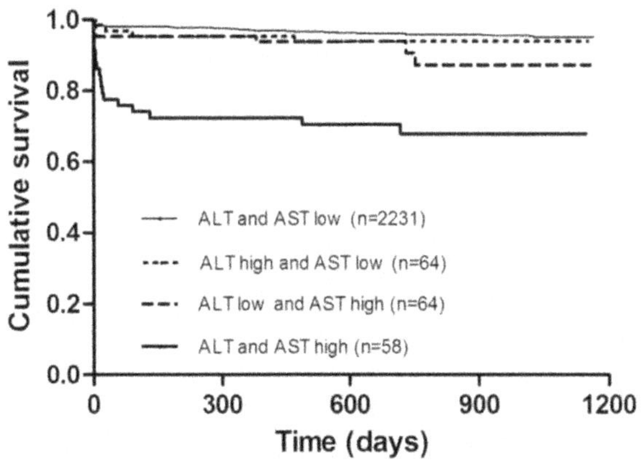

Fig. 2 Kaplan-Meier analysis. All-cause mortality according to combinations generated by having low or high values for ALT and AST. ALT and AST were defined low if under 95th percentage, high if above 95th percentage. ALT 95th percentage value = 125 unit/L, AST 95th percentage value = 492 unit/L

contribute to the liver injury [2, 4, 27, 28]. We excluded patients with chronic hepatitis to exclude liver injury derived from hepatic disorders. The infarct-related artery only strategy for patients with multivessel arteries disease presenting with STEMI in our center minimize potential impact of different strategies of complete vs. culprit-only revascularization [29]. The primary infarct-related coronary artery in patients with ALT ≥ 95th percentage was LAD. Our findings support LAD occlusion as the factor most closely associated with left ventricular ejection fraction and with measures of left ventricular regional hypofunction, especially caused by proximal LAD [30, 31].

The liver has high metabolic activity and perfusion rate, and acute circulatory changes, such as cardiogenic shock resulting from an acute myocardial infarction, directly influence hepatic blood flow [32–34]. Every 10 mmHg drop in arterial pressure decreases the hepatic blood flow by approximately 10% [33, 35]. Circulatory failure triggers compensatory mechanisms in the liver by increasing oxygen extraction from the blood up to 95%, which results in hepatocellular dysfunction and elevation of AST/ALT [36]. The assessment for the presence and severity of circulatory failure were assessed by the Killip classification through physical examination, which showed the serum level of ALT and AST were high along with the increasing of the grade of Killip classification. Because hypoxic injury to the liver is a reversible subclinical condition accounting for over 50% of dramatic serum aminotransferase activity identified in hospital admissions [37], our results demonstrating the predictive value of ALT and AST for short-term, but not long-term, all-cause mortality were not surprising. The influences of genetics on the ethnic and environmental factors, the dosage of prescription drugs, adherence to therapy and cardiac rehabilitation all had important roles on the long-term overall cardiovascular risk. Unless for ALT and AST levels ≥95th percentage, the all-cause mortality at 1 month and 2 years post-procedure both significantly increased.

Study limitations

This study had several limitations. This was an observational study based on data from a single center and the population belonging to a single ethnic group which located in an agricultural province of Northeast China with 52% of participants living in the countryside. The crude death rate of coronary heart disease is significantly different form urban citizens and rural residents in China [38]. The proportion of rural population may influence the result and the data may not reflect the general population of STEMI patients; however, compared to a multicenter study, this study design could be an advantage. The patients' data were imputed electronically by a relatively constant group of attending physicians. The severity and location of coronary lesions were based on visual assessments by the same operators. Ticagrelor was not available during the study period in our center which avoided different P2Y12 inhibitors affecting AST and ALT levels. The overall strategic management of patients, including PCI technique and device used during the procedure, were more homogeneous than would be in a multi-centered study. Second, we performed only a single measurement of ALT and AST for most patients admitted to our center. We tried to exclude patients with conditions potentially associated with liver cell damage, and we also excluded 5% of patients who did not have complete evaluation of liver enzymes at admission. Those limitations are balanced by our continuous admission and, in particular, by the avoidance of ascertainment bias that occurs in clinical studies of selected patients. Third, the results of our multivariate analysis may be biased due to the potential impact of important factors that are not available in our database. Fourth, validation of the cause of death was reported only in a portion of our cohort. Due to culture and social reasons, some patients' families did not know the exact cause of death.

Conclusions

In summary, to our knowledge, this is the first study to investigate the value of serum transaminases in patients with STEMI treated with primary PCI. Elevated transaminases significant correlated with Killip classification, pre-TIMI flow, infarct-related coronary artery, and cardiac troponin I. Moreover, the all-cause mortality at short- and long-term post-procedure was significantly increased in patients with levels of AST and ALT ≥95th percentage.

Abbreviations

ALP: Alkaline phosphatase; ALT: Alanine transaminase; AST: Aspartate aminotransferase; CKMB: Creatine kinase MB; GGT: γ-glutamyl transpeptidase; HDL-C: High-density lipoprotein cholesterol; LAD: Left anterior descending artery; LCX: Left circumflex coronary artery; LDL-C: Low-density lipoprotein cholesterol; NT-proBNP: N-terminal pro-brain natriuretic peptide; PCI: Percutaneous coronary intervention; RCA: Right coronary artery; ROC-AUC: Receiver operating characteristic area under the curve; STEMI: ST-segment elevation myocardial infarction; TC: Total cholesterol; TG: Triglyceride; TIMI: Thrombolysis-in-myocardial-infarction; Tn I: Cardiac troponin I

Acknowledgements

We thank Rose Mikulski who performed English language revision.

Funding

This work was supported by the funds from National Natural Science Foundation of China (81573230).

Authors' contributions

LQ and MG made main contribution to design of the study, drafted the manuscript, and performed the statistical analysis and participated. YC and YZ performed data collection and helped to draft the manuscript and make the statistical analysis. WHZ and LW participated in the design and coordination of the study and participated in the data collection. All authors have read and approved the final manuscript.

Competing interests

The authors declare that they have no competing interests.

Author details

[1]The Cardiovascular Center, the First Hospital of Jilin University, 71 Xinmin Street, Changchun 130021, China. [2]Laboratory for Cardiovascular Diseases, Institute of Translational Medicine, the First Hospital of Jilin University, Changchun, China. [3]Key Laboratory for Cardiovascular Mechanism of Traditional Chinese Medicine, the First Hospital of Jilin University, Changchun, China.

References

1. Poelzl G, Ess M, Mussner-Seeber C, et al. Liver dysfunction in chronic heart failure: prevalence, characteristics and prognostic significance. Eur J Clin Invest. 2012;42:153–63.
2. Batin P, Wickens M, McEntegart D, et al. The importance of abnormalities of liver function tests in predicting mortality in chronic heart failure. Eur Heart J. 1995;16:1613–8.
3. Allen LA, Felker GM, Pocock S, et al. Liver function abnormalities and outcome in patients with chronic heart failure: data from the Candesartan in Heart Failure: Assessment of Reduction in Mortality and Morbidity (CHARM) program. Eur J Heart Fail. 2009;11:170–7.
4. Alvarez AM, Mukherjee D. Liver abnormalities in cardiac diseases and heart failure. Int J Angiol. 2011;20:135–42.
5. Fouad YM, Yehia R. Hepato-cardiac disorders. World J Hepatol. 2014;6:41–54.
6. Yun KE, Shin CY, Yoon YS, et al. Elevated alanine aminotransferase levels predict mortality from cardiovascular disease and diabetes in Koreans. Atherosclerosis. 2009;205:533–7.

7. Kunutsor SK, Apekey TA, Seddoh D, et al. Liver enzymes and risk of all-cause mortality in general populations: a systematic review and meta-analysis. Int J Epidemiol. 2014;43:187–201.
8. Lee TH, Kim WR, Benson JT, et al. Serum aminotransferase activity and mortality risk in a United States community. Hepatology. 2008;47:880–7.
9. Prati D, Taioli E, Zanella A, et al. Updated definitions of healthy ranges for serum alanine aminotransferase levels. Ann Intern Med. 2002;137:1–10.
10. Lee JK, Shim JH, Lee HC, et al. Estimation of the healthy upper limits for serum alanine aminotransferase in Asian populations with normal liver histology. Hepatology. 2010;51:1577–83.
11. Al-hamoudi W, Ali S, Hegab B, et al. Revising the upper limit of normal for levels of serum alanine aminotransferase in a Middle Eastern population with normal liver histology. Dig Dis Sci. 2013;58:2369–75.
12. Hochholzer W, Neumann FJ. The new 2015 ESC Guidelines for the management of acute coronary syndromes in patients presenting without persistent ST-segment elevation. Dtsch Med Wochenschr. 2016;141:782–5.
13. Killip 3rd T, Kimball JT. Treatment of myocardial infarction in a coronary care unit. A two year experience with 250 patients. Am J Cardiol. 1967;20:457–64.
14. Thygesen K, Alpert JS, Jaffe AS, et al. Third universal definition of myocardial infarction. Eur Heart J. 2012;33:2551–67.
15. Steg PG, James SK, Atar D, et al. ESC Guidelines for the management of acute myocardial infarction in patients presenting with ST-segment elevation. Eur Heart J. 2012;33:2569–619.
16. O'Gara PT, Kushner FG, Ascheim DD, et al. 2013 ACCF/AHA guideline for the management of ST-elevation myocardial infarction: a report of the American College of Cardiology Foundation/American Heart Association Task Force on Practice Guidelines. Circulation. 2013;127:e362–425.
17. Moon J, Kang W, Oh PC, et al. Serum transaminase determined in the emergency room predicts outcomes in patients with acute ST-segment elevation myocardial infarction who undergo primary percutaneous coronary intervention. Int J Cardiol. 2014;177:442–7.
18. Ruhl CE, Everhart JE. Elevated serum alanine aminotransferase and gamma-glutamyltransferase and mortality in the United States population. Gastroenterology. 2009;136:477–485.e411.
19. Koehler EM, Sanna D, Hansen BE, et al. Serum liver enzymes are associated with all-cause mortality in an elderly population. Liver Int. 2014;34:296–304.
20. Masoudkabir F, Karbalai S, Vasheghani-Farahani A, et al. The association of liver transaminase activity with presence and severity of premature coronary artery disease. Angiology. 2011;62:614–9.
21. Cagli K, Basar FN, Tok D, et al. How to interpret liver function tests in heart failure patients? Turk J Gastroenterol. 2015;26:197–203.
22. Moller S, Bernardi M. Interactions of the heart and the liver. Eur Heart J. 2013;34:2804–11.
23. Kavoliuniene A, Vaitiekiene A, Cesnaite G. Congestive hepatopathy and hypoxic hepatitis in heart failure: a cardiologist's point of view. Int J Cardiol. 2013;166:554–8.
24. Ladue JS, Wroblewski F. The significance of the serum glutamic oxalacetic transaminase activity following acute myocardial infarction. Circulation. 1955;11:871–7.
25. Tapper EB, Sengupta N, Bonder A. The incidence and outcomes of ischemic hepatitis: a systematic review with meta-analysis. Am J Med. 2015;128:1314–21.
26. Saner FH, Heuer M, Meyer M, et al. When the heart kills the liver: acute liver failure in congestive heart failure. Eur J Med Res. 2009;14:541–6.
27. Samsky MD, Patel CB, DeWald TA, et al. Cardiohepatic interactions in heart failure: an overview and clinical implications. J Am Coll Cardiol. 2013;61:2397–405.
28. van Deursen VM, Damman K, Hillege HL, et al. Abnormal liver function in relation to hemodynamic profile in heart failure patients. J Card Fail. 2010;16:84–90.
29. Moretti C, D'Ascenzo F, Quadri G, et al. Management of multivessel coronary disease in STEMI patients: a systematic review and meta-analysis. Int J Cardiol. 2015;179:552–7.
30. Stadius ML, Maynard C, Fritz JK, et al. Coronary anatomy and left ventricular function in the first 12 hours of acute myocardial infarction: the Western Washington Randomized Intracoronary Streptokinase Trial. Circulation. 1985;72:292–301.
31. Brener SJ, Witzenbichler B, Maehara A, et al. Infarct size and mortality in patients with proximal versus mid left anterior descending artery occlusion: the Intracoronary Abciximab and Aspiration Thrombectomy in Patients With Large Anterior Myocardial Infarction (INFUSE-AMI) trial. Am Heart J. 2013;166:64–70.
32. Nikolaou M, Parissis J, Yilmaz MB, et al. Liver function abnormalities, clinical profile, and outcome in acute decompensated heart failure. Eur Heart J. 2013;34:742–9.
33. Naschitz JE, Slobodin G, Lewis RJ, et al. Heart diseases affecting the liver and liver diseases affecting the heart. Am Heart J. 2000;140:111–20.
34. Denis C, De Kerguennec C, Bernuau J, et al. Acute hypoxic hepatitis ('liver shock'): still a frequently overlooked cardiological diagnosis. Eur J Heart Fail. 2004;6:561–5.
35. Jolobe OM. Jaundice as a presentation of heart failure. J R Soc Med. 2005;98:532.
36. Eipel C, Abshagen K, Vollmar B. Regulation of hepatic blood flow: the hepatic arterial buffer response revisited. World J Gastroenterol. 2010;16:6046–57.
37. Emmanuel A, Inns S. Lecture notes in gastroenterology and hepatology. 1st ed. Blackwell Pub; 2011.
38. Hu SS, Kong LZ, Gao RL, et al. Outline of the report on cardiovascular disease in China, 2010. Biomed Environ Sci. 2012;25:251–6.

10

Association of silent hypoglycemia with cardiac events in non-diabetic subjects with acute myocardial infarction undergoing primary percutaneous coronary interventions

Jian-wei Zhang and Yu-jie Zhou*

Abstract

Background: Some studies have shown that hypoglycemic episodes in diabetic patients might be associated with increased cardiovascular events. It is not clear whether episodes of silent hypoglycemia had greater prognostic value on cardiac events compared with normoglycemia or hyperglycemia in non-diabetic patients, so the aim of this study was to investigate the association of silent hypoglycemia and cardiac events in non-diabetic patients with acute ST-segment elevation myocardial infarction (STEMI) who underwent primary percutaneous coronary intervention (p-PCI).

Methods: We enrolled non-diabetic patients with STEMI who underwent p-PCI and whose clinical and laboratory data were collected. Interstitial glucose values were recorded using a continuous glucose monitoring system (CGMS), and Holter monitoring was recorded for 3 days in parallel. Cardiac ischemia and ventricular arrhythmia was evaluated.

Results: Based on the inclusion and exclusion criteria, we enrolled 164 STEMI patients undergoing p-PCI for final analysis. A total of 280 episodes of silent hypoglycemia (CGMS glucose <70 mg/dl) were recorded. Episodes of silent cardiac ischemia were recorded in 50 of 280 hypoglycemic episodes. The incidence of silent cardiac ischemia during hypoglycemia was significantly higher than the incidence during both hyperglycemia and normoglycemia($P < 0.01$). Moreover, we found a significantly higher frequency of ventricular extrasystoles (VESs) or nonsustained ventricular tachycardias (NSVTs) in patients with silent hypoglycemia. The average number of events of silent cardiac ischemia was also significantly increased in the silent hypoglycemia group (0.91 ± 0.82 vs. 0.35 ± 0.54, $P < 0.01$) compared with either hyperglycemia or normoglycemia group.

Conclusions: Hypoglycemia was frequent and most of the time asymptomatic in non-diabetic patients with STEMI undergoing p-PCI. Silent hypoglycemia was associated with silent cardiac ischemia. STEMI patients with silent hypoglycemia had a significantly higher frequency of VESs or NSVTs.

Keywords: ST-segment elevation myocardial infarction, Primary percutaneous coronary interventions, Continuous glucose monitoring system, Silent hypoglycemia

* Correspondence: azzyj12@163.com
Department of Cardiology, Beijing Anzhen Hospital, Capital Medical University, Beijing Institute of Heart Lung and Blood Vessel Disease, the Key Laboratory of Remodeling-related Cardiovascular Disease, Ministry of Education, Beijing 100029, China

Background

Glycemic management in subjects with acute myocardial infarction (AMI) remains controversy. The general consensus in present is that hyperglycemia (>10 mmol/L) and hypoglycemia (<3.9 mmol/L) should be avoided for critically ill patients [1]. AMI patients with hypoglycemia appeared to have worse outcomes [2–4]. Pinto et al. [3] thought an admission blood glucose <4.5 mmol/L had a 3-fold increased rate of adverse outcomes in patients with ST-segment elevation myocardial infarction (STEMI). Moreover, a previous study showed that spontaneous hypoglycemia was associated with a 2-fold increased in-hospital mortality in AMI patients [4]. Many studies [5, 6] showed that hypoglycemia was common in patients with type 2 diabetes and the vast majority of hypoglycemic episodes were asymptomatic and occurred at night. Moreover, with the use of continuous glucose monitoring systems (CGMS), which could monitor hypoglycemia conveniently, by simultaneously equipping subjects with CGMS and Holter monitoring, Chow et al. [5] revealed that hypoglycemia was associated with possible ischemic changes and various cardiac arrhythmias, suggesting that these events could be interconnected.

Previous studies have focused on the prognostic effects of iatrogenic hypoglycemia in diabetic patients. However, there have been few studies examining hypoglycemia-induced arrhythmias and cardiac ischemia in non-diabetic patients with STEMI undergoing primary percutaneous coronary intervention (p-PCI). Our previous study have approved that the use of CGMS was feasible and safety in STEMI subjects undergoing p-PCI Therefore, with the use of CGMS and Holter monitoring in parallel, the aim of this study was to investigate the association of silent hypoglycemia and cardiac events in non-diabetic subjects with STEMI who underwent p-PCI.

Methods

Study design and patient population

This study was conducted from January 2012 to November 2013. After admission, information about previous clinical history, cardiovascular risk factors, and medication were collected. Moreover, laboratory and echocardiography data were recorded. The inclusion criteria were as follows: 1) confirmed admission diagnosis of STEMI and undergoing p-PCI; 2) admission glucose <22.2 mmol/l and no history of diabetes; and 3) written informed consent. The exclusion criteria included: 1) a history of hepatic or renal impairment or of other diseases that could influence glucose metabolism,including malnutrition and cancer; and 2) a history of diabetes, cardiac pacing,or ventricular arrhythmia. The study protocol was approved by the Medical Ethics Committee of Beijing Anzhen Hospital, Beijing Daxing Hospital, Capital Medical University.

Definition of hypoglycemia and hyperglycemia

Silent hypoglycemia was defined by no typical symptoms of hypoglycemia being noted, but the plasma glucose concentration was <3.9 mmol/l (70 mg/dl) [7].

Hyperglycemia (stress hyperglycemia) was defined as a plasma glucose concentration of at least 10 mmol/l (180 mg/dl) [8, 9].

CGMS and holter

All of the patients were equipped with CGMS (Medtronic Mini-Med, USA) and were monitored for 72 consecutive hours after p-PCI. A CGMS sensor was inserted in the abdominal subcutis and was calibrated every 6 h according to the manufacturer's indications. blood glucose levels of each patient was examined by a self-monitoring of blood glucose (SMBG) device (Medisafe Mini, Terumo, Japan) at least 4 times per day. The sensor measures interstitial glucose every 10 s and records the mean values at 5-min intervals. The sensor remained in place for 3 days for the collection of data, having been adapted from previously established criteria for optimal accuracy of the CGMS [10, 11].

Holter was used to monitor for cardiac ischemia and arrhythmia simultaneously. Continuous glucose and Holter monitoring was performed over a period of 72 h. The CGMS and Holter were removed after 72 h.

The Holter monitoring recordings were read by a cardiologist, and the glucose monitoring results were read by an endocrinologist, both of whom were blinded to the other's results.

Definitions of cardiac ischemia and ventricular arrhythmia

Silent cardiac ischemia was defined as no typical symptoms of chest pain being noted, but ischemic ECG abnormalities were recorded. Ischemic ECG abnormalities included ST-segment depression and T-wave abnormalities. ST-segment abnormalities indicative of ischemia were defined as flat or down-sloping segment depressions with ST-J depression of ≥1.0 mm in ≥2 adjacent leads. T-wave abnormalities indicative of ischemia were defined as any negative or biphasic T-wave in ≥2 contiguous leads [12].

Ventricular arrhythmia included ventricular extrasystoles (VESs), couplets, triplets, and ventricular tachycardias (VTs).

All of the cardiac event data were adjudicated by an experienced cardiovascular physician blinded to the clinical details and outcomes.

Statistical analysis

CGM parameters were analyzed using Medtronic MiniMed CGMS software, version 3.0. The data are presented as frequencies and percentages for categorical variables and as the mean ± SD for continuous variables. We used the χ^2 test to compare the categorical variables, and the 2-sample t test for continuous variables. Hypoglycemic and hyperglycemic episodes were compared with episodes of silent cardiac ischemia or typical angina. Hypoglycemic and hyperglycemic episodes occurring within the preceding 30 min of an ischemic event were noted [13]. Statistical analysis was performed using the Yates-corrected χ^2 test. A P value <0.05 (two-sided) was considered significant. The data were analyzed with SPSS software, version 21.0 (Chicago, Illinois, USA).

Results

Based on the inclusion and exclusion criteria, we enrolled 172 STEMI patients undergoing p-PCI, and six cases were excluded for final analysis due to CGMS signal interruption or failure to meet the accuracy requirements. Two cases with symptomatic hypoglycemia were also excluded. Data from the remaining 164 subjects (115 men and 49 women) were incorporated into the statistical analysis.

Table 1 provides the basic characteristics and CGMS features of the study patients. The mean number of episodes of hypoglycemia per patient was 1.7 ± 1.8, and the mean number of episodes of hyperglycemia per patient was 2.4 ± 2.7. The mean duration of hypoglycemia per patient was 1.6 ± 3.0 h, and the mean duration of hyperglycemia per patient was 2.5 ± 3.9 h.

A total of 280 episodes of silent hypoglycemia (CGMS glucose <70 mg/dl) were recorded. Episodes with silent cardiac ischemia were recorded in 50 out of 280 hypoglycemic episodes. Episodes with typical angina were found in 23 of 280 hypoglycemic episodes (Table 2). Hyperglycemia (CGMS glucose >180 mg/dl) occurred a total of 473 times. Of these 473 episodes of hyperglycemia, 32 silent cardiac ischemia was noted, and 20 episodes of typical angina occurred. There were seven episodes of silent cardiac ischemia and five episodes of typical angina during normoglycemia (Table 2). The difference between the frequency of silent cardiac ischemia during hypoglycemia and the frequency during both hyperglycemia and normoglycemia was statistically significant ($P < 0.01$). The difference between the frequency of typical angina episodes with silent hypoglycemia and with both hyperglycemia and normoglycemia was also statistically significant ($P < 0.01$) (Table 2).

Table 3 shows the relationship between silent hypoglycemia and cardiac events over 3 days of parallel recording. Three patients were excluded due to frequent malignant arrhythmia, which was treated with medication intervention or electroversion. We divided the whole study population into a silent hypoglycemia group ($n = 55$) and non-silent hypoglycemia group ($n = 105$). Mean QTc, as well as couplets per patient, triplets per patient, and SVTs (sustained ventricular tachycardias) per patient, was not different; however, we found a significantly higher frequency of VESs or NSVTs (nonsustained ventricular tachycardias) in patients with silent hypoglycemia. Moreover, the average number of silent cardiac ischemia was significantly higher in the silent hypoglycemia group (0.91 ± 0.82 vs. 0.35 ± 0.54, $P < 0.01$).

Table 1 Clinical characteristics at baseline and CGMS features of study participants

Parameter	value
Subject number	164
Age (years)	53 ± 15
Males	115(70)
BMI, kg/m^2	24.7 ± 4.1
LVEF, %	54.2 ± 7.4
HbA1c (%)	5.1 ± 1.0
Glycated albumin (%)	12.8 ± 4.6
Oral beta-blocker therapy(n,%)	135(82.3)
Risk factors (n,%)	
Hyperlipidemia	61(37.2)
Hypertension	65(39.6)
Current smoking	76(46.3)
Family history	21(13)
Obesity	35(21)
CGMS parameters	
MBG(mmol/l)	6.6 ± 0.8
MAGE (mmol/l)	2.8 ± 1.6
SDBG(mmol/l)	1.4 ± 0.5
The number of Mean episodes of hypoglycemia per patient	1.7 ± 1.8
The numberof Mean episodes of hyperglycemia per patient	2.4 ± 2.7
Mean duration of hypoglycemia per patient (h)	1.6 ± 3.0
Mean duration of hyperglycemia per patient (h)	2.5 ± 3.9
Angiographic data (n,%)	
Single vessel	71(43.3)
Double vessels	50(30.5)
Triple vessels	43(26.2)
Main stem involved	20(12)
Multivessel	93(57)

Data given as mean ± SD or n (%)
BMI body mass index, *LVEF* left ventricularejectionfraction, *HbA1c* Hemoglobin A1c, *MBG* Mean blood glucose, *MAGE* the mean amplitude of glycemic excursions, *SDBG* the standard deviation of blood glucose values

Discussion

It is commonly accepted knowledge that CGMS can detect a significantly greater number of hypoglycemic episodes than repeated capillary blood glucose testing. Several studies have reported that the incidence of hypoglycemia in non-diabetic patients was rare [14–16]. However, non-diabetic hypoglycemia was common in critical care settings [17, 18]. With the use of CGMS, Chow et al. [5] found that in diabetic subjects hypoglycemia was frequently asymptomatic and may increase the risk of arrhythmias. In our study, we also found that hypoglycemia

Table 2 CGMS and Holter monitoring abnormalities

	Total episodes	Episodes with silent cardiac ischemia	Episodes with typical angina
Silent Hypoglycemia	280	50*	23*
Normoglycemia	N/A	7 *	5*
Hyperglycemia	473	32 *	20*

*P < 0.01

was frequent and most of the time asymptomatic in non-diabetic patients with STEMI undergoing p-PCI in the cardiac intensive care unit.

Recent studies have shown that symptomatic severe and mild hypoglycemia were associated with increased cardiovascular events [19, 20]. However, the impact of silent hypoglycemia on cardiac adverse events in AMI patients remains unclear. Based on the availability of CGMS, combined with continuous ECG monitoring, which makes it possible to examine the relationships between hypoglycemia and cardiac adverse events, Cyrus Desouza et al. [13] found that silent hypoglycemia was more likely to be associated with cardiac ischemia than normoglycemia and hyperglycemia in diabetic patients. In our study we also found that silent hypoglycemia was associated with silent cardiac ischemia. Our results indicated that AMI patients with silent hypoglycemia might be associated with poorer outcomes

Our investigations of parallel recording of CGMS and ECG revealed a high incidence of both silent hypoglycemia episodes and silent ventricular arrhythmias in non-diabetic patients with STEMI undergoing p-PCI. However, symptomatic hypoglycemia and severe symptomatic ventricular arrhythmias were rare. Previous studies [21, 22] have also shown that the incidence of serious arrhythmias was very low in AMI patients after successful early revascularization. Moreover, in our study we detected a significantly higher frequency of VESs and NSVTs in patients with silent hypoglycemia. The incidence of SVTs in non-diabetic patients with STEMI undergoing p-PCI was very low. These silent ventricular arrhythmias occurred more often at night than during daytime. Our foundings are similar to those of previous studies [5, 6].

Some potential mechanisms of which hypoglycemia might lead to myocardial ischemia and arrhythmias have been listed: increasing sympathetic activity which can induce vasoconstriction and platelet aggregation and consequently ischemia [23],a rise in some markers of endothelial dysfunction, such as VIII factor,von Willebrand factor, interleukins, cytokines levels, and increases in endothelin-1 and reactive oxygen species [24–26]; a prolongation in QT-segment,activation of the sympathoadrenal system and the production of proarrhythmogenic catecholamines, which can cause ventricular arrhythmias [23, 27, 28].

Following the use of CGMS, silent hypoglycemia could be conveniently monitored. Although the prognostic value of silent hypoglycemia in AMI patients remains controversial, it might be an important predictor of cardiac events after AMI. Further studies are needed to investigate the mechanisms, prognostic value and therapeutic strategies.

There were several limitations to this study. First, the number of patients was relatively small so that comparisons of some subgroups might be lack of power to detect significant differences for selected variables. Second, many of the AMI patients were on β-blockers, which can mask catecholamine-induced symptoms and increase episodes of silent hypoglycemia and silent ischemia. Third, the results of CGMS sometimes are unstable; moreover, this was an observational study and reflected only a possible association of silent hypoglycemia and cardiac events. Hence, the results of the present study should be interpreted with caution.

Conclusions

Hypoglycemia was frequent and, most of the time, asymptomatic in non-diabetic patients with STEMI

Table 3 Relationship between silent hypolycemia and cardiac events during 3 days of parallel recording

	Silent hypolycemia ($n = 55$)	No Silent hypolycemia ($n = 106$)	P
Silent cardiac ischemia	0.91 ± 0.82	0.35 ± 0.54	0.001
Mean QTc(ms)	391.4 ± 55.3	384.6 ± 51.7	0.441
VESs per patient(n)	4681 ± 6784	2685 ± 4378	0.048
Couplets per patient(n)	28.4 ± 58.1	20.7 ± 50.3	0.384
Triplets per patient(n)	3.4 ± 7.2	2.1 ± 6.4	0.244
NSVTs per patient(n)	2.8 ± 5.7	1.1 ± 3.5	0.043
SVTs per patient(n)	0.11 ± 0.37	0.06 ± 0.23	0.337

VESs ventricular extrasystoles, *VTs* ventricular tachycardias, *NSVTs* nonsustained ventricular tachycardias, *SVTs* sustained ventricular tachycardias undergoing p-PCI. Silent hypoglycemia was associated with silent cardiac ischemia. AMI patients with silent hypoglycemia had a significantly higher frequency of VESs or NSVTs.

Abbreviations

BMI: body mass index; CGMS: continuous glucose monitoring system; FBG: fasting blood glucose; LVEF: left ventricular ejection fraction; MACE: major adverse cardiac event; MBG: mean blood glucose; NSVTs: nonsustained ventricular tachycardias; p-PCI: primary percutaneous coronary intervention; SDBG: standard deviation of blood glucose values; SMBG: self-monitoring of blood glucose; STEMI: ST-segment elevation myocardial infarction; SVTs: sustained ventricular tachycardias; VESs: ventricular extrasystoles; VTs: ventricular tachycardias.

Competing interests

The authors declare that they have no competing interests.

Authors' contribution

YZ and JZ designed the experiments; JZ performed the experiments; YZ and JZ analyzed the experimental results and wrote the manuscript. Both authors read and approved the final manuscript.

Acknowledgements

The authors wish to thank all of the study participants. This work was supported by the Beijing Municipal High-Level Talent Foundation of the Health System (No. 2011-1-5), the Beijing Municipal Administration of Hospitals Clinical Medicine Development of Special Funding Support (code: ZY201303) and the National Key Clinical Specialty Construction Project. We thank Dr. Shu-jun Cao and Dr. Xiao-wei Yu for their suggestions regarding our study, the patient volunteers for their participation, and our study nurses Bao-ling Zheng and Ya-juan Liu for their skills and devotion to patient care.

References

1. Mesotten D, Preiser JC, Kosiborod M. Glucose management incritically ill adults and children. Lancet Diabetes Endocrinol. 2015;3(9):723–33.
2. Svensson AM, McGuire DK, Abrahamsson P, Dellborg M. Association between hyper- and hypoglycaemia and 2 year all-cause mortality risk in diabetic patients with acute coronary events. Eur Heart J. 2005;26:1255–61.
3. Pinto DS, Skolnick AH, Kirtane AJ, Murphy SA, Barron HV, Giugliano RP, Cannon CP, Braunwald E, Gibson M. U-shaped relationship of blood glucose with adverse outcomes among patients with ST-segment elevation myocardial infarction. J Am Coll Cardiol. 2005;46:178–80.
4. Kosiborod M, Inzucchi SE, Goyal A, Krumholz HM, Masoudi FA, Xiao L, Spertus JA. Relationship between spontaneous and iatrogenic hypoglycemia and mortality in patients hospitalized with acute myocardial infarction. JAMA. 2009;301:1556–64.
5. Chow E, Bernjak A, Williams S, et al. Risk of cardiac arrhythmias during hypoglycemia in patients with type 2 diabetes and cardiovascular risk. Diabetes. 2014;63(5):1738–47. doi:10.2337/db13-0468.
6. Hay LC, Wilmshurst EG, Fulcher G. Unrecognized hypo- and hyperglycemia in well-controlled patients with type 2 diabetes mellitus: the results of continuous glucose monitoring. Diabetes Technol Ther. 2003;5:19–26.
7. Seaquist ER, Anderson J, Childs B, et al. Hypoglycemia and diabetes: a report of a workgroup of the american diabetes association and the endocrine society. Diabetes Care. 2013;36:1384–95.
8. Gwilt DJ, Petri M, Lamb P, Nattrass M, Pentecost BL. Effect of intravenous insulin infusion on mortality among diabetic patients after myocardial infarction. Br Heart J. 1984;51:626–30.
9. Lynch M, Gammage MD, Lamb P, Nattrass M, Pentecost BL. Acute myocardial infarction in diabetic patients in the thrombolytic era. Diabet Med. 1994;11:162–5.
10. Mastrototaro JJ. The MiniMed continuous glucose monitoring system[J]. Diabetes Technol Ther. 2000;2(1, Supplement 1):13–8.
11. Gross TM, Mastrototaro JJ. Efficacy and reliability of the continuous glucose monitoring system[J]. Diabetes Technol Ther. 2000;2(1, Supplement 1):19–26.
12. Wagner GS, Macfarlane P, Wellens H, Josephson M, Gorgels A, Mirvis DM, Pahlm O, Surawicz B, Kligfield P, Childers R, Gettes LS, Bailey JJ, Deal BJ, Gorgels A, Hancock EW, Kors JA, Mason JW, Okin P, Rautaharju PM, van HG. AHA/ACCF/HRS recommendations for the standardization and interpretation of the electrocardiogram: part VI: acute ischemia/infarction: a scientific statement from the American Heart Association Electrocardiography and Arrhythmias Committee, Council on Clinical Cardiology; the American College of Cardiology Foundation; and the Heart Rhythm Society: endorsed by the International Society for Computerized Electrocardiology. Circulation. 2009;119:e262–70.
13. Desouza C, Salazar H, Cheong B, et al. Association of Hypoglycemia and Cardiac Ischemia A study based on continuous monitoring[J]. Diabetes Care. 2003;26(5):1485–9.
14. Kagansky N, Levy S, Rimon E, Cojocaru L, Fridman A, Ozer Z, Knobler H. Hypoglycemia as a predictor of mortality in hospitalized elderly patients. Arch Intern Med. 2003;163:1825–9.
15. Mannucci E, Monami M, Mannucci M, Chiasserini V, Nicoletti P, Gabbani L, Giglioli L, Masotti G, Marchionni N. Incidence and prognostic significance of hypoglycemia in hospitalized non-diabetic elderly patients. Aging Clin Exp Res. 2006;18:446–51.
16. Nirantharakumar K, Marshall T, Hodson J, et al. Hypoglycemia in non-diabetic in-patients: clinical or criminal? PLoS ONE. 2012;7:e40384.
17. Anabtawi A, Hurst M, Titi M, Patel S, Palacio C, Rajamani K. Incidence of hypoglycemia with tight glycemic control protocols: a comparative study. Diabetes Technol Ther. 2010;12:635–9.
18. Krinsley JS, Schultz MJ, Spronk PE, Harmsen RE, van Braam HF, van der Sluijs JP, Melot C, Preiser JC. Mild hypoglycemia is independently associated with increased mortality in the critically ill. Crit Care. 2011;15:R173.
19. Hsu PF, Sung SH, Cheng HM, et al. Association of clinical symptomatic hypoglycemia with cardiovascular events and total mortality in type 2 diabetes: a nationwide population-based study. Diabetes Care. 2013;36:894–900.
20. Yancy CW, Jessup M, Bozkurt B, et al. Writing Committee Members. 2013 ACCF/AHA guideline for the management of heart failure: a report of the American College of Cardiology Foundation/American Heart Association Task Force on practice guidelines. Circulation. 2013;128:e240–327.
21. Rahimi K, Watzlawek S, Thiele H, Secknus MA, Hayerizadeh BF, Niebauer J, et al. Incidence, time course, and predictors of early malignant ventricular arrhythmias after non-ST-segment elevation myocardial infarction in patients with early invasive treatment. Eur Heart J. 2006;27(14):1706–11.
22. Wildi K, Cuculi F, Twerenbold R, Marxer T, Rubini Gimenez M, Reichlin T, et al. Incidence and timing of serious arrhythmias after early revascularization in non ST-elevation myocardial infarction. Eur Heart J Acute Cardiovasc Care. 2015;4(4):359–64.
23. Sanon VP, Sanon S, Kanakia R, et al. Hypoglycemia from a cardiologist's perspective[J]. Clin Cardiol. 2014;37(8):499–504.
24. Lee SA, Cho SJ, Jeong MH, et al. Hypoglycemia at admission in patients with acute myocardial infarction predicts a higher 30-day mortality in patients with poorly controlled type 2 diabetes than in well-controlled patients. Diabetes Care. 2014;37:2366–73.
25. Rana OA, Byrne CD, Greaves K. Intensive glucose control and hypoglycaemia: a new cardiovascular risk factor? Heart. 2014;100:21–7.
26. Desouza CV, Bolli GB, Fonseca V. Hypoglycemia, diabetes, and cardiovascular events. Diabetes Care. 2010;33:1389–94.
27. Stahn A, Pistrosch F, Ganz X, Teige M, Koehler C, Bornstein S, et al. Relationship between hypoglycemic episodes and ventricular arrhythmias in patients with type 2 diabetes and cardiovascular diseases: silent hypoglycemias and silent arrhythmias. Diabetes Care. 2014;37(2):516–20.
28. Clark AL, Best CJ, Fisher SJ. Even silent hypoglycemia induces cardiac arrhythmias. Diabetes. 2014;63(5):1457–9.

11

Abdominal aortic peripheral intervention to facilitate intra-aortic balloon pump support during high risk percutaneous coronary intervention

See W Low[1], Justin Z Lee[2] and Kwan S Lee[3*]

Abstract

Background: The use of intra-aortic balloon pump (IABP) via the trans-femoral approach has been established for hemodynamic support in patients undergoing high-risk percutaneous coronary intervention (PCI). However, there are various challenges associated with its use, especially in patients with aortoiliac occlusive arterial disease.

Case presentation: We describe a case of high-risk PCI with IABP support complicated by intra-procedural detection of severe abdominal aortic stenosis that was successfully overcome with angioplasty of the stenotic lesion.

Conclusions: Our report highlights distal abdominal aortic stenosis as a potential barrier to successful PCI with IABP support, and angioplasty as an effective means to overcome it.

Keywords: Abdominal aortic stenosis, Intra aortic balloon pump, Percutaneous coronary intervention

Background

The use of intra-aortic balloon pump (IABP) is a well–recognized technique for hemodynamic support in patients undergoing high-risk percutaneous coronary intervention (PCI) [1]. The trans-femoral approach has been the preferred percutaneous access for IABP insertion. However, this approach has its own challenges, particularly in patients with severe occlusive arterial disease [2]. We describe a case of high-risk PCI with IABP support complicated by intra-procedural detection of severe abdominal aortic stenosis, and the approach we used to overcome it.

Case presentation

A 68-year-old man with history of coronary artery disease, ischemic cardiomyopathy, diabetes mellitus, primary prevention automated implantable cardioverter defibrillator (AICD), polio, obesity and systolic heart failure presented to our institution with increasing ischemic chest pain for three days. He was found to have a non-ST segment elevation myocardial infarction with decompensated heart failure with ejection fraction of 24%, as well as acute kidney injury secondary to cardiorenal syndrome. This was also complicated by sustained slow ventricular tachycardia (VT), which caused further decompensation.

A decision was made to perform emergency cardiac catheterization with possible PCI. No good radial pulses were palpable. Secondary to his underdeveloped lower extremities from polio, obesity and faint femoral pulses, micropuncture technique under fluoroscopic guidance was used to obtain retrograde right common femoral arterial access, with placement of a 6-French sheath. Selective left coronary angiography was performed with a JL4 catheter, revealing a distal left main into ostial left anterior descending artery (LAD) 70% in-stent restenosis (ISR) lesion which gave rise to a small diagonal after which the LAD was chronically occluded, and a chronically occluded circumflex (Figure 1). This resulted in significant hypotension from severe ischemia and the development of cardiogenic shock. Distal abdominal aortography was performed using a 6-French JR4 catheter with bilateral iliofemoral runoff to determine if he was a candidate for Impella (Abiomed, Danvers, Massachusetts) percutaneous left ventricular assist

* Correspondence: klee@shc.arizona.edu
[3]3950 S Country Club Road, Suite 200, Tucson, AZ 85714, USA
Full list of author information is available at the end of the article

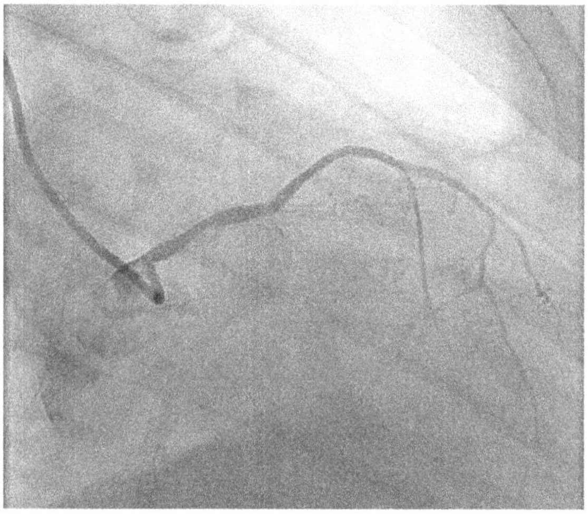

Figure 1 Coronary angiography before PCI showing 70% in-stent restenosis (arrow) of the distal left main coronary artery extending into the LAD with chronic occlusion of ostial circumflex and mid LAD just after origin of small first diagonal.

device or IABP support and to outline the course of his femoral artery for contralateral groin access (Figure 2). Utilizing micropuncture technique, left common femoral arterial access was gained with placement of an 8-French sheath. A 40cc Datascope IABP was advanced via the left common femoral access into the appropriate position, with difficulty during initial wiring with the 0.028" wire secondary to a distal abdominal aortic lesion (Figure 3). IABP support was commenced at 1:1 ratio with vasopressor and inotropic support. From the right common femoral access site, a 0.035" J-wire or angled Glide wire (Terumo Interventional Systems, Somerset, New Jersey) could not get pass the abdominal aortic lesion with the IABP in situ. Thus, the distal abdominal aortic lesion was crossed with a 0.014" Runthrough coronary guidewire (Terumo Interventional Systems, Somerset, New Jersey) and the lesion was dilated with a Viatrec (Abbott, Abbott Park, Illinois) 7.0 × 40 mm balloon to 7 atm for 30 seconds serially (Figure 4). A 5-French Glidecath was then used to exchange the Runthrough for an exchange length 0.035" J-wire in the ascending aorta. A 6-French JR4 was used to perform the selective right coronary angiography. Intravenous heparin was used as the procedural anticoagulant. The left main was engaged with a 6-French EBU 3.5 side hole guide, providing good support. The diagonal was wired with 0.014" Runthrough guidewire and the left main into ostial LAD ISR was directly stented with a Xience Xpedition 2.5 × 15 mm drug eluting stent (DES) (Abbott, Abbott Park, Illinois) to 20 atm for 10 seconds (Figure 5). Subsequently a NC Trek (Abbott, Abbott Park, Illinois) 3.0 × 12 mm balloon was used to post-dilate to 24 atm for 10 seconds.

Post PCI, he developed recurrent slow VT and this was cardioverted with anti-tachycardia pacing via his implantable cardiac defibrillator (ICD). His right coronary artery (RCA) was then engaged with a 6-French AR1 guide with side holes and the posterolateral branch (PLB) was wired with the Runthrough guidewire. Overlapping Xience Xpedition 2.25 × 18 mm and 2.5 × 12 mm

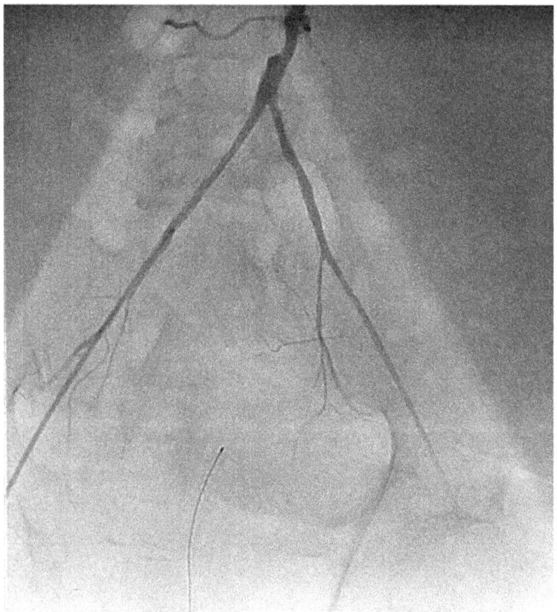

Figure 2 Distal abdominal aortic angiography with bilateral iliofemoral runoff showing distal abdominal aortic, focal 80% eccentric stenosis with patent, small caliber bilateral ilio-femoral arterial system, excluding possible use of Impella percutaneous left ventricular assist device via femoral approach.

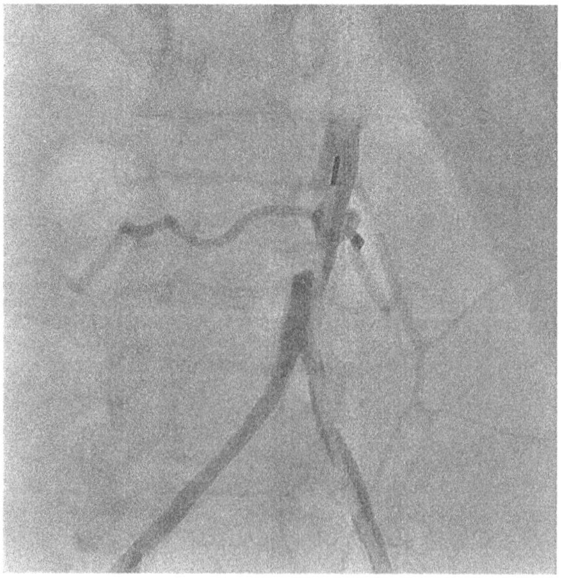

Figure 3 Post insertion of IABP in the abdominal aorta, showing limited space for possible adjacent guide catheter passage.

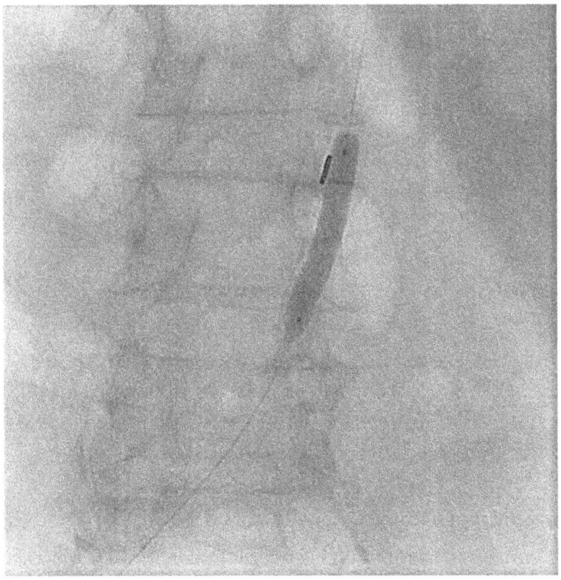

Figure 4 Angioplasty of abdominal aortic stenosis with IABP in-situ utilizing Viatrec 7.0 × 40 mm balloon.

DES were deployed into the distal right, followed by proximally overlapping Xience Xpedition 3.0 × 38 mm and 3.0 × 15 mm DES for his mid to ostial ISR (Figure 6). Final coronary angiographic images were obtained.

Distal abdominal aortography digital subtraction angiography (DSA) was then performed with the AR1 guide and repeat dilatation was then performed with an Armada 9.0 × 80 mm balloon (Abbott, Abbott Park, Illinois) to 12 atm for 30 seconds. Secondary to concerns about limb ischemia, the IABP and 8-French sheath were both removed

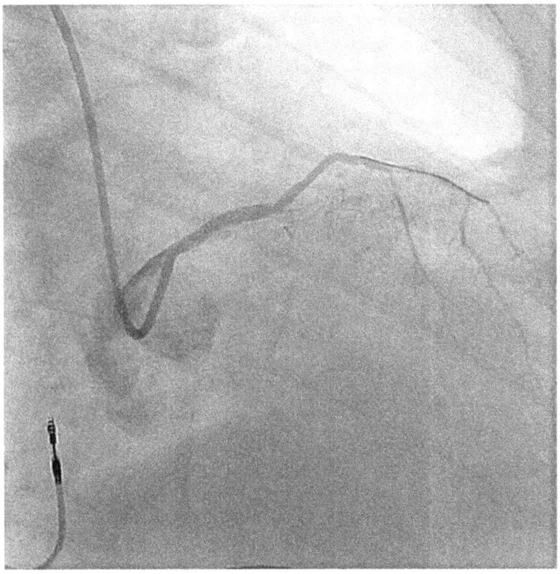

Figure 5 Post PCI of the left main coronary artery with placement of Xience Xpedition 2.5 × 15 mm DES.

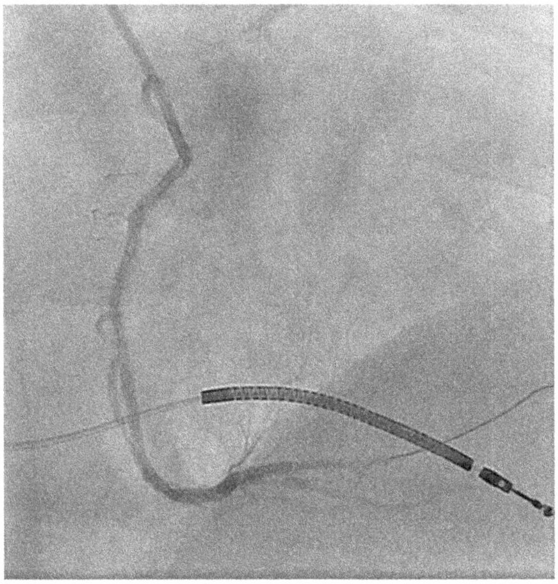

Figure 6 Post PCI of the RCA, distally with placement of overlapping Xience Xpedition 2.25 × 18 mm and 2.5 × 12 mm DES and proximally with overlapping Xience Xpedition 3.0 × 38 mm and 3.0 × 15 mm DES.

and manual pressure was held for 30 minutes for hemostasis. He made a good initial clinical recovery without any acute post-procedural complications such as bleeding requiring blood transfusion or pseudo-aneurysm. However, he had continued deterioration of his renal function due to acute tubular injury from his previous episodes of hypotension and cardiorenal syndrome, to the point where dialysis was required. The patient and family decided against dialysis after several days, and the patient subsequently succumbed to his renal failure.

Discussion

We describe a case of angioplasty of severe abdominal aortic stenosis to facilitate successful emergency high-risk PCI with IABP support complicated by intra-procedural detection of the abdominal aortic stenosis. To our knowledge, no similar case report has been published. The benefit of IABP for hemodynamic support has been established in patients undergoing high risk PCI [1], complicated by cardiogenic shock [3]. The common preferred site for percutaneous insertion of IABP is the common femoral artery, and the distal end of the catheter is advanced and positioned in the proximal descending aorta. Consequentially, peripheral aortoiliac vascular disease has been described as a relative contraindication to IABP insertion, although several approaches have been described to overcome utilizing peripheral interventional techniques especially with iliac disease [4-6].

Abdominal aortic stenosis has an overall incidence of 1 in 62,500 [7]. The treatment of abdominal aortic stenosis ranges from surgical therapy, with aortoiliac endarterectomy or aortobifemoral bypass, to endovascular therapy, with balloon angioplasty or stenting [8]. In our case, we discovered the abdominal aortic stenosis during emergency high-risk PCI after having difficulty with passing the 0.032" J-wire through a section of the distal abdominal aorta with the IABP in-situ. We proceeded with angioplasty of the stenosis, which allowed for passing of the J-wire over the lesion with the IABP in-situ.

Other methods of IABP insertion include trans-radial, trans-axillary, trans-brachial method, and trans-aortic method. Burack at al's and H'Doubler et al's have reported the use of transaxillary or transaortic approach. However, in patients who are hemodynamically unstable, this approach is not appropriate, as it requires general anesthesia and surgical procedures [9,10]. We selected the trans-femoral approach over the trans-radial approach because of the critical emergent need for IABP support and the lack of palpable radial pulses in our patient. There is limited data on the superiority of trans-radial approach in critical situation. In the RADIAL PUMP UP trial, it is shown that the use of transradial approach in high risk patients who is undergoing PCI and requires IABP support is associated with fewer thirty days net adverse clinical events (NACEs) of postprocedural bleeding, cardiac death, myocardial infarction, target lesion revascularization and stroke, mainly because of lower access-related bleeding events although there is no significant differences in the hospital stay length [11]. In a retrospective study, the use of transbrachial versus transfemoral was compared and it only showed the use of transbrachial to have reduced bedrest time (0 minutes vs 340.0 ± 104.9 minutes; $P < .001$) and duration of hospital stay (1.4 ± 0.6 days vs 5.4 ± 7.1 days; $P = .04$) [12]. The use of transbrachial approach has not been widely reported as the small diameter of the brachial artery requires smaller devices and has the potential to increase the vascular compromise to the distal vasculature.

The most common complications of IABP use are vascular complications such as ischemia, vascular obstruction and hemorrhage [13,14]. Established risk factors for bleeding in patients with IABP includes female gender, peripheral vascular disease, diabetes, body surface area (<1.65 m^2), age (>75 years), and aggressive anticoagulant regimens (eg, glycoprotein IIb/IIIa inhibitor) [15]. Our patient is a 68-year-old man with multiple risk factors namely, history of coronary artery disease, diabetes mellitus, obesity and systolic heart failure. However, he did not suffer from any post-procedural bleeding complications.

The data on the use of IABP in patients post myocardial infarction with cardiogenic shock remains inconclusive. IABP SHOCK-II trial was the first large-scale multicenter randomized trial of balloon pump–supported early revascularization in AMI complicated by cardiogenic shock. No significant differences in the 30-day mortality and secondary outcomes were found. Although the timing, clinical scenarios and conditions which IABP demonstrates its beneficial effects remain unclear and despite the randomized controlled trial data suggesting no IABP-supported revascularization in post-myocardial infarction cardiogenic shock patients, the IABP insertion should still be tailored to the clinical condition of the patient and the caution of the operating physician [16].

Conclusions

This report highlights severe distal abdominal aortic stenosis as potential challenge faced when attempting PCI with IABP support via the trans-femoral approach, and the utilization of angioplasty of the stenosis as a means to overcome it.

Consent

Written informed consent was obtained from the patient's next of kin for publication of this case report and any accompanying images. A copy of the written consent is available for review by the Editor of this journal.

Abbreviations

IABP: Intra-aortic balloon pump; PCI: Percutaneous coronary intervention; AICD: Automated implantable cardioverter defibrillator; VT: Ventricular tachycardia; LAD: Left anterior descending artery; ISR: In-stent restenosis; DES: Drug eluting stent; ICD: Implantable cardiac defibrillator; RCA: Right coronary artery; DSA: Digital subtraction angiography.

Competing interests

The authors declare that they have no competing interests.

Authors' contributions

SWL drafted the manuscript. JL integrated the data and revised the manuscript. KL revised critically for important intellectual content and final approval of manuscript submitted. All authors read and approved the final manuscript.

Author details

[1]Department of Cardiovascular Diseases, University of Arizona South Campus, 2800 E Ajo Way, Tucson, AZ 85713, USA. [2]Department of Internal Medicine, University of Arizona, 1501 N Campbell Ave, RM 6336, Tucson, AZ 85724, USA. [3]3950 S Country Club Road, Suite 200, Tucson, AZ 85714, USA.

References

1. Perera D, Stables R, Clayton T, De Silva K, Lumley M, Clack L, et al. Long-term mortality data from the balloon pump-assisted coronary intervention study (BCIS-1): a randomized, controlled trial of elective balloon counterpulsation during high-risk percutaneous coronary intervention. Circulation. 2013;127(2):207–12. Jan 15 PubMed.
2. Colyer Jr WR, Burket MW, Ansel GM, Ramee SR, Minor RL, Gibson CM, et al. Intra-aortic balloon pump placement following aorto-iliac angioplasty and stent placement. Catheter Cardiovasc Interv. 2002;55(2):163–8. PubMed.
3. Iqbal J, Serruys PW. Revascularization strategies for patients with stable coronary artery disease. J Intern Med. 2014;276(4):336–51. PubMed.
4. Marcu CB, Donohue TJ, Ferneini A, Ghantous AE. Intraaortic balloon pump insertion through the subclavian artery. Subclavian Artery Insertion IABP Heart Lung Circ. 2006;15(2):148–50. PubMed.
5. Toktas F, Yavuz S, Eris C, Surer S. Transaortic intra-aortic balloon pump catheter insertion through a separate saphenous vein graft in patients with severe aortoiliac disease. The Sci World J. 2014;2014:247803. PubMed Pubmed Central PMCID: 3910074.

6. Rubino AS, Onorati F, Serraino F, Renzulli A. Safety and efficacy of transbrachial intra-aortic balloon pumping with the use of 7-Fr catheters in patients undergoing coronary bypass surgery. Interact Cardiovasc Thorac Surg. 2009;9(1):135–7. PubMed.
7. Park TC, Hamre DW, Porter JM. Nonatherosclerotic causes of lower extremity claudication. Ann Vasc Surg. 1992;6(6):541–9. PubMed.
8. Delis KT, Gloviczki P. Middle aortic syndrome: from presentation to contemporary open surgical and endovascular treatment. Perspect Vasc Surg Endovasc Ther. 2005;17(3):187–203. PubMed.
9. Burack JH, Uceda P, Cunningham Jr JN. Transthoracic intraaortic balloon pump: a simplified technique. Ann Thorac Surg. 1996;62(1):299–301. PubMed.
10. H'Doubler Jr PB, H'Doubler WZ, Bien RC, Jansen DA. A novel technique for intraaortic balloon pump placement via the left axillary artery in patients awaiting cardiac transplantation. Cardiovasc Surg. 2000;8(6):463–5. PubMed.
11. Romagnoli E, De Vita M, Burzotta F, Cortese B, Biondi-Zoccai G, Summaria F, et al. Radial versus femoral approach comparison in percutaneous coronary intervention with intraaortic balloon pump support: the RADIAL PUMP UP registry. Am Heart J. 2013;166(6):1019–26. PubMed.
12. Fujii T, Masuda N, Ijichi T, Kamiyama Y, Tanaka S, Nakazawa G, et al. Feasibility of 6 Fr intra-aortic balloon pumping via the femoral or brachial approach. J Invasive Cardiol. 2012;24(12):641–4. PubMed.
13. Kumbasar SD, Semiz E, Sancaktar O, Yalcinkaya S, Deger N. Mechanical complications of intra-aortic balloon counterpulsation. Int J Cardiol. 1999;70(1):69–73. Jul 1 PubMed.
14. Mackenzie DJ, Wagner WH, Kulber DA, Treiman RL, Cossman DV, Foran RF, et al. Vascular complications of the intra-aortic balloon pump. Am J Surg. 1992;164(5):517–21. PubMed.
15. Parissis H, Soo A, Al-Alao B. Intra aortic balloon pump: literature review of risk factors related to complications of the intraaortic balloon pump. J Cardiothorac Surg. 2011;6:147. PubMed Pubmed Central PMCID: 3216865.
16. Patterson T, Perera D, Redwood SR. Intra-aortic balloon pump for high-risk percutaneous coronary intervention. Circ Cardiovasc Interv. 2014;7(5):712–20.

12

Major adverse cardiac events and mortality in chronic obstructive pulmonary disease following percutaneous coronary intervention

Pravesh Kumar Bundhun[1], Chakshu Gupta[2] and Guang Ma Xu[3*]

Abstract

Background: We aimed to systematically compare Major Adverse Cardiac Events (MACEs) and mortality following Percutaneous Coronary Intervention (PCI) in patients with and without Chronic Obstructive Pulmonary Diseases (COPD) through a meta-analysis.

Methods: Electronic databases (Cochrane library, EMBASE and Medline/PubMed) were searched for English publications comparing in-hospital and long-term MACEs and mortality following PCI in patients with a past medical history of COPD. Statistical analysis was carried out by Revman 5.3 whereby Odds Ratio (OR) and 95% Confidence Intervals (CI) were considered the relevant parameters.

Results: A total number of 72,969 patients were included (7518 patients with COPD and 65,451 patients without COPD). Results of this analysis showed that in-hospital MACEs were significantly higher in the COPD group with OR: 1.40, 95% CI: 1.19–1.65; $P = 0.0001$, $I^2 = 0\%$. Long-term MACEs were still significantly higher in the COPD group with OR: 1.58, 95% CI: 1.38–1.81; $P = 0.00001$, $I^2 = 29\%$. Similarly, in-hospital and long-term mortality were significantly higher in patients with COPD, with OR: 2.25, 95% CI: 1.78–2.85; $P = 0.00001$, $I^2 = 0\%$ and OR: 2.22, 95% CI: 1.33–3.71; $P = 0.002$, $I^2 = 97\%$ respectively. However, the result for the long-term death was highly heterogeneous.

Conclusion: Since in-hospital and long-term MACEs and mortality were significantly higher following PCI in patients with versus without COPD, COPD should be considered a risk factor for the development of adverse clinical outcomes following PCI. However, the result for the long-term mortality was highly heterogeneous warranting further analysis.

Keywords: Chronic obstructive pulmonary diseases, Percutaneous coronary intervention, Mortality, Major adverse cardiac events

* Correspondence: guangmaxudr@163.com
[3]Department of Cardiology, The People's Hospital of Guangxi Zhuang Autonomous Region, Nanning, Guangxi 530021, People's Republic of China
Full list of author information is available at the end of the article

Background

In this new era of 2016–2017, where the total number of smokers has increased drastically among the youngsters and the older population of males and females (smoking cigarettes began at a very young age, female smokers are on the rise, and passive smokers are becoming more and more common), Chronic Obstructive Pulmonary Diseases (COPD) might soon overcome other major worldwide causes of death [1, 2]. Even though this severe chronic respiratory disease is known from decades, limited data are available on patients who suffer coronary co-morbidities and who are candidates for Percutaneous Coronary Intervention (PCI).

Among the few researches which were undertaken, controversies have already been observed among COPD patients who underwent PCI. Insights from the National Heart, Lung and Blood Institute Dynamic Registry showed COPD to be associated with higher Major Adverse Cardiac Events (MACEs) and mortality rates following PCI [3]. In contrast, in a research which was carried out in a hospital in Taiwan, the authors concluded that COPD was not an independent predictor of major adverse clinical outcomes in patients with STEMI following PCI [4]. This same study also unexpectedly showed no difference in hospital mortality between COPD and non-COPD patients following PCI.

Therefore, we aimed to systematically compare MACEs and mortality following PCI, in patients with and without COPD, through a meta-analysis.

Methods

Data sources and search strategies

Electronic databases (Cochrane library, EMBASE and Medline/PubMed) were searched for English publications related to COPD and PCI by typing the following words or phrases each at a time:

(a) Chronic obstructive pulmonary disease and percutaneous coronary intervention
(b) COPD and PCI
(c) COPD and coronary angioplasty
(d) COPD and myocardial infarction

If an article appeared to be fully relevant, its reference list was also checked for any suitable study.

Inclusion criteria

Studies which satisfied the inclusion criteria were those studies that:

(a) Were randomized trials or observational studies which compared PCI in patients with versus without COPD.
(b) Reported either MACEs or death among their clinical outcomes.
(c) Involved data which were relevant to this current analysis.

Exclusion criteria

Studies were excluded if:

(a) They were other types of studies apart from randomized trials or observational studies.
(b) They did not involve patients with COPD.
(c) They did not report either MACEs or mortality among their clinical endpoints.
(d) They were either duplicates or involved the same cohort or trial.

Definitions, outcomes and follow ups

COPD was defined differently in different studies. COPD, as defined in each of the study has been listed in Table 1.

The main outcomes which were analyzed included:

(a) MACEs which consisted of death, myocardial infarction (MI), repeated revascularization or another clinical outcome.
(b) Mortality (all-cause death)
(c) MI
(d) Coronary revascularization (CR)

Follow up periods included:

- In-hospital follow up
- A longer follow up period greater than one year.

The definitions of the outcomes were listed in Table 2 and the reported outcomes and follow up periods were summarized in Table 3.

Data extraction and review

The following data were extracted by two independent reviewers (PKB and CG):

(a) Author names;
(b) Publication year;
(c) Types of study;
(d) Year of patients' enrollment;
(e) Number of patients with COPD;
(f) Number of patients without COPD;
(g) Outcomes reported in each study;
(h) The follow up periods;
(i) The baseline characteristics of the patients (those with and without COPD) including the mean age, percentage of male patients, percentage of patients suffering from hypertension, dyslipidemia, diabetes mellitus and current smokers;

Table 1 Definitions of chronic obstructive pulmonary disease within the different studies

Studies	Definitions
Almagro 2015	COPD was defined as a post-bronchodilator forced expiratory volume in the 1st second (FEV1)/forced vital capacity (FVC) ratio < 0.70.
Berger 2004	COPD was defined by the requirement of chronic bronchodilator therapy or a forced expiratory volume in 1 s < 75% of the predicted value or a room air pO2 < 60 or a pCO2 > 50.
Campo 2013	A patient was considered to have COPD combining different sources of data: i) documented history of hospital admission for COPD; ii) treatment with pharmacologic therapies specific for COPD (e.g., inhaled steroids, inhaled anticholinergics, inhaled β-agonists or theophylline).
Enriquez 2011	COPD was defined as a history or presence of physician-diagnosed COPD. Additionally, the patients were required to be on chronic pharmacologic therapy and/or have an FEV_1 < 75% of predicted value.
Jatene 2016	The presence of COPD was determined clinically by local investigators, based on history, clinical presentation, previous examinations, and medications, recorded as COPD in the case report form at enrollment.
Konecny 2010	Very severe COPD was defined as an FEV 1 /FVC ratio ≤ 70% and an FEV 1 ≤ 30% predicted, severe COPD as an FEV 1/FVC ratio ≤ 70% and an FEV 1 between 30% and 50% predicted, and mild-to-moderate COPD as an FEV 1/FVC ratio ≤ 70 and an FEV 1 > 50% predicted.
Nishiyama 2009	A patient was considered to have COPD if it was listed as a comorbid condition in our database and its diagnosis was confirmed by a simple test called spirometry. Such a diagnosis should be considered in any patient who has symptoms of cough, sputum production, or dyspnea (difficult or labored breathing), and/or a history of exposure to risk factors for the disease. In cases where spirometry is unavailable, the diagnosis of COPD should be made using all available tools. Clinical symptoms and signs such as abnormal shortness of breath and increased forced expiratory time can be used to arrive at the diagnosis.
Selvaraj 2005	The diagnosis of COPD was based on the clinical history or obtained from chart review and recorded as a co-morbidity in the database.
Sung 2013	COPD was defined according to one of the following criteria: (1) Information on COPD status was obtained by reviewing chart record of the need for pharmacologic therapy using bronchodilator agent; (2) Past history of a 1-s forced expiratory volume < 70% of the predicted value (by pulmonary function test); (3) Physical examination (by auscultation) showed expiratory wheezing and further confirmed by blood gas and chest radiograph (i.e., emphysematous change); or (4) Current use of bronchodilators prior to acute myocardial infarction.
Zhang 2012	A diagnosis of COPD should be considered in any patient who has symptoms of cough, sputum production, or dyspnea, and/or a history of exposure to risk factors for the disease. The diagnosis is confirmed by spirometry. The presence of a postbronchodilator FEV1 < 80% of the predicted value in combination with an FEV1/FVC < 70% confirms the presence of airflow limitation that is not fully reversible. Where spirometry is unavailable, the diagnosis of COPD should be made using all available tools.

Abbreviations: *COPD* chronic obstructive pulmonary disease, *FEV* forced expiratory volume, *FVC* forced vital capacity

(j) Number of events in the study (COPD) as well as the control (non-COPD) groups.

Any disagreement which followed were discussed carefully with each other. However, any unsolved issue was further discussed by the third author (GMX) and a final decision was made by him. In this meta-analysis, the PRISMA guideline was followed [5].

The Newcastle Ottawa Scale (NOS) was used to assess the methodological quality of the studies (non-randomized studies) and NOS has been refined based on expertise and experience whereby it was used in several projects [6].

This NOS consists of eight items, which have been categorized in three different groups: selection, comparability, and outcome or exposure. These three groups involved several sub-items whereby 'stars' were given if

Table 2 Definition of outcomes and follow-up periods

Outcomes	Definitions
Major adverse cardiac events (MACEs)	Defined as a combination of several outcomes including death, MI and revascularization
Death	Defined as all-cause mortality, that is, mortality due to any medical reason including cardiac and non-cardiac
Myocardial infarction (MI)	Defined as re-infarction that occurred post percutaneous coronary intervention based on two or more of the following: 1. Typical chest pain, 2. ECG showing ST-T or Q wave changes, 3. Increase in serum enzyme (creatinine kinase, lactate dehydrogenase or troponin), 4. New wall motion abnormalities on ultrasound
Coronary revascularization (CR)	Defined as repeated revascularization in the coronary arteries resulting in re-stenosis
In-hospital follow-up	Defined as the follow-up period during their hospital stay (≤ 1 month)
Long-term follow-up	Defined as the follow-up period of one or more years

Abbreviations: *ECG* electrocardiogram

Table 3 Reported outcomes and follow up periods

Studies	Outcomes	Follow up period
Almagro 2015 [8]	Death	3 years
Berger 2004 [9]	MACEs, MI	In-hospital
Campo 2013 [10]	Death, MI, CR	In-hospital and 3 years
Enriquez 2011 [3]	Death, MI, MACEs, CR	In-hospital and 1 year
Jatene 2016 [11]	Death, MACEs, MI, CR	2 years
Konecny 2010 [12]	Death, MI	10 years
Nishiyama 2009 [13]	Death, MACEs, MI	In-hospital, 1–4 years
Selvaraj 2005 [14]	Death, MI	In-hospital
Sung 2013 [4]	MACEs	1 year
Zhang 2012 [15]	Death, MI, MACEs, CR	In-hospital

Abbreviations: *MACEs* major adverse cardiac events, *MI* myocardial infarction, *CR* coronary revascularization

these items were present. Each item deserved one star, however, a maximum of 2 stars could be given for comparability.

Selection included (maximum 4 stars): representativeness of the exposed cohort, selection of the non-exposed cohort, ascertainment of exposure, demonstrating the fact that any outcome of interest was not present at the beginning of the study.

Comparability included (maximum 2 stars): comparability of the cohorts on the basis of the design or analysis.

Outcome included (maximum 3 stars): assessment of the outcome, longer duration of the follow up, adequacy of follow-up of cohorts.

NOS assessment involved a minimum number of zero star to a maximum number of nine stars depending on the quality of the study being assessed. The total number of scores allotted were listed in Table 4.

Statistical analysis

Statistical analysis was carried out by the latest version of Revman software (5.3) whereby odds ratio (OR) and 95% confidence intervals (CI) were considered relevant.

Table 4 Study assessment using the Newcastle Ottawa Scale

Studies	Stars allocated following NOS assessment	No of stars (n)
Almagro 2015	*******	7
Berger 2004	******	6
Campo 2013	********	8
Enriquez 2011	*******	7
Konecny 2010	********	8
Nishiyama 2009	*******	7
Selvaraj 2005	******	6
Sung 2013	******	6
Zhang 2012	******	6

Abbreviations: *NOS* Newcastle Ottawa scale

During the subgroup analysis, heterogeneity [7] was assessed by the Q statistic test focusing on the *P* value with a cut-off point of 0.05. A *P* value less or equal to 0.05 was considered statistically significant or else, the result was considered insignificant.

Heterogeneity was also dependent on the I^2 test. A low heterogeneity was denoted by a low percentage of I^2 whereas an increasing percentage denoted an increasing heterogeneity.

The decision to use a fixed effects model ($I^2 < 50\%$) or a random effects model ($I^2 > 50\%$) was also dependent upon the I^2 value.

Publication bias was visually estimated through funnel plots.

Sensitivity analyses were also carried out by the exclusion method (each study was excluded one by one and a new analysis was carried out each time).

Ethical Board Review approval was not required.

Results

Flow of study selection

Figure 1 represents the process of the study selection. In all, a total number of 138 publications was obtained through the electronic search. After a careful assessment of the titles and a close check of the abstracts, 112 articles were eliminated (not related to the idea of this research). Twenty-six full text articles were assessed for eligibility. Further articles were deselected since they were either case studies (2), letter to editors (1), they did not report the relevant endpoints (3), they were duplicates (8) or they were associated with the same trial or cohort (2). Finally, 10 studies [3, 4, 8–15] were selected for this analysis.

General features of the studies which were included

A total number of 72,969 patients were included (7518 patients with COPD and 65,451 patients without COPD) in this analysis. Most of the studies were observational studies and the enrollment period of the patients ranged from 1997 to 2011 (Table 5).

Baseline features of the studies which were included

Baseline features have been summarized in Table 6. A mean age ranging from 66.1 to 70.0 in the COPD group and 60.9 to 66.0 in the non-COPD group were observed. Most of the patients were males with a percentage above 50% in each study. The percentage of patients with co-morbidities such as hypertension, dyslipidemia, and diabetes mellitus has been listed in Table 6. Current smokers were slightly higher in the COPD group compared to the non-COPD group. Overall, almost no significant difference was observed in the baseline features of the patients in both of the groups.

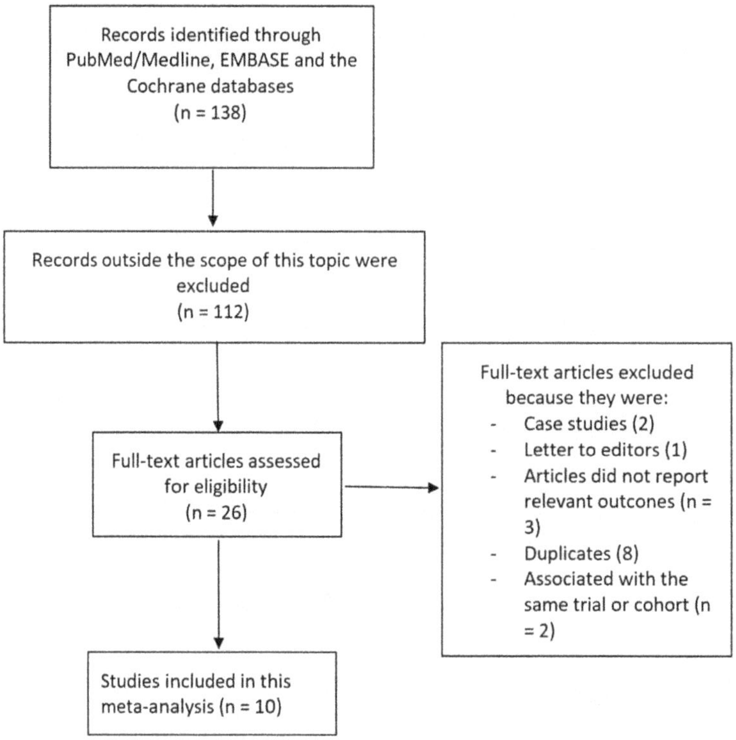

Fig. 1 Flow diagram representing the study selection

MACEs following PCI in patients with COPD versus patients without COPD

Results of this analysis showed that in-hospital MACEs were significantly higher in the COPD group with OR: 1.40, 95% CI: 1.19–1.65; P = 0.0001, I^2 = 0%. It was also observed that this result might have been influenced by the study Selvaraj 2005. Therefore, another analysis was carried out with the exclusion of study Selvaraj 2005. This time, even if in hospital MACEs were higher in the COPD group with OR: 1.21, 95% CI: 0.92–1.59; P = 0.17, I^2 = 0%, the result was not statistically significant. Results illustrating in-hospital MACEs have been represented in Fig. 2.

When MACEs were analyzed during a longer follow up period, MACEs were significantly higher in the COPD group with OR: 1.58, 95% CI: 1.38–1.81; P = 0.00001, I^2 = 29%. This time, it came to our attention that the result might have been influenced by study Enriquez 2011. Therefore, when study Enriquez 2011 was excluded and another analysis was conducted,

Table 5 General features of the studies which were included

Studies	Patients enrollment period	Types of study	No of patients with COPD (n)	No of patients without COPD (n)	Total no of patients (n)
Almagro 2015	2011	Observational	33	100	133
Berger 2004	1998–1999	Observational	183	4101	4284
Campo 2013	2003–2009	Observational	2032	9086	11,118
Enriquez 2011	1997–2006	Observational	860	10,048	10,908
Jatene 2016	-	RCT	283	4322	4605
Konecny 2010	2005–2008	Observational	2001	12,345	14,346
Nishiyama 2009	2000–2002	Observational	240	9632	9872
Selvaraj 2005	1997–2003	Observational	1117	9877	10,994
Sung 2013	2002–2011	Observational	124	1430	1554
Zhang 2012	2006–2011	Observational	645	4510	5155
Total (*n*)			7518	65,451	72,969

Abbreviations: *COPD*chronic obstructive pulmonary disease, *RCT*randomized controlled trial

Table 6 Baseline features of the patients

Studies	Age (yrs)	Males (%)	Ht (%)	Ds (%)	Cs (%)	DM (%)
	+/−	+/−	+/−	+/−	+/−	+/−
Almagro 2015	67.5/61.6	84.8/76.0	69.7/69.0	66.7/62.0	18.2/17.0	36.4/27.0
Berger 2004	66.1/63.3	56.0/69.0	71.0/70.0	–	30.0/22.0	30.0/27.0
Campo 2013	70.0/65.0	66.0/74.0	70.0/61.0	46.8/48.3	24.0/27.0	21.8/20.9
Enriquez 2011	66.8/63.2	57.0/66.1	78.1/69.7	67.0/70.0	30.9/24.4	36.9/30.2
Jatene 2016	67.8/63.0	75.6/76.7	74.6/63.6	67.8/63.0	42.4/33.8	24.4/16.8
Konecny 2010	69.9/66.0	72.0/70.0	74.0/70.0	73.0/76.0	30.0/17.0	26.0/24.0
Nishiyama 2009	–	82.5/70.4	62.5/69.2	–	43.8/35.7	31.7/39.0
Selvaraj 2005	67.6/64.1	62.0/71.1	75.1/71.6	17.2/20.1	27.0/18.0	37.2/30.5
Sung 2013	68.5/60.9	85.5/81.2	54.8/55.6	39.5/42.3	37.1/34.5	32.3/36.2
Zhang 2012	68.4/64.7	73.0/71.0	75.0/71.0	65.0/63.0	38.0/29.0	25.0/22.0

Abbreviations: *yrs*. years, *Ht* hypertension, *Ds* dyslipidemia, *Cs* current smoking, *DM*diabetes mellitus, '+': *COPD* '-': no COPD

MACEs still significantly favored non-COPD with OR: 1.90, 95% CI: 1.46–2.48; P = 0.00001, I^2 = 0% during this longer follow up period. Results showing MACEs during the longer follow up have been illustrated in Fig. 3.

Mortality following PCI in COPD versus non-COPD

When mortality was analyzed, in-hospital death was significantly higher in patients with COPD, with OR: 2.25, 95% CI: 1.78–2.85; P = 0.00001, I^2 = 0% (Fig. 4).

During a longer follow up period, mortality was still significantly higher in the COPD group with OR: 2.22, 95% CI: 1.33–3.71; P = 0.002, I^2 = 97%. However, even if it was fully relevant to the literature, this long-term result was highly heterogeneous (Fig. 5).

Other outcomes following PCI in patients with versus without COPD

Other clinical outcomes were also analyzed. Our results showed that in-hospital MI and CR were not significantly different with OR: 1.06, 95% CI: 0.82–1.36; P = 0.67, I^2 = 0% and OR: 1.32, 95% CI: 0.95–1.81; P = 0.09, I^2 = 13% respectively (Fig. 6).

When a longer follow up was considered, MI and CR were still not significantly different with OR: 1.37, 95%

	COPD		No COPD			Odds Ratio
Study or Subgroup	Events	Total	Events	Total	Weight	M-H, Fixed, 95% CI
1.1.1 Major Adverse Cardiac Events						
Berger2004	5	183	123	4101	3.4%	0.91 [0.37, 2.25]
Enriquez2011	47	860	442	10048	22.1%	1.26 [0.92, 1.71]
Nishiyama2009	7	240	235	9632	3.7%	1.20 [0.56, 2.58]
Selvaraj2005	114	1117	680	9877	41.6%	1.54 [1.25, 1.89]
Subtotal (95% CI)		**2400**		**33658**	**70.8%**	**1.40 [1.19, 1.65]**
Total events	173		1480			
Heterogeneity: Chi² = 2.27, df = 3 (P = 0.52); I² = 0%						
Test for overall effect: Z = 4.00 (P < 0.0001)						
1.1.2 Major Adverse Cardiac Events (excluding study Selvaraj2005)						
Berger2004	5	183	123	4101	3.4%	0.91 [0.37, 2.25]
Enriquez2011	47	860	442	10048	22.1%	1.26 [0.92, 1.71]
Nishiyama2009	7	240	235	9632	3.7%	1.20 [0.56, 2.58]
Subtotal (95% CI)		**1283**		**23781**	**29.2%**	**1.21 [0.92, 1.59]**
Total events	59		800			
Heterogeneity: Chi² = 0.44, df = 2 (P = 0.80); I² = 0%						
Test for overall effect: Z = 1.36 (P = 0.17)						
Total (95% CI)		**3683**		**57439**	**100.0%**	**1.35 [1.17, 1.55]**
Total events	232		2280			
Heterogeneity: Chi² = 3.55, df = 6 (P = 0.74); I² = 0%						
Test for overall effect: Z = 4.11 (P < 0.0001)						
Test for subgroup differences: Chi² = 0.83, df = 1 (P = 0.36), I² = 0%						

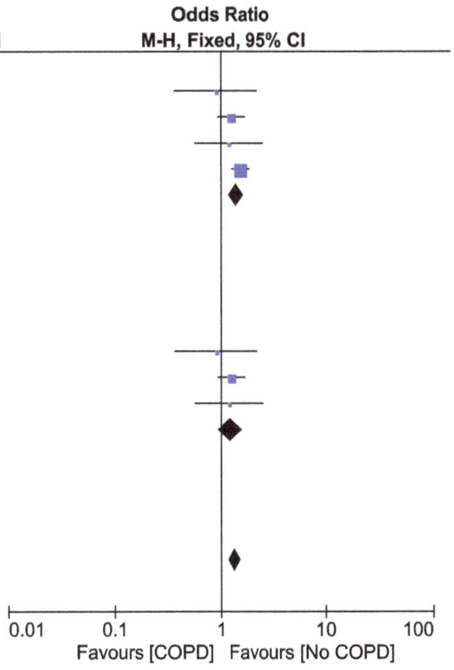

Fig. 2 In-hospital major adverse cardiac events reported in patients with versus without COPD

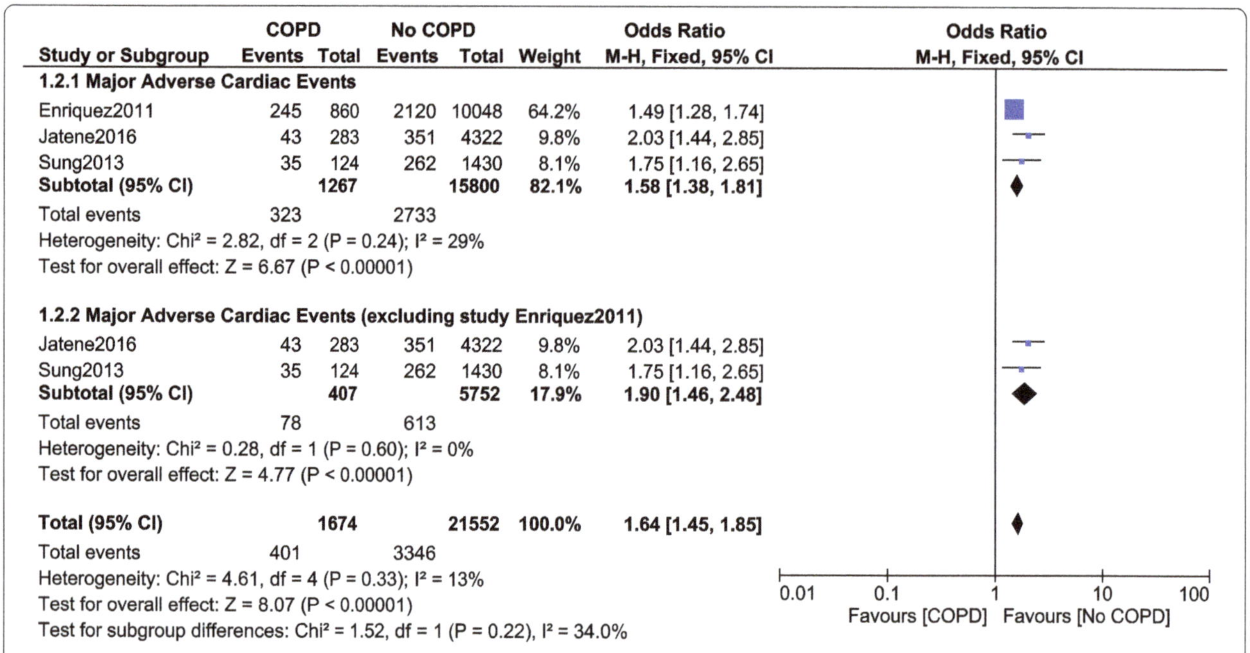

COPD
No COPD
Odds Ratio
Odds Ratio
Study or Subgroup Events Total Events Total Weight M-H, Fixed, 95% CI M-H, Fixed, 95% CI
1.2.1 Major Adverse Cardiac Events
Enriquez2011 245 860 2120 10048 64.2% 1.49 [1.28, 1.74]
Jatene2016 43 283 351 4322 9.8% 2.03 [1.44, 2.85]
Sung2013 35 124 262 1430 8.1% 1.75 [1.16, 2.65]
Subtotal (95% CI) 1267 15800 82.1% 1.58 [1.38, 1.81]
Total events 323 2733
Heterogeneity: Chi² = 2.82, df = 2 (P = 0.24); I² = 29%
Test for overall effect: Z = 6.67 (P < 0.00001)
1.2.2 Major Adverse Cardiac Events (excluding study Enriquez2011)
Jatene2016 43 283 351 4322 9.8% 2.03 [1.44, 2.85]
Sung2013 35 124 262 1430 8.1% 1.75 [1.16, 2.65]
Subtotal (95% CI) 407 5752 17.9% 1.90 [1.46, 2.48]
Total events 78 613
Heterogeneity: Chi² = 0.28, df = 1 (P = 0.60); I² = 0%
Test for overall effect: Z = 4.77 (P < 0.00001)
Total (95% CI) 1674 21552 100.0% 1.64 [1.45, 1.85]
Total events 401 3346
Heterogeneity: Chi² = 4.61, df = 4 (P = 0.33); I² = 13%
Test for overall effect: Z = 8.07 (P < 0.00001)
Test for subgroup differences: Chi² = 1.52, df = 1 (P = 0.22), I² = 34.0%
0.01 0.1 1 10 100
Favours [COPD] Favours [No COPD]

Fig. 3 Long-term major adverse cardiac events reported in patients with versus without COPD

CI: 0.92–2.04; $P = 0.12$, $I^2 = 19\%$ and OR: 1.15, 95% CI: 0.90–1.46; $P = 0.26$, $I^2 = 0$ respectively (Fig. 7).

Analysis including patients with COPD which was confirmed by a spirometry test

Another subgroup analysis was carried out including patients with COPD defined based on a spirometry test. In-hospital mortality was still significantly higher in patients with COPD with OR: 1.79, 95% CI: 1.17–2.73; $P = 0.007$, $I^2 = 0\%$. However, MACEs and MI were not significantly different with OR: 1.21, 95% CI: 0.92–1.59; $P = 0.17$, $I^2 = 0\%$ and OR: 1.26, 95% CI: 0.79–1.99; $P = 0.33$, $I^2 = 0\%$ respectively as shown in Fig. 8.

In addition, long-term death in this particular subgroup of patients was not significantly different with OR: 2.05, 95% CI: 0.90–4.68; $P = 0.09$, $I^2 = 98\%$ as shown in Fig. 9.

Sensitivity analyses obtained consistent results. Table 7 summarized the overall results of this analysis.

Publication bias

Based on the funnel plots obtained (Figs. 10 and 11), there was only little evidence of publication bias among the studies which assessed most of the clinical endpoints.

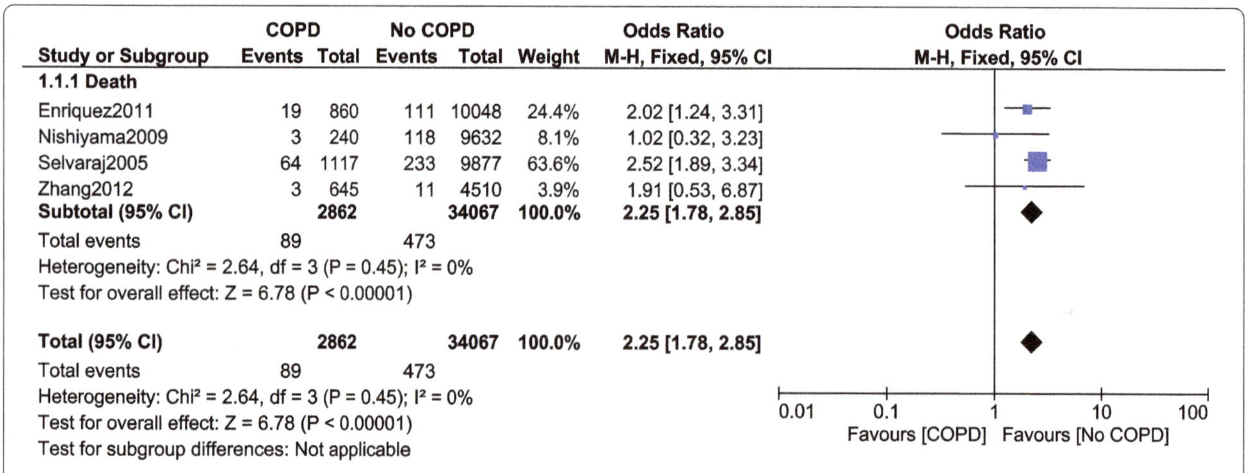

COPD
No COPD
Odds Ratio
Odds Ratio
Study or Subgroup Events Total Events Total Weight M-H, Fixed, 95% CI M-H, Fixed, 95% CI
1.1.1 Death
Enriquez2011 19 860 111 10048 24.4% 2.02 [1.24, 3.31]
Nishiyama2009 3 240 118 9632 8.1% 1.02 [0.32, 3.23]
Selvaraj2005 64 1117 233 9877 63.6% 2.52 [1.89, 3.34]
Zhang2012 3 645 11 4510 3.9% 1.91 [0.53, 6.87]
Subtotal (95% CI) 2862 34067 100.0% 2.25 [1.78, 2.85]
Total events 89 473
Heterogeneity: Chi² = 2.64, df = 3 (P = 0.45); I² = 0%
Test for overall effect: Z = 6.78 (P < 0.00001)
Total (95% CI) 2862 34067 100.0% 2.25 [1.78, 2.85]
Total events 89 473
Heterogeneity: Chi² = 2.64, df = 3 (P = 0.45); I² = 0%
Test for overall effect: Z = 6.78 (P < 0.00001)
Test for subgroup differences: Not applicable
0.01 0.1 1 10 100
Favours [COPD] Favours [No COPD]

Fig. 4 In-hospital mortality reported in patients with versus without COPD

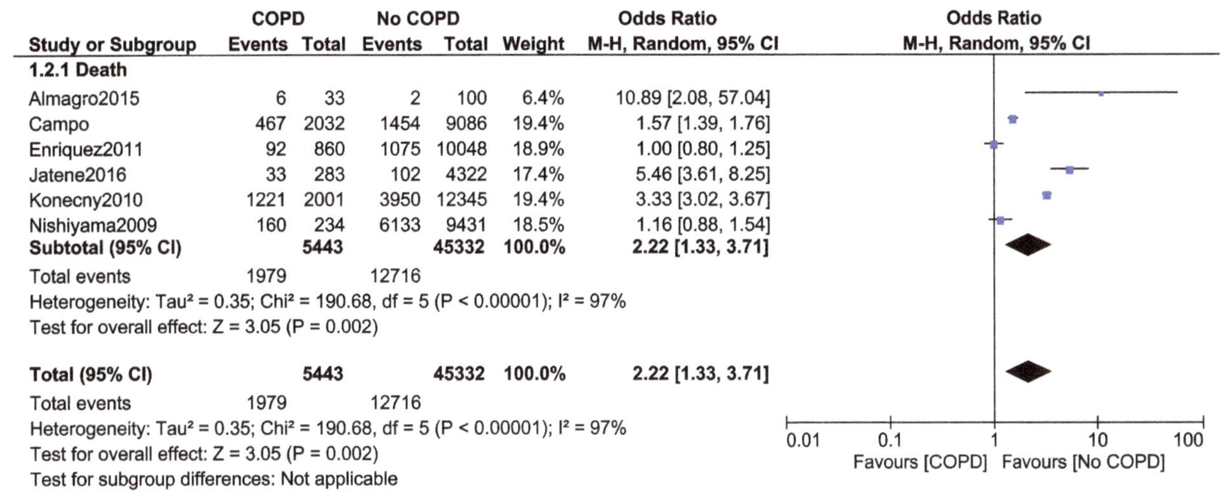

COPD
No COPD
Odds Ratio
Odds Ratio
Study or Subgroup Events Total Events Total Weight M-H, Random, 95% CI
M-H, Random, 95% CI
1.2.1 Death
Almagro2015 6 33 2 100 6.4% 10.89 [2.08, 57.04]
Campo 467 2032 1454 9086 19.4% 1.57 [1.39, 1.76]
Enriquez2011 92 860 1075 10048 18.9% 1.00 [0.80, 1.25]
Jatene2016 33 283 102 4322 17.4% 5.46 [3.61, 8.25]
Konecny2010 1221 2001 3950 12345 19.4% 3.33 [3.02, 3.67]
Nishiyama2009 160 234 6133 9431 18.5% 1.16 [0.88, 1.54]
Subtotal (95% CI) 5443 45332 100.0% 2.22 [1.33, 3.71]
Total events 1979 12716
Heterogeneity: Tau² = 0.35; Chi² = 190.68, df = 5 (P < 0.00001); I² = 97%
Test for overall effect: Z = 3.05 (P = 0.002)
Total (95% CI) 5443 45332 100.0% 2.22 [1.33, 3.71]
Total events 1979 12716
Heterogeneity: Tau² = 0.35; Chi² = 190.68, df = 5 (P < 0.00001); I² = 97%
Test for overall effect: Z = 3.05 (P = 0.002)
Test for subgroup differences: Not applicable
0.01 0.1 1 10 100
Favours [COPD] Favours [No COPD]

Fig. 5 Long-term mortality reported in patients with versus without COPD

Discussion

Since the total number of patients with COPD is on the rise, this analysis aimed to compare MACEs and mortality following PCI in patients with and without COPD. Results of this analysis showed in-hospital as well as long-term MACEs to be higher in COPD patients following coronary angioplasty. Mortality was also significantly higher during the in-hospital and longer follow-up periods. However, other clinical outcomes which were analyzed (MI and CR) were not significantly different between these 2 groups of patients.

Several studies have shown an association of cardiovascular diseases with COPD. Cardiovascular diseases accounts for a high portion of mortality in such chronic pulmonary patients. A recent systematic review summarizing the existing data regarding subclinical cardiovascular events in patients with COPD on the base of identifying screening strategies in such patients showed a high subclinical burden of coronary artery disease in these chronic pulmonary patients [16]. Other studies have shown carotid-intima media thickness to significantly increase in patients with COPD suffering from

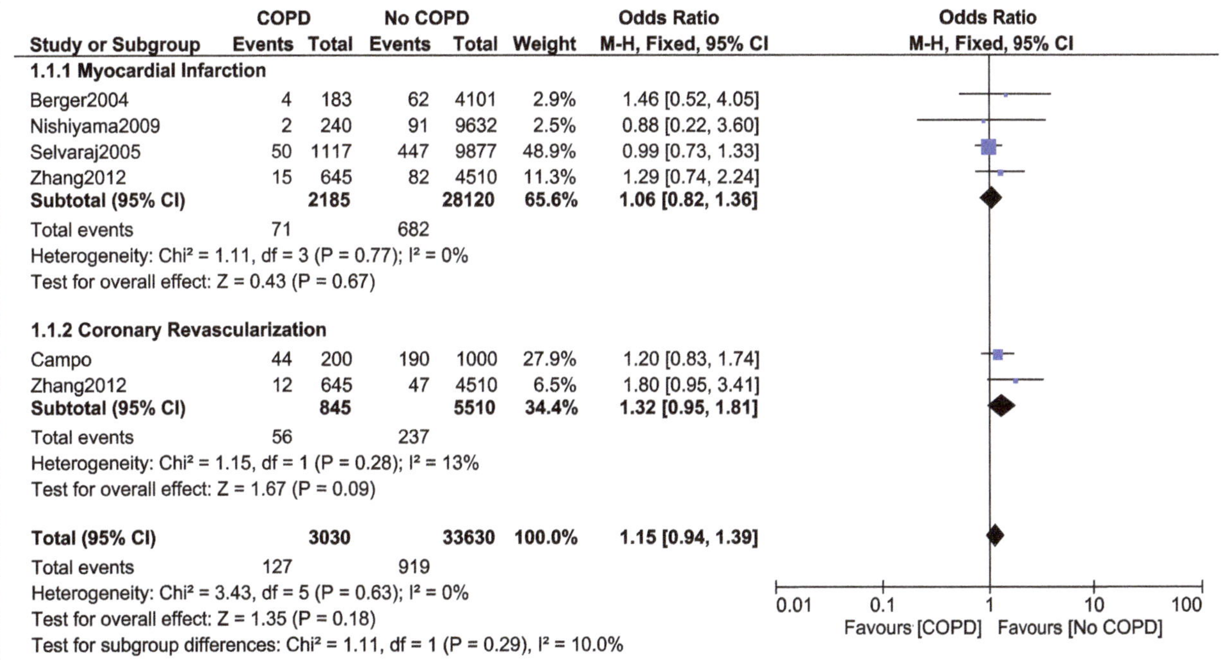

COPD
No COPD
Odds Ratio
Odds Ratio
Study or Subgroup Events Total Events Total Weight M-H, Fixed, 95% CI
M-H, Fixed, 95% CI
1.1.1 Myocardial Infarction
Berger2004 4 183 62 4101 2.9% 1.46 [0.52, 4.05]
Nishiyama2009 2 240 91 9632 2.5% 0.88 [0.22, 3.60]
Selvaraj2005 50 1117 447 9877 48.9% 0.99 [0.73, 1.33]
Zhang2012 15 645 82 4510 11.3% 1.29 [0.74, 2.24]
Subtotal (95% CI) 2185 28120 65.6% 1.06 [0.82, 1.36]
Total events 71 682
Heterogeneity: Chi² = 1.11, df = 3 (P = 0.77); I² = 0%
Test for overall effect: Z = 0.43 (P = 0.67)
1.1.2 Coronary Revascularization
Campo 44 200 190 1000 27.9% 1.20 [0.83, 1.74]
Zhang2012 12 645 47 4510 6.5% 1.80 [0.95, 3.41]
Subtotal (95% CI) 845 5510 34.4% 1.32 [0.95, 1.81]
Total events 56 237
Heterogeneity: Chi² = 1.15, df = 1 (P = 0.28); I² = 13%
Test for overall effect: Z = 1.67 (P = 0.09)
Total (95% CI) 3030 33630 100.0% 1.15 [0.94, 1.39]
Total events 127 919
Heterogeneity: Chi² = 3.43, df = 5 (P = 0.63); I² = 0%
Test for overall effect: Z = 1.35 (P = 0.18)
Test for subgroup differences: Chi² = 1.11, df = 1 (P = 0.29), I² = 10.0%
0.01 0.1 1 10 100
Favours [COPD] Favours [No COPD]

Fig. 6 Other in-hospital outcomes reported in patients with versus without COPD

Study or Subgroup	COPD Events	COPD Total	No COPD Events	No COPD Total	Weight	Odds Ratio M-H, Fixed, 95% CI
1.2.1 Myocardial Infarction						
Enriquez2011	18	300	230	4500	17.2%	1.19 [0.72, 1.94]
Jatene2016	10	283	82	4322	6.2%	1.89 [0.97, 3.69]
Subtotal (95% CI)		**583**		**8822**	**23.4%**	**1.37 [0.92, 2.04]**
Total events	28		312			
Heterogeneity: Chi² = 1.23, df = 1 (P = 0.27); I² = 19%						
Test for overall effect: Z = 1.56 (P = 0.12)						
1.2.2 Coronary Revascularization						
Enriquez2011	55	300	689	4500	44.9%	1.24 [0.92, 1.68]
Jatene2016	30	283	452	4322	31.7%	1.02 [0.69, 1.50]
Subtotal (95% CI)		**583**		**8822**	**76.6%**	**1.15 [0.90, 1.46]**
Total events	85		1141			
Heterogeneity: Chi² = 0.64, df = 1 (P = 0.42); I² = 0%						
Test for overall effect: Z = 1.13 (P = 0.26)						
Total (95% CI)		**1166**		**17644**	**100.0%**	**1.20 [0.98, 1.47]**
Total events	113		1453			
Heterogeneity: Chi² = 2.55, df = 3 (P = 0.47); I² = 0%						
Test for overall effect: Z = 1.75 (P = 0.08)						
Test for subgroup differences: Chi² = 0.57, df = 1 (P = 0.45), I² = 0%						

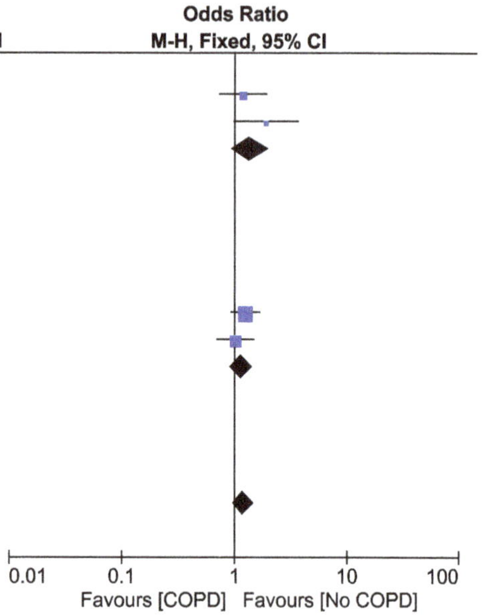

Fig. 7 Other long-term outcomes reported in patients with versus without COPD

Study or Subgroup	COPD Events	COPD Total	No COPD Events	No COPD Total	Weight	Odds Ratio M-H, Fixed, 95% CI
1.1.1 Major Adverse Cardiac Events						
Berger2004	5	183	123	4101	7.2%	0.91 [0.37, 2.25]
Enriquez2011	47	860	442	10048	46.3%	1.26 [0.92, 1.71]
Nishiyama2009	7	240	235	9632	7.8%	1.20 [0.56, 2.58]
Subtotal (95% CI)		**1283**		**23781**	**61.3%**	**1.21 [0.92, 1.59]**
Total events	59		800			
Heterogeneity: Chi² = 0.44, df = 2 (P = 0.80); I² = 0%						
Test for overall effect: Z = 1.36 (P = 0.17)						
1.1.2 Death						
Enriquez2011	19	860	111	10048	12.0%	2.02 [1.24, 3.31]
Nishiyama2009	3	240	118	9632	4.0%	1.02 [0.32, 3.23]
Zhang2012	3	645	11	4510	1.9%	1.91 [0.53, 6.87]
Subtotal (95% CI)		**1745**		**24190**	**17.9%**	**1.79 [1.17, 2.73]**
Total events	25		240			
Heterogeneity: Chi² = 1.16, df = 2 (P = 0.56); I² = 0%						
Test for overall effect: Z = 2.69 (P = 0.007)						
1.1.3 Myocardial Infarction						
Berger2004	4	183	62	4101	3.6%	1.46 [0.52, 4.05]
Nishiyama2009	2	240	91	9632	3.1%	0.88 [0.22, 3.60]
Zhang2012	15	645	82	4510	14.1%	1.29 [0.74, 2.24]
Subtotal (95% CI)		**1068**		**18243**	**20.8%**	**1.26 [0.79, 1.99]**
Total events	21		235			
Heterogeneity: Chi² = 0.33, df = 2 (P = 0.85); I² = 0%						
Test for overall effect: Z = 0.97 (P = 0.33)						
Total (95% CI)		**4096**		**66214**	**100.0%**	**1.32 [1.08, 1.62]**
Total events	105		1275			
Heterogeneity: Chi² = 4.57, df = 8 (P = 0.80); I² = 0%						
Test for overall effect: Z = 2.67 (P = 0.008)						
Test for subgroup differences: Chi² = 2.41, df = 2 (P = 0.30), I² = 16.9%						

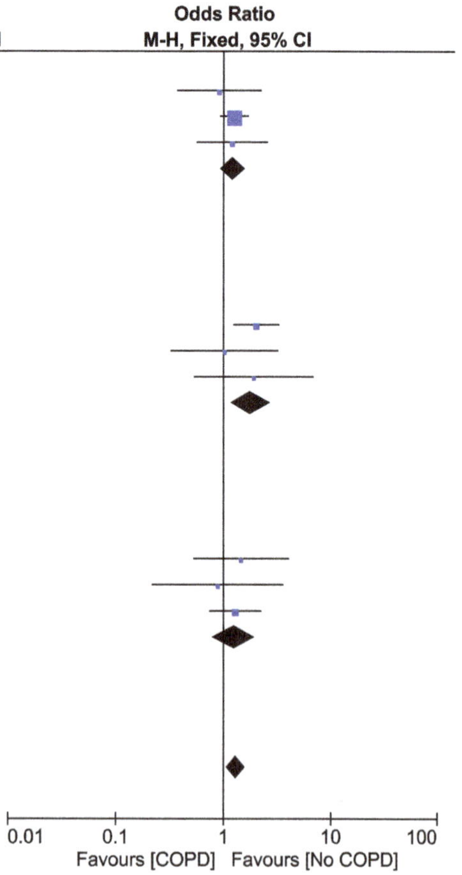

Fig. 8 In-hospital outcomes reported in patients with versus without COPD (defined with respect to the spirometry test)

Study or Subgroup	COPD Events	COPD Total	No COPD Events	No COPD Total	Weight	Odds Ratio M-H, Random, 95% CI
1.2.1 Death						
Almagro2015	6	33	2	100	13.5%	10.89 [2.08, 57.04]
Enriquez2011	92	860	1075	10048	28.8%	1.00 [0.80, 1.25]
Konecny2010	1221	2001	3950	12345	29.3%	3.33 [3.02, 3.67]
Nishiyama2009	160	234	6133	9431	28.5%	1.16 [0.88, 1.54]
Subtotal (95% CI)		**3128**		**31924**	**100.0%**	**2.05 [0.90, 4.68]**
Total events	1479		11160			
Heterogeneity: Tau² = 0.60; Chi² = 128.48, df = 3 (P < 0.00001); I² = 98%						
Test for overall effect: Z = 1.70 (P = 0.09)						
Total (95% CI)		**3128**		**31924**	**100.0%**	**2.05 [0.90, 4.68]**
Total events	1479		11160			
Heterogeneity: Tau² = 0.60; Chi² = 128.48, df = 3 (P < 0.00001); I² = 98%						
Test for overall effect: Z = 1.70 (P = 0.09)						
Test for subgroup differences: Not applicable						

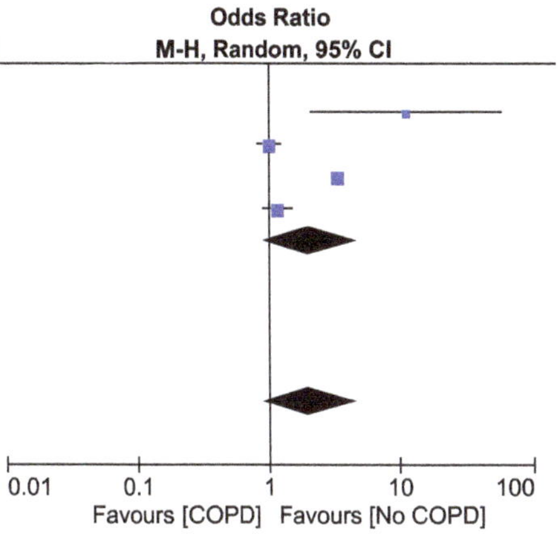

Fig. 9 Long-term mortality reported in patients with versus without COPD (defined with respect to the spirometry test)

coronary artery disease [17]. Recent research has also shown COPD to also be very prevalent in European patients with atrial fibrillation, and these patients were at a higher risk of several cardiovascular complications and death [18].

Well, to support the results of this current analysis, a study involving 1 of 3 tertiary medical centers in New York City showed COPD to be independently associated with long-term mortality following PCI [9]. Another study published by Selvaraj et al. and including 10,994 patients also showed a higher in-hospital and long-term mortality to be associated with COPD [14]. In addition, Insights from the National Heart, Lung and Blood Institute Dynamic Registry also showed worse prognosis in patients with COPD following PCI [3]. The authors even concluded that a lower rate of guidelines recommended class I medications which were prescribed at discharge might be hugely responsible for such higher death rates. Our results were further supported by the REAL registry [10].

Table 7 Results of this analysis

Outcomes analyzed	No of studies included	OR with 95% CI	*P* value	I^2 (%)
In-hospital follow up				
MACEs	4	1.40 [1.19–1.65]	0.0001	0
MACEs	3	1.21 [0.92–1.59]	0.17	0
Death	4	2.25 [1.78–2.85]	0.00001	0
MI	4	1.06 [0.82–1.36]	0.67	0
CR	2	1.32 [0.95–1.81]	0.09	13
Above 1 year follow up				
MACEs	3	1.58 [1.38–1.81]	0.00001	29
MACEs	2	1.90 [1.46–2.48]	0.00001	0
Death	6	2.22 [1.33–3.71]	0.002	97
MI	2	1.37 [0.92–2.04]	0.12	19
CR	2	1.15 [0.90–1.46]	0.26	0

Abbreviations: *MACEs* major adverse cardiac events, *MI* myocardial infarction, *CR* coronary revascularization, *OR* odds ratio, *CI* confidence intervals

Nevertheless, a few studies did not report significantly high post-angioplasty MACEs or mortality associated with COPD. The study published by Sung et al. which aimed to report the incidence and prognostic outcome in COPD patients with acute coronary syndrome (NSTEMI) showed COPD not to be an independent predictor of short and medium-term major adverse clinical outcomes in such patients following PCI [4].

Finally, according to our observations, it is recommended that special care and strict medical adherence have to be considered when managing COPD patients following PCI to avoid or reduce re-admission to the hospital, exacerbation of the obstructive disease, or any increase in mortality or MACEs following PCI. An overview of the pharmacological challenges facing physicians in the management of patients with concomitant cardiovascular disease and COPD strongly suggests that evidence-based treatment in such cases should not be changed [19]. In daily practice in clinics, obtaining the optimal titration of cardiovascular and respiratory drugs is a vital element. Early identification of co-morbidities and counselling about the harm of cigarette smoking might help to improve prognosis in such patients.

Novelty

This research contributes to a novel aspect in clinical medicine due to the fact that it is the first meta-analysis of COPD versus non-COPD and PCI. The larger population size might also contribute to its novelty. In addition, a low level of heterogeneity which was obtained among several subgroups which were analyzed could represent another new feature of this analysis.

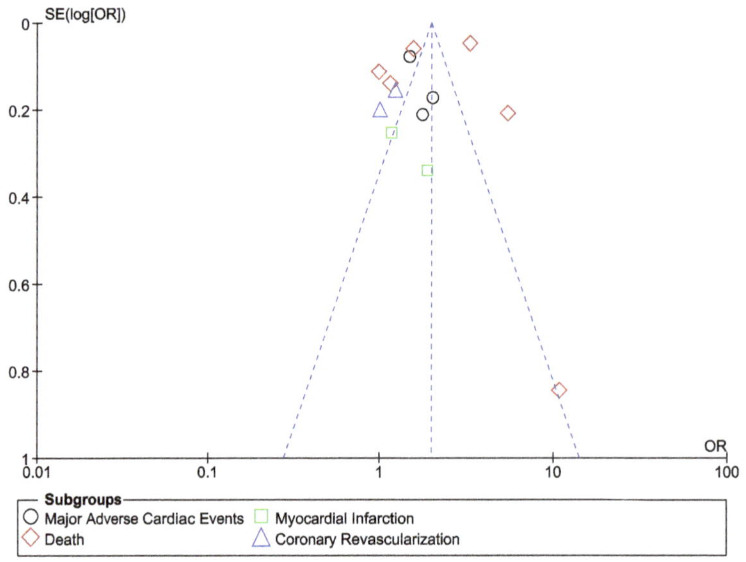

Fig. 10 Funnel plot showing publication bias

Limitations

Limitations of this research were:

- Even though a large number of patients was used, this number might still be small compared to other studies outside this scope.
- Most of the studies which were included were observational studies with heterogeneous data. Therefore, the subgroup analyzing long-term mortality involved a very high level of heterogeneity.
- In addition, different studies had different follow-up periods further contributing to this high level of heterogeneity when analyzing long-term mortality.
- When other clinical outcomes (MI and CR) were analyzed, in some cases, the number of patients were adjusted to avoid the influence of studies with larger number of patients. This might also have affect the results for other clinical outcomes.

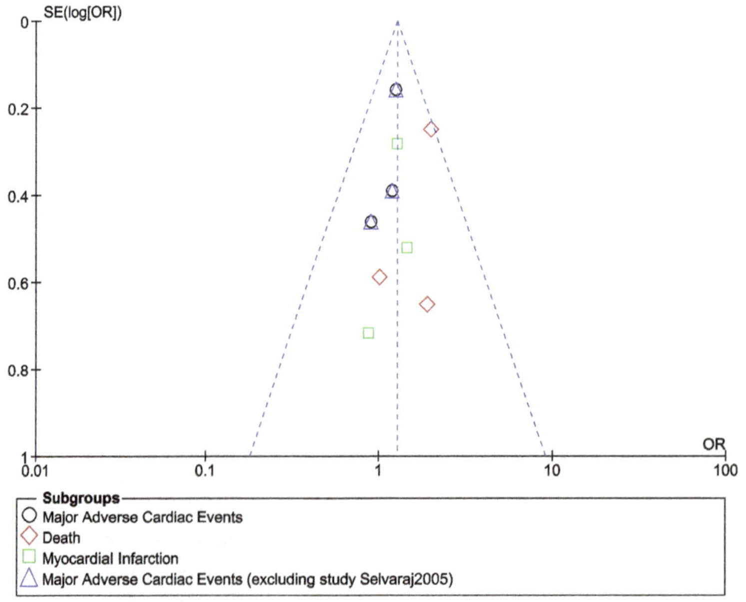

Fig. 11 Funnel plot showing publication bias

– Important endpoints were not reported in all the studies. A few studies reported MACEs while others reported mortality. Therefore, only a few studies were available for comparison during the subgroup analysis.

Conclusion

Since in-hospital and long-term MACEs and mortality were significantly higher following PCI in patients with versus without COPD, COPD should be considered a risk factor for the development of adverse clinical outcomes following PCI. However, the result for the long-term mortality was highly heterogeneous warranting further analysis.

Abbreviations

COPD: Chronic obstructive pulmonary disease; MACEs: Major adverse cardiac events; PCI: Percutaneous coronary intervention

Acknowledgements

Not applicable.

Funding

There was no external source of funding for this research.

Authors' contributions

PKB, CG and GMX were responsible for the conception and design, acquisition of data, analysis and interpretation of data, drafting the initial manuscript and revising it critically for important intellectual content. PKB wrote the final manuscript. All authors read and approved the final manuscript.

Competing interests

The authors declare that they have no competing interests.

Author details

[1]Institute of Cardiovascular Diseases, the First Affiliated Hospital of Guangxi Medical University, Nanning, Guangxi 530027, People's Republic of China. [2]Guangxi Medical University, Nanning, Guangxi 530027, People's Republic of China. [3]Department of Cardiology, The People's Hospital of Guangxi Zhuang Autonomous Region, Nanning, Guangxi 530021, People's Republic of China.

References

1. Parasuramalu BG, Huliraj N, Prashanth Kumar SP, Gangaboraiah RMNR, Srinivasa Babu CR. Prevalence of chronic obstructive pulmonary disease and its association with tobacco smoking and environmental tobacco smoke exposure among rural population. Indian J Public Health. 2014 Jan-Mar; 58(1):45–9.
2. Burney P, Jithoo A, Kato B, Janson C, Mannino D, Nizankowska-Mogilnicka E, Studnicka M, Tan W, Bateman E, Koçabas A, Vollmer WM, Gislason T, Marks G, Koul PA, Harrabi I, Gnatiuc L, Buist S, Burden of obstructive lung disease (BOLD) study. Chronic obstructive pulmonary disease mortality and prevalence: the associations with smoking and poverty–a BOLD analysis. Thorax. 2014 May;69(5):465–73.
3. Enriquez JR, Parikh SV, Selzer F, Jacobs AK, Marroquin O, Mulukutla S, Srinivas V, Holper EM. Increased adverse events after percutaneous coronary intervention in patients with COPD: insights from the National Heart, Lung, and Blood Institute dynamic registry. Chest. 2011 Sep;140(3):604–10.
4. Sung PH, Chung SY, Sun CK, Yang CH, Chen SM, Hang CL, Chen CJ, Yeh KH, Chen YL, Wu CJ, Chang HW, Tsai TH, Yip HK. Impact of chronic obstructive pulmonary disease on patient with acute myocardial infarction undergoing primary percutaneous coronary intervention. Biom J. 2013 Nov-Dec;36(6):274–81.
5. Liberati A, Altman DG, Tetzlaff J, et al. The PRISMA statement for reporting systematic reviews and meta-analyses of studies that evaluate healthcareinterventions: explanation and elaboration. BMJ. 2009;339:b2700.
6. Wells GA, Shea B, O'Connell D, Peterson J, Welch V, Losos M, et al. The Newcastle-Ottawa Scale (NOS) for assessing the quality if nonrandomized studies in meta-analyses. http://www ohrica/programs/clinical_ epidemiology/oxford htm 2009 [cited 2009 Oct 19]; Available from: URL: http://www.ohri.ca/programs/clinical_epidemiology/oxford.htm
7. Higgins JP, Thompson SG, Deeks JJ. Measuring inconsistency in meta-analyses. BMJ. 2003 Sep 6;327(7414):557–60.
8. Almagro P, Lapuente A, Pareja J, Yun S, Garcia ME, Padilla F, Heredia JL, De la Sierra A, Soriano JB. Yip HKpulmonary disease after percutaneous coronary intervention: a prospective study. Int J Chron Obstruct Pulmon Dis. 2015 Jul 16;10:1353–61.
9. Berger JS, Sanborn TA, Sherman W, Brown DL. Effect of chronic obstructive pulmonary disease on survival of patients with coronary heart disease having percutaneous coronary intervention. Am J Cardiol. 2004 Sep 1;94(5):649–51.
10. Campo G, Guastaroba P, Marzocchi A, Santarelli A, Varani E, Vignali L, Sangiorgio P, Tondi S, Serenelli C, De Palma R, Saia F. Impact of COPD on long-term outcome after ST-segment elevation myocardial infarction receiving primary percutaneous coronary intervention. Chest. 2013 Sep;144(3):750–7.
11. Jatene T, Biering-Sørensen T, Nochioka K, Mangione FM, Hansen KW, Sørensen R, Jensen JS, Jørgensen PG, Jeger R, Kaiser C, Pfisterer M, Galatius S, BASKET-PROVE Investigators. Frequency of Cardiac Death and Stent Thrombosis in Patients With Chronic Obstructive PulmonaryDisease Undergoing Percutaneous Coronary Intervention (from the BASKET-PROVE I and II Trials). Am J Cardiol. 2016 Sep 29. Epub.
12. Konecny T, Somers K, Orban M, Koshino Y, Lennon RJ, Scanlon PD, Rihal CS. Interactions between COPD and outcomes after percutaneous coronary intervention. Chest. 2010 Sep;138(3):621–7.
13. Nishiyama K, Morimoto T, Furukawa Y, Nakagawa Y, Ehara N, Taniguchi R, Ozasa N, Saito N, Hoshino K, Touma M, Tamura T, Haruna Y, Shizuta S, Doi T, Fukushima M, Kita T, Kimura T. Chronic obstructive pulmonary disease–an independent risk factor for long-term cardiac and cardiovascular mortality in patients with ischemic heart disease. Int J Cardiol. 2010 Aug 20;143(2):178–83.
14. Selvaraj CL, Gurm HS, Gupta R, Ellis SG, Bhatt DL. Chronic obstructive pulmonary disease as a predictor of mortality in patients undergoing percutaneous coronary intervention. Am J Cardiol. 2005 Sep 15;96(6):756–9.
15. Zhang JW, Zhou YJ, Yang Q, Yang SW, Nie B, Xu XH. Impact of chronic obstructive pulmonary diseases on outcomes and hospital days after percutaneouscoronary intervention. Angiology. 2013 Aug;64(6):430–4.
16. Ye C, Younus A, Malik R, Roberson L, Shaharyar S, Veledar E, Ahmad R, Ali SS, Latif MA, Maziak W, Feiz H, Aneni E, Nasir K. Subclinical cardiovascular disease in patients with chronic obstructive pulmonary disease: a systematic review. QJM. 2016 Aug 18.
17. Köseoğlu C, Kurmuş Ö, Ertem AG, Çolak B, Bilen E, İpek G, Durmaz T, Keleş T, Bozkurt E. Association between carotid intima-media thickness and presence of coronary artery disease in chronic obstructive pulmonary disease patients. Anatol J Cardiol. 2016 Aug;16(8):601–7.
18. Proietti M, Laroche C, Drozd M, Vijgen J, Cozma DC, Drozdz J, Maggioni AP, Boriani G, Lip GY, EORP-AF investigators. Impact of chronic obstructive pulmonary disease on prognosis in atrial fibrillation: a report from the EURObservational research Programme pilot survey on atrial fibrillation (EORP-AF) general registry. Am Heart J. 2016 Nov;181:83–91.

13

Arterial stiffness in patients with coronary artery disease: relation with in-stent restenosis following percutaneous coronary intervention

Zrinko Prskalo[1], Ivica Brizić[1*], Darko Markota[1], Ivica Markota[1], Mladen Boban[3], Monika Tomic[2] and Boris Starcevic[4]

Abstract

Background: Coronary artery disease (CAD) is one of the most important issues in modern medicine due to its high mortality and prevalence. An early detection and prevention can reduce morbidity and mortality. Arterial stiffness is a potent and independent predictor of CAD. We aimed to investigate the arterial stiffness in CAD patients undergoing the coronary angiography. Also, we investigated a possible correlation between arterial stiffness and in-stent restenosis (ISR), an important limitation of percutaneous coronary intervention (PCI).

Methods: The study included 160 patients undergoing coronary angiography, treated either with PCI or with CABG. The pulse wave velocity (PWV) and augmentation index (AIx) were measured by the Arteriograph.

Results: PWV in the CAD group (12.24 ± 2.78 m/s) was significantly higher compared to the control group (8.27 ± 1.89 m/s). PWV in ISR and left main (LM) stenosis group (14.03 ± 3.15 and 13.89 ± 2.95 m/s) was significantly higher compared to the control and CAD groups. Peripheral and central AIx were significantly higher in CAD group (1.38 ± 30.63 % and 38.35 ± 15.52 %) than in control group (−11.35 ± 26.74 % and 26.91 ± 10.62 %). Patients with LM stenosis have significantly higher values of peripheral and central AIx (23.37 ± 23.77 % and 49.71 ± 12.02 %) than the CAD and ISR group.

Conclusions: The study confirmed a positive correlation between arterial stiffness measures, PWV and AIx, and CAD. Also, this study showed the correlation between PWV and ISR which can help to select more appropriate stent.

Keywords: Vascular stiffness, Coronary artery disease, Coronary restenosis

Background

Coronary artery disease (CAD) is one of the most important issues in modern medicine due to high prevalence and mortality. Both, the prevention and treatment of CAD in recent decades have been improved, however, CAD remains the first inductor of morbidity and mortality in humans [1]. An early detection and prevention of CAD is very important and can reduce morbidity and mortality. Numerous epidemiological and clinical studies showed a positive correlation between CAD and male gender, high blood pressure, diabetes, smoking, physical inactivity, and hyperlipidemia [2]. In addition to these traditional risk factors, the arterial stiffness defined as a direct measure - aortic pulse wave velocity (PWV) and an indirect parameter - augmentation index (AIx), is a strong and independent predictor of CAD and adverse cardiovascular events [3, 4]. The majority of the current research, investigating correlation between arterial stiffness and CAD was of observational or epidemiological nature [5, 6]. Only few clinical studies showed a direct correlation between PWV and CAD diagnosed by coronary angiography [7, 8].

Treatment of CAD could involve pharmacotherapy, percutaneous coronary interventions (PCI), and surgical revascularization. All methods are associated with some limitations and disadvantages. In the past few decades

* Correspondence: ibrizic@gmail.com
[1]Department of Cardiology, University Hospital Mostar, Bijeli Brijeg bb, 88 000 Mostar, Bosnia and Herzegovina
Full list of author information is available at the end of the article

the development of PCI, atherectomy, with bare-metal (BMS) and drug eluting stents (DES) has made a significant progress in the management of CAD [1]. The most important limitation of PCI is thrombosis and in-stent restenosis (ISR). The incidence of ISR after a BMS implantation is 20–25 % in the first 6 months [9]. The development of DES contributed to a significant reduction of the ISR, as it decreased the incidence rate of ISR in only 5–10 % cases [10–12]. However, the rate of DES use is lower than 10 % in most countries due to the high cost. The incidence of DES implantation in developing countries, such as ours, is smaller than an average rate, because of its higher cost.

Factors that contribute to ISR are not fully understood. Cassese et al. showed that diabetes mellitus, multiple lesions, small vessels, multiple stents, smaller final stent lumen diameter and stent design are predictors for ISR [11, 13]. Some previous studies established a link between arterial stiffness and ISR. Ueda et al. found a correlation between AIx in the ascending aorta and ISR [14]. Also, Nakayama et al. showed a correlation between pulse pressure and ISR [15]. Recently, Mahfouz et al. described a correlation between arterial stiffness measured with ultrasonography and ISR [16].

In this study we aimed to investigate the correlation between CAD assessed by coronary angiography graded by SYNTAX score and arterial stiffness measured by Arteriograph, a simple, inexpensive, reproducible and investigator-independent method. Also, we investigated the correlation between ISR and aortic PWV and Aix.

Methods

The study included 160 patients with CAD who underwent an elective coronary angiography in the Department of Invasive Cardiology of Clinical Hospital Mostar from 1st April 2014 to 1st October 2014. The control group consisted of 59 sex and age-matched healthy people. All subjects in the control group underwent the clinical examination, ECG, stress test, echocardiography, measuring of arterial stiffness and laboratory testing. All those subjects had a clear medical history. The CAD group excluded subjects with atrial fibrillation, acute coronary syndrome, and with significant valvular disease. All CAD patients had previous concordant non-invasive findings for CAD and experienced angina pectoris. They received an appropriate treatment (statines, beta blockers, ACE inhibitors and aspirin) in accordance with the guidelines for CAD [17]. Out of a total number of CAD patients, 102 were treated with PCI and 58 underwent heart surgery. During the next 6 months 23 patients had ISR in BMS. All patients who underwent PCI had dual antiplatelet therapy, aspirin and clopidogrel. The study was conducted in accordance with the Helsinki Declaration and approved by the Ethics Committee of the University Hospital Mostar. All subjects gave written informed consent to participate in this study.

Coronary angiography and SYNTAX score

All patients underwent routine coronary angiography using the Judkins technique on digitized coronary angiography equipment (Shimadzu, Kyoto, Japan). Coronary angiograms were computerized and assessed by two experienced angiographers who were blinded to the results of arterial stiffness measurements. A significant CAD was defined as at least 50 % or more stenosis. ISR was defined as >50 % diameter stenosis at the stent site.

The SYNTX score is a semi-quantitative angiographic tool to determine the extent of CAD [18]. The algorithm contains of 12 questions referring to the coronary anatomy and total number and extent of coronary artery lesions. The SYNTAX score was calculated for each coronary lesion producing a ≥50 % luminal obstruction in vessels with a diameter of 1.5 mm or more. Patients were divided according to 2-year rates of major adverse coronary events as low (0–22), intermediate (23–32), and high (≥33) risk group. The SYNTAX score was calculated with a computer-based questionnaire program.

Measurements of arterial stiffness

Arterial stiffness was measured by an oscillometric non-invasive device Arteriograph (TensioMed, Budapest, Hungary). The device detects and processes oscillations on the upper-arm positioned cuff by a special high fidelity sensor during a complete occlusion of brachial artery. Simultaneously with the parameters of arterial stiffness (PWV (m/s) an AIx (%), the device also recorded systolic and diastolic blood pressures and heart rate [19].

Twenty-four hours prior to the examination subjects were asked to refrain from exercise, fruits, vegetables, dietary supplements, tea, alcoholic beverages, and caffeine containing foods. Also, 12 hours before measurement of arterial stiffness patients did not take any drugs. All experiments were carried out in a quiet, temperature controlled room maintained around 24 °C and were started at 8 a.m. The subjects had rested quietly for 15 min in the supine position before the measurement.

Statistics

Data are expressed as mean ± SD. Statistical analyses were performed using GraphPad Instat and GraphPad Prism (San Diego, CA USA). All variables were normalized before data statistical analyses on age, heart rate and blood pressure. One-way ANOVA test was used to evaluate changes in AIx and PWV. When statistical significance was reached by ANOVA (P <0.05), Bonferroni test was used for the post hoc analysis.

Results

In this study we investigated the association of arterial stiffness with CAD and correlation between degrees of CAD measured by SYNTAX score. We found a strong correlation between CAD and arterial stiffness, but no association between degrees of the CAD with the parameters of arterial stiffness. From CAD group we extracted CABG, PCI, left main (LM) stenosis and ISR groups.

The general characteristics of control, CAD, ISR and LM stenosis groups are shown in Table 1. In the control and all experimental groups the male sex was dominant. Also, in the CAD, ISR and LM stenosis group, patients were slightly older with higher mean arterial pressure.

Aortic PWV in the CAD group (12.24 ± 2.78 m/s) was significantly higher compared to the control group (8.27 ± 1.89 m/s) (P <0.05). Also, PWV of an ISR and LM stenosis group (14.03 ± 3.15 and 13.89 ± 2.95 m/s) was significantly higher than in the control and CAD group (P <0.05) (Fig. 1).

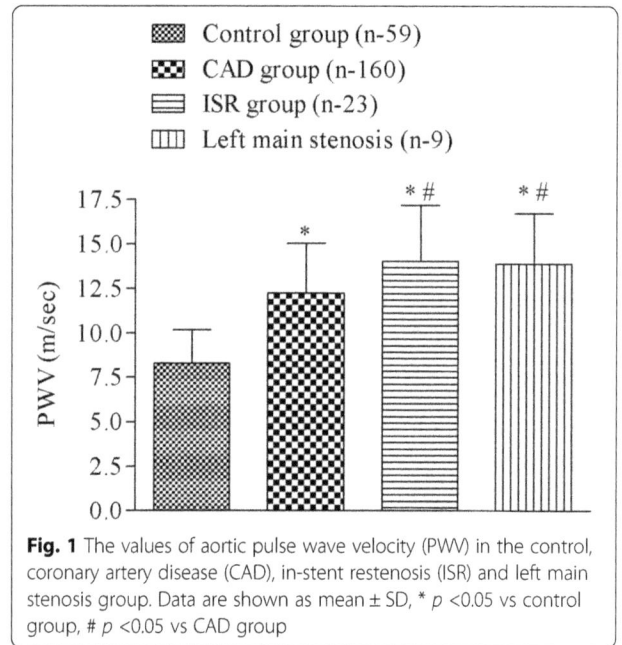

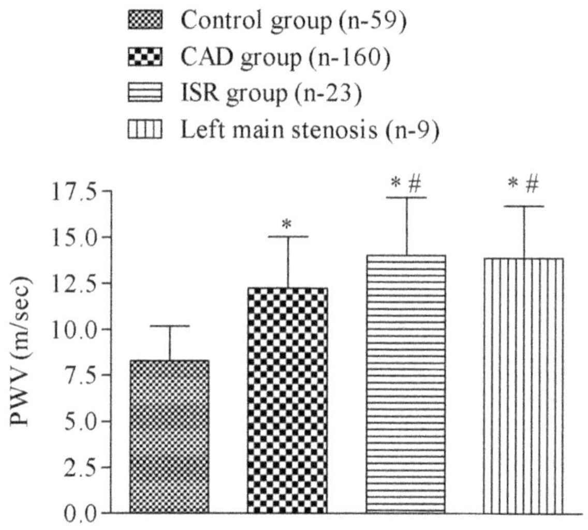

Fig. 1 The values of aortic pulse wave velocity (PWV) in the control, coronary artery disease (CAD), in-stent restenosis (ISR) and left main stenosis group. Data are shown as mean ± SD, * p <0.05 vs control group, # p <0.05 vs CAD group

The central AIx in the CAD, ISR and LM stenosis group (38.35 ± 15.52, 39.71 ± 13.97 and 49.71 ± 12.02 %, respectively) was significantly higher compared to the control group (26.91 ± 10.62 %) (P <0.05). Also, central AIx of an LM stenosis group was significantly higher than in the CAD and ISR group (P <0.05) (Fig. 2).

The peripheral AIx in the CAD, ISR and LM stenosis group (1.38 ± 30.63 and 4.09 ± 27.60 and 23.37 ± 23.77 %, respectively) was significantly higher compared to the control group (−11.35 ± 26.74 %) (P <0.05). Also, peripheral AIx of an LM stenosis group was significantly higher than in the CAD and ISR group (P <0.05) (Fig. 3).

The SYNTAX score was significantly higher in patients who were referred for CABG and patients with LM stenosis (34.62 ± 12.46 and 36.78 ± 16.47) compared

Table 1 General characteristics of control, CAD and ISR groups

	Control group (*n*-58)	CAD group (*n*-160)	ISR group (*n*-23)	LM stenosis group (*n*-9)
Age (year)	59.5 ± 5.4	61.5 ± 4.8	62.1 ± 6.1	63.8 ± 8.4
Male *n* (%)	43 (72.9)	115 (71.7)	22 (95.7)	9 (100)
Female *n* (%)	16 (27.1)	45 (28.3)	1 (4.3)	0 (0)
Smoking *n* (%)	21 (35.6)	82 (51.3)	8 (34.8)	6 (66.6)
Cholesterol (mmol/L)	5.59 ± 1.45	5.38 ± 1.33	5.06 ± 1.56	5.45 ± 1.73
LDL (mmol/L)	3.84 ± 0.78	3.66 ± 0.51	3.58 ± 0.68	3.78 ± 1.44
HDL (mmol/L)	1.02 ± 0.43	1.08 ± 0.25	1.13 ± 0.58	1.06 ± 0.29
Triglycerides (mmol/L)	2.12 ± 0.91	1.92 ± 0.77	1.84 ± 0.98	1.79 ± 0.43
Heart rate (beats/min)	65.7 ± 6.1	64.1 ± 4,2	65.1 ± 9,7	64.7 ± 8,9
Mean blood pressure (mm Hg)	101.3 ± 5.6	104.6 ± 6,5	105.7 ± 8.9	106.1 ± 9.6
Diabetes mellitus *n* (%)	0.0 (0.0)	25 (15.7)	3 (13.0)	0 (0)
Glucose blood level (mmol/L)	5.17 ± 0.67	5.71 ± 1.73	8.23 ± 0.72	5.34 ± 0.89
Renal failure *n* (%)	0.0 (0.0)	6 (3.75)	1 (4.3)	1 (11,1)
Creatinine (μmol/L)	94.22 ± 22.96	98.30 ± 26.04	143	109.78 ± 32.12
SYNTAX scores		25.27 ± 4.1	19.33 ± 6.9	36.78 ± 14.47
Multiple stents *n* (%)		14 (16.1)	4 (17.3)	
Stent diameter (mm)		3.01 ± 0.78	3.09 ± 0.93	
Length of stent (mm)		18.4 ± 0.58	18.1 ± 2.42	

Data are shown as mean value ± SD
CAD coronary artery disease, *HDL* low-density lipoprotein, *ISR* in-stent restenosis, *LM* left main, *LDL* high-density lipoprotein, *SD* standard deviation

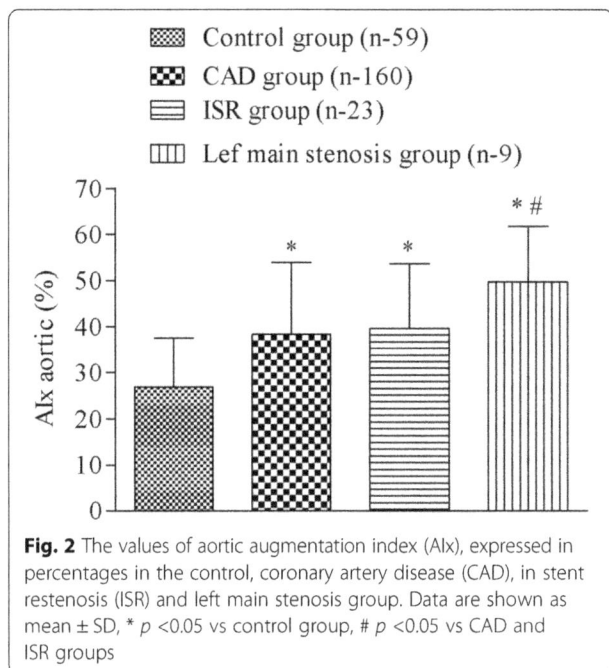

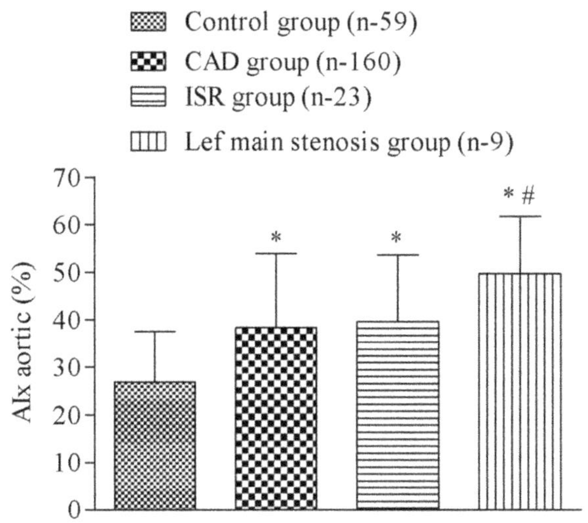

Fig. 2 The values of aortic augmentation index (AIx), expressed in percentages in the control, coronary artery disease (CAD), in stent restenosis (ISR) and left main stenosis group. Data are shown as mean ± SD, * *p* <0.05 vs control group, # *p* <0.05 vs CAD and ISR groups

to the PCI and ISR group (17.63 ± 9.77 and 19.33 ± 6.9) (P <0.05). Among patients treated with PCI and patients who underwent CABG we did not find a difference in the parameters of arterial stiffness (CABG *vs* PCI group; PWV 12.23 ± 2.93 *vs* 12.26 ± 2.68 m/s; central Aix 37.93 ± 14.36 *vs* 38.47 ± 15.39 %; peripheral AIx 1.35 ± 28.32 *vs* 1.57 ± 30.38 %) (Additional file 1).

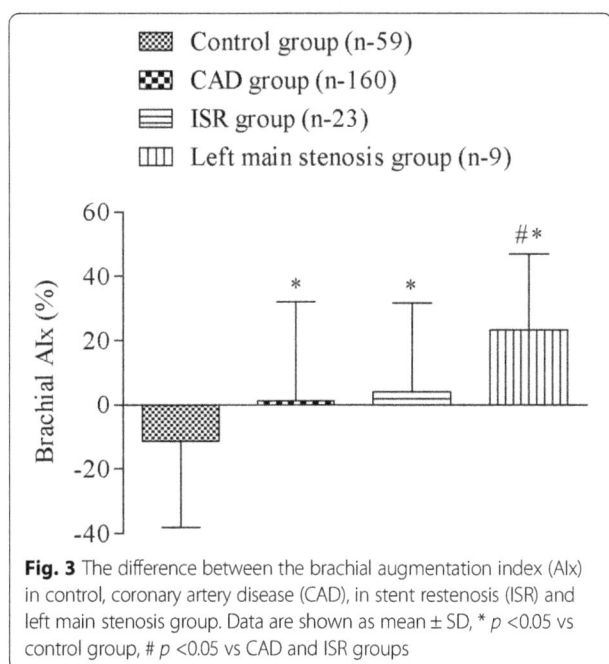

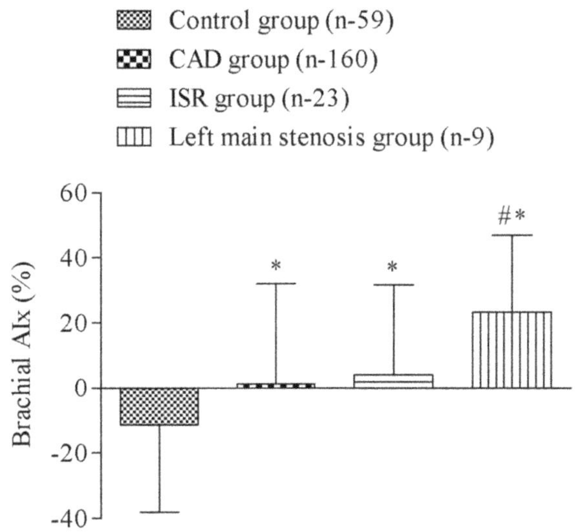

Fig. 3 The difference between the brachial augmentation index (AIx) in control, coronary artery disease (CAD), in stent restenosis (ISR) and left main stenosis group. Data are shown as mean ± SD, * *p* <0.05 vs control group, # *p* <0.05 vs CAD and ISR groups

Discussion

In this study we showed a positive correlation between arterial stiffness parameters and CAD proved with coronary angiography. Also, our study showed the correlation between PWV and ISR.

Some previous studies showed the correlation between arterial stiffness and CAD [20–22]. In the most of them CAD was proved with non-invasive methods. Several studies demonstrated the correlation between CAD examined with coronary angiography and arterial stiffness. Liu et al. showed positive correlation between arterial stiffness measured by Sphygmocor and CAD proved with multi slice computed tomography coronary angiography [23]. Imanishi et al. concluded that high brachial–ankle PWV is an independent predictor for the presence of CAD, especially in men [24]. Contrary to our investigation, the arterial stiffness in the mentioned studies was proved with different devices and at different blood vessels or coronary artery disease was not identified at coronary angiography. Only one study investigated the correlation between CAD and PWV measured by Arteriograph. Similar to our study, they found the positive correlation between CAD examined with coronary angiography and arterial stiffness [7]. However, despite high differences between PWV and AIx in the control and CAD group, we also did not find the correlation between the CAD grades (defined by SYNTAX score) with PWV and AIx. But still, in this study we proved a correlation between arterial stiffness and left main stenosis. However, Cho et al. showed the correlation between AIx and the grade of CAD in patients aged less than 65 years, but not in the older ones [25]. The correlation was not found in patients above 65 years. In our opinion, it is not realistic to expect that even this method can determine the level of CAD. Also, the measuring of arterial elasticity is developed in order to asses an increased cardiovascular risk but some other specific methods should be used to confirm and prove CAD.

Furthermore, we investigated a correlation between ISR and arterial stiffness. The correlation between PWV and ISR was found, but not between AIx and ISR. Arterial stiffness is strongly dependent on the balance of two major proteins, elastin and collagen [26]. Normally, there is a tightly regulated balance between synthesis and degradation of these two proteins. Therefore, if there is an increased collagen production and reduced degradation in the whole vascular system, arterial stiffness will be increased and more likely an ISR will occur [27]. After the stent insertion some inflammatory changes in the coronary artery wall such as endothelial degradation, macrophage infiltration and smooth muscle cell proliferation could occur. Also, the inflammation in arteries increases the extracellular matrix proteins and collagen synthesis contributing to the ISR [28, 29]. BMS causes neointimal hyperplasia after implantation and leads to ISR and reintervention in more than 20 % of patients by 6 months [10, 11]. Similarly to our study, Ueda et al. showed the correlation between aortic stiffness and restenosis after balloon angioplasty [30]. However, mechanisms including collagen turnover in ISR and restenosis after balloon angioplasty are different. Stenting causes an even greater increase in collagen accumulation compared with balloon angioplasty [28, 31, 32]. Accordingly, the same author showed the correlation between aortic AIx and ISR [14], although the correlation between Aix and ISR was not found in our study. Recently, Mahfouz et al. proved the association of ISR and arterial elasticity [16]. All studies that have found a correlation between the extent of ISR and arterial stiffness were performed with various devices and methods. All results can contribute to a better understanding of ISR and help to make a decision considering stent implantation. In the cases of high PWV and other risks factors for ISR a cardiologist may be guided to implant DES. Moreover, this could be very useful in a cath lab with limited finances.

Conclusion

Our results confirm the importance of measuring arterial elasticity in patients with CAD predisposition. Also, we have found that an elevated PWV is associated with ISR suggesting its measuring before the procedure which contributes for a better selection of the stent implant. This study confirms the value of Arteriograph in cardiovascular risk assessment as a broadly applicable method for screening the general population.

Abbreviations

ACE, angiotensin-converting-enzyme; AIx, augmentation index; BMS, bare-metal stent; CABG, coronary artery bypass graft; CAD, coronary artery disease; DES, drug eluting stent; ISR, in-stent restenosis; LAD, left anterior descending artery; LM, left main; PCI, percutaneous coronary intervention; PWV, pulse wave velocity

Funding

This work was supported by the grant from the Ministry of Science, Education, and Sports of the Federation of Bosnia and Herzegovina.

Authors' contributions

ZP contributed to the study design, analysis and interpretation of data, drafting manuscript, and made coronary angiographies. IB contributed to the study design, data collection, analysis and interpretation of data, drafting manuscript, and made coronary angiography. DM made coronary angiographies and SYNTAX score. IM made coronary angiographies and PWV measurements. MB was involved in drafting the manuscript and revising it critically for important intellectual content. MT participate in the design of the study and performed the statistical analysis. BS made coronary angiography and SYNTAX score. All authors critically revised the manuscript and added important intellectual content. All authors read and approved the final manuscript.

Competing interests

The authors declare that they have no competing interest.

Author details

[1]Department of Cardiology, University Hospital Mostar, Bijeli Brijeg bb, 88 000 Mostar, Bosnia and Herzegovina. [2]Department of Nephrology, University Hospital Mostar, Mostar, Bosnia and Herzegovina. [3]Department of Pharmacology, University of Split, Split, Croatia. [4]Department of Cardiology, University Hospital Dubrava, Zagreb, Croatia.

References

1. Bonnefoy E, Kirkorian G. Mortality of myocardial infarction. Ann Cardiol Angeiol (Paris). 2011;60:311–6.
2. De Backer G, Ambrosioni E, Borch-Johnsen K, Brotons C, Cifkova R, Dallongeville J, et al. European guidelines on cardiovascular disease prevention in clinical practice. Third Joint Task Force of European and Other Societies on Cardiovascular Disease Prevention in Clinical Practice. Eur Heart J. 2003;24:1601–10.
3. Shirwany NA, Zou MH. Arterial stiffness: a brief review. Acta Pharmacol Sin. 2010;31:1267–76.
4. Weber T, Auer J, O'Rourke MF, Kvas E, Lassnig E, Berent R, et al. Arterial stiffness, wave reflections, and the risk of coronary artery disease. Circulation. 2004;109:184–9.
5. Vlachopoulos C, Aznaouridis K, Stefanadis C. Prediction of cardiovascular events and all-cause mortality with arterial stiffness: a systematic review and meta-analysis. J Am Coll Cardiol. 2010;55:1318–27.
6. Laurent S, Boutouyrie P, Asmar R, Gautier I, Laloux B, Guize L, et al. Aortic stiffness is an independent predictor of all-cause and cardiovascular mortality in hypertensive patients. Hypertension. 2001;37:1236–41.
7. Gaszner B, Lenkey Z, Illyes M, Sarszegi Z, Horvath IG, Magyari B, et al. Comparison of aortic and carotid arterial stiffness parameters in patients with verified coronary artery disease. Clin Cardiol. 2012;35:26–31.
8. Kim HJ, Nam JS, Park JS, Cho M, Kim CS, Ahn CW, et al. Usefulness of brachial-ankle pulse wave velocity as a predictive marker of multiple coronary artery occlusive disease in Korean type 2 diabetes patients. Diabetes Res Clin Pract. 2009;85:30–4.
9. Morice MC, Serruys PW, Sousa JE, Fajadet J, Ban Hayashi E, Perin M, et al. A randomized comparison of a sirolimus-eluting stent with a standard stent for coronary revascularization. N Engl J Med. 2002;346:1773–80.
10. Babapulle MN, Joseph L, Belisle P, Brophy JM, Eisenberg MJ. A hierarchical Bayesian meta-analysis of randomised clinical trials of drug-eluting stents. Lancet. 2004;364:583–91.
11. Cassese S, Byrne RA, Tada T, Pinieck S, Joner M, Ibrahim T, et al. Incidence and predictors of restenosis after coronary stenting in 10 004 patients with surveillance angiography. Heart. 2014;100:153–9.
12. Moses JW, Kipshidze N, Leon MB. Perspectives of drug-eluting stents: the next revolution. Am J Cardiovasc Drugs. 2002;2:163–72.
13. Milewski K, Zurakowski A, Pajak J, Pajak-Zielinska E, Liszka L, Buszman PP, et al. Comparison of thin-strut cobalt-chromium stents and stainless steel stents in a porcine model of neointimal hyperplasia. Med Sci Monit. 2010;16:40–4.
14. Ueda H, Hayashi T, Tsumura K, Yoshimaru K, Nakayama Y, Yoshikawa J. The timing of the reflected wave in the ascending aortic pressure predicts restenosis after coronary stent placement. Hypertens Res. 2004;27:535–40.
15. Nakayama Y, Tsumura K, Yamashita N, Yoshimaru K, Hayashi T. Pulsatility of ascending aortic pressure waveform is a powerful predictor of restenosis after percutaneous transluminal coronary angioplasty. Circulation. 2000;101:470–2.
16. Mahfouz RA, Abdulmoneim A, Abduo M, Elawady W. The relation of aortic stiffness and in-stent restenosis in patients undergoing percutaneous coronary stenting. Echocardiography. 2013;30:582–7.
17. Fraker Jr TD, Fihn SD, Chronic Stable Angina Writing C, American College of C, American Heart A, Gibbons RJ, et al. 2007 chronic angina focused update of the ACC/AHA 2002 guidelines for the management of patients with chronic stable angina: a report of the American College of Cardiology/American Heart Association Task Force on Practice Guidelines Writing Group to develop the focused update of the 2002 guidelines for the management of patients with chronic stable angina. J Am Coll Cardiol. 2007;50:2264–74.
18. Sianos G, Morel MA, Kappetein AP, Morice MC, Colombo A, Dawkins K, et al. The SYNTAX Score: an angiographic tool grading the complexity of coronary artery disease. EuroIntervention. 2005;1:219–27.
19. Baulmann J, Schillings U, Rickert S, Uen S, Dusing R, Illyes M, et al. A new oscillometric method for assessment of arterial stiffness: comparison with tonometric and piezo-electronic methods. J Hypertens. 2008;26:523–8.

20. Yamashina A, Tomiyama H, Arai T, Hirose K, Koji Y, Hirayama Y, et al. Brachial-ankle pulse wave velocity as a marker of atherosclerotic vascular damage and cardiovascular risk. Hypertens Res. 2003;26:615–22.
21. Liao J, Farmer J. Arterial stiffness as a risk factor for coronary artery disease. Curr Atheroscler Rep. 2014;16:387.
22. Ede H, Erkoc MF, Okur A, Erbay AR. Impaired aortic elasticity and diastolic functions are associated with findings of coronary computed tomographic angiography. Med Sci Monit. 2014;20:2061–8.
23. Liu CS, Li CI, Shih CM, Lin WY, Lin CH, Lai SW, et al. Arterial stiffness measured as pulse wave velocity is highly correlated with coronary atherosclerosis in asymptomatic patients. J Atheroscler Thromb. 2011;18:652–8.
24. Imanishi R, Seto S, Toda G, Yoshida M, Ohtsuru A, Koide Y, et al. High brachial-ankle pulse wave velocity is an independent predictor of the presence of coronary artery disease in men. Hypertens Res. 2004;27:71–8.
25. Cho SW, Kim BK, Kim JH, Byun YS, Goh CW, Rhee KJ, et al. Non-invasively measured aortic wave reflection and pulse pressure amplification are related to the severity of coronary artery disease. J Cardiol. 2013;62:131–7.
26. Zieman SJ, Melenovsky V, Kass DA. Mechanisms, pathophysiology, and therapy of arterial stiffness. Arterioscler Thromb Vasc Biol. 2005;25:932–43.
27. Strauss BH, Robinson R, Batchelor WB, Chisholm RJ, Ravi G, Natarajan MK, et al. In vivo collagen turnover following experimental balloon angioplasty injury and the role of matrix metalloproteinases. Circ Res. 1996;79:541–50.
28. Chung IM, Gold HK, Schwartz SM, Ikari Y, Reidy MA, Wight TN. Enhanced extracellular matrix accumulation in restenosis of coronary arteries after stent deployment. J Am Coll Cardiol. 2002;40:2072–81.
29. Osherov AB, Gotha L, Cheema AN, Qiang B, Strauss BH. Proteins mediating collagen biosynthesis and accumulation in arterial repair: novel targets for anti-restenosis therapy. Cardiovasc Res. 2011;91:16–26.
30. Ueda H, Nakayama Y, Tsumura K, Yoshimaru K, Hayashi T, Yoshikawa J. Inflection point of ascending aortic waveform is a powerful predictor of restenosis after percutaneous transluminal coronary angioplasty. Am J Hypertens. 2002;15:823–6.
31. Farb A, Sangiorgi G, Carter AJ, Walley VM, Edwards WD, Schwartz RS, et al. Pathology of acute and chronic coronary stenting in humans. Circulation. 1999;99:44–52.
32. Li C, Cantor WJ, Nili N, Robinson R, Fenkell L, Tran YL, et al. Arterial repair after stenting and the effects of GM6001, a matrix metalloproteinase inhibitor. J Am Coll Cardiol. 2002;39:1852–8.

Prognostic significance of endothelial dysfunction in patients undergoing percutaneous coronary intervention in the era of drug-eluting stents

Motoki Kubo[1], Toru Miyoshi[1*], Hiroki Oe[2], Yuko Ohno[1], Kazufumi Nakamura[1] and Hiroshi Ito[1]

Abstract

Background: Endothelial function is a prognostic predictor in patients undergoing percutaneous coronary intervention (PCI). However, in an era with widespread use of drug-eluting stents, the clinical relevance of endothelial dysfunction on restenosis in patients undergoing PCI has not been fully evaluated.

Methods: This study included 80 patients with stable angina pectoris. Flow-mediated dilation (FMD) of the brachial artery was examined 1 week after PCI. Patients were retrospectively followed-up for an average of 21 months after PCI. The primary endpoints included cardiac death, nonfatal myocardial infarction, stroke, coronary revascularization, and critical limb ischemia.

Results: A drug-eluting stent was used in 58 patients and a cardiovascular event was recorded in 34 patients during follow-up. The incidence of all cardiovascular diseases was significantly greater in the low FMD (median FMD <4.2 %) than the high FMD (median FMD ≥4.2 %) group (60 % vs. 25 %, p <0.01). Furthermore, the incidence of coronary revascularization was significantly higher in the low than the high FMD group ($p = 0.02$), while the incidence of in-stent restenosis did not differ between the two groups. Cox regression analysis showed that low FMD was an independent predictor of cardiovascular events (hazard ratio: 2.77, 95 % confidence interval: 1.23 to 6.19, $p = 0.01$).

Conclusions: Impaired brachial artery FMD independently predicts long-term cardiovascular events after PCI in the era of drug-eluting stents.

Keywords: Endothelial function, Stable angina pectoris, Restenosis, Percutaneous coronary intervention

Background

Endothelial dysfunction leads to the initiation of atherosclerosis and is linked to many risk factors that predispose individuals to atherosclerosis [1–3]. Noninvasive ultrasound assessment of brachial artery flow-mediated dilation (FMD) has emerged as a method for studying nitric-oxide-dependent endothelial function [4]. Although reproducible FMD measurements require careful attention to training, technique, and analysis [5], previous studies have shown that FMD is a predictor of future cardiovascular events in populations with coronary risk factors [6, 7], and in patients with established coronary artery disease (CAD) [8, 9].

Percutaneous coronary intervention (PCI) with stenting is currently an effective and widespread treatment for patients with CAD. Although in-stent restenosis is a limitation of PCI, the use of drug-eluting stents (DES) has dramatically reduced the risk of restenosis [10]. Previous studies have shown that impaired FMD is a predictor of in-stent restenosis and cardiovascular events in patients undergoing PCI [11–14]. However, the use of DES modifies the association between endothelial function and in-stent restenosis because a drug released from the stent struts strongly suppresses the re-growth of endothelial cells onto stent struts [15]. Owing to the widespread use of DES in PCI, the association between impaired endothelial function and prognosis in patients undergoing PCI, including in-stent restenosis, needs to be re-evaluated.

* Correspondence: miyoshit@cc.okayama-u.ac.jp
[1]Department of Cardiovascular Medicine, Okayama University Graduate School of Medicine, Dentistry and Pharmaceutical Sciences, Okayama, Japan

We investigated whether early assessment of FMD predicts cardiovascular events, including in-stent restenosis, in patients undergoing PCI in the era of DES.

Methods

Study patients

This study enrolled 80 patients from among 138 consecutive patients with stable angina who were admitted to Okayama University Hospital for PCI and joined a cardiac rehabilitation program from August 2008 to February 2014. Patients who had angiographic documentation of organic stenosis of >70 % of at least one major coronary artery and had PCI successfully performed were eligible. Patients were excluded based on the presence of any of the following criteria: 1) acute coronary syndrome; 2) prior myocardial infarction; 3) history of stroke; 4) New York Heart Association functional classification ≥ III; 5) left main trunk disease; 6) left ventricular ejection fraction on echocardiography <40 %; 7) malignant disease; 8) chronic hepatic disease; 9) chronic inflammatory diseases; 10) chronic renal failure (serum creatinine levels >2.0 mg/dl); and 11) other serious systemic diseases. This study was approved by the institutional ethics committee of Okayama University Hospital. Written informed consent was provided by all of the patients before the study. The investigation conformed to the principles outlined in the Declaration of Helsinki.

Study protocol

Measurement of FMD was performed in the morning after an overnight fast in the same manner at 1 week after PCI. All vasodilators were withdrawn 24 h before the FMD measurements. After PCI, all patients had individualized, optimized therapies, including medications and lifestyle changes, to reduce risk factors for CAD according to the American College of Cardiology/American Heart Association guidelines [16]. Levels of serum lipids, hemoglobin A1c, malondialdehyde-modified low-density lipoprotein (LDL) cholesterol, C-reactive protein, and adiponectin were measured, as described previously [17]. Patients were then retrospectively followed after PCI.

PCI

PCI was performed with conventional techniques by the femoral or radial approach under systemic heparinization, and oral administration of aspirin and ticlopidine. The stent type and inflation pressure were chosen at the discretion of the physicians, who were blinded to the study protocol and the data regarding FMD. Procedural success was defined as reduction of stenosis to <30 % residual narrowing, with improvement of ischemic symptoms and without major in-hospital complications, such as death, emergency bypass surgery, or myocardial infarction (defined as >5 times increase in cardiac troponin T levels). After PCI, patients received aspirin (100 mg/day) indefinitely and ticlopidine (200 mg/day) or clopidogrel (75 mg/day) for at least 9 months. Original stented target lesion revascularization was defined as repeated PCI, and was performed in the presence of in-stent restenosis and any symptoms or objective signs of myocardial ischemia.

Measurements of FMD in the brachial artery

FMD was assessed as a parameter of vasodilation according to the guidelines for ultrasound assessment [4]. Using a 10-MHz linear-array transducer probe (Unex Company Ltd., Nagoya, Japan), longitudinal images of the brachial artery at baseline were recorded with a stereotactic arm, and measurements of the arterial diameter were made after supine rest for ≥5 min. The diameter of the artery was measured, then suprasystolic compression (50 mmHg higher than systolic blood pressure) was performed at the right forearm for 5 min. Measurements of the arterial diameter were made continuously from 30 s after cuff release. Maximum vasodilation was then evaluated from the change in arterial diameter after release of occlusion. An experienced technician blinded to the clinical data of the study participants measured FMD and intra- and inter-observer correlation coefficients were high (>0.9) [18].

Follow-up study

The primary endpoints included cardiac death, nonfatal myocardial infarction, coronary revascularization, critical limb ischemia, and stroke. The time to the first primary endpoint was evaluated retrospectively. The definition and assessment of endpoints were based on the statement from the American College of Cardiology/American Heart Association Task Force [19]. Myocardial infarction was defined as type 1 or type 2 myocardial infarction according to the Third Universal Definition of Myocardial Infarction [20]. All elective coronary revascularizations were undertaken only if the invasive fractional flow reserve of a coronary lesion was 0.80 or less [21]. Stroke included both ischemic and hemorrhagic types. Peripheral vascular intervention was documented in a Report of the American College of Cardiology/American Heart Association Task Force on Clinical Data Standards [20]. Critical limb ischemia needs emergency vascular intervention. Therefore, we included critical limb ischemia as a cardiovascular endpoint in this study. Data regarding primary and secondary outcomes were carefully collected from clinical charts and the diagnosis was confirmed by an investigator who was blinded to FMD data.

Statistical analysis

Data are expressed as the mean ± standard deviation or number (percentage). The frequencies and continuous values between the two groups of patients were compared using the chi-square test and the Student's t test, respectively. Kaplan–Meier analysis of event-free survival during follow-up was performed on the basis of the cut-off value of FMD. The association of FMD with future events was assessed by Cox proportional hazards analysis. The data were initially analyzed using a univariate model with covariates, including FMD and other potential confounders that were significantly different between patients with and without events. Multivariate Cox proportional hazards analysis was then applied using covariates that showed $p < 0.1$ in the univariate Cox proportional hazards analysis. Based on previous studies [11–14], we estimated that the incidence of cardiovascular events, including restenosis, in this study would be lower than that in previous studies because of the high use of DES. With an estimated event rate in patients with low versus high FMD of 30 % versus 4 %, respectively, a population of 80 patients would be needed to detect this difference with $\alpha = 0.05$ and a power of 0.80. $p < 0.05$ was considered statistically significant. Statistical analysis was performed using SPSS 17.0 for Windows (SPSS Inc., Chicago, IL, USA).

Results

A flow diagram of this study is shown in Fig. 1. Of 632 patients who underwent PCI from August 2008 to February 2014, we excluded 494 patients without FMD data. Of the 138 remaining patients, 58 patients were excluded because of acute coronary syndrome ($n = 24$), coronary artery bypass graft ($n = 16$), FMD measured over 1 week after PCI ($n = 16$), and lost to follow-up ($n = 2$). Finally, 80 patients were analyzed.

The clinical characteristics of patients with and without an event are shown in Table 1. In this study, 56.3 % of patients had diabetes mellitus and 43.8 % had renal insufficiency. All of the patients were divided into two groups: the high FMD group (FMD ≥4.2 %, $n = 40$) and the low FMD group (FMD <4.2 %, $n = 40$), according to the median value of FMD. Patients with low FMD had lower high-density lipoprotein (HDL) cholesterol levels than those with high FMD ($p = 0.04$). Patients with low FMD tended to have greater body mass index and higher triglyceride levels than those with high FMD. There was no difference in prescription rates for angiotensin-converting enzyme (ACE) inhibitors and angiotensin II

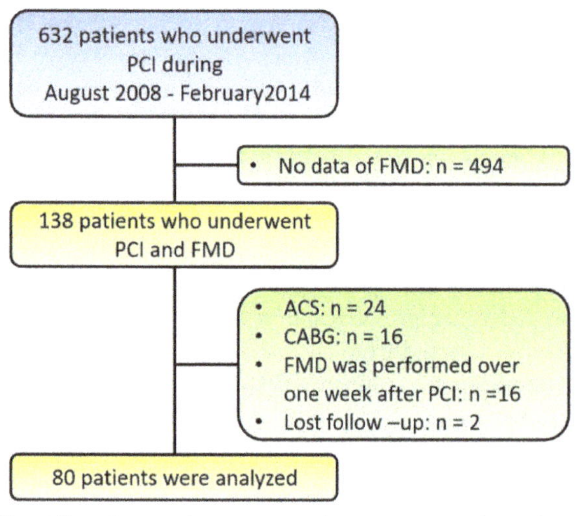

Fig. 1 Flow diagram showing patients' acceptance into the study

Table 1 Clinical characteristics in patients with FMD <4.2 % and ≥4.2 %

	FMD <4.2 % (*n* = 40)	FMD ≥ 4.2 % (*n* = 40)	p
Age (years)	69.5 ± 7.1	69.4 ± 7.3	0.96
Female gender, n (%)	34 (85.0)	30 (75.0)	0.26
Body mass index	25.1 ± 3.4	23.6 ± 3.3	0.06
Diabetes mellitus, n (%)	23 (57.5)	22 (55.0)	0.82
Hypertension, n (%)	27 (65.7)	27 (67.5)	1.00
Dyslipidemia, n (%)	22 (55.0)	31 (77.5)	0.03
Current smoking, n (%)	10 (25.0)	11 (27.5)	0.80
Chronic renal insufficiency, n (%)	16 (40.0)	19 (47.5)	0.50
Previous PCI, n (%)	5 (12.5)	10 (25.0)	0.15
Previous myocardial infarction, n (%)	2 (5.0)	2 (5.0)	1.00
HDL cholesterol (mg/dl)	43.8 ± 11.2	49.3 ± 12.3	0.04
LDL cholesterol (mg/dl)	87.8 ± 28.1	88.1 ± 24.6	0.96
Triglycerides (mg/dl)	142.9 ± 73.6	113.7 ± 61.6	0.06
MDA-LDL cholesterol	97.9 ± 36.8 (*n* = 33)	82.2 ± 32.0 (*n* = 27)	0.62
Adiponectin	11.3 ± 5.2	12.0 ± 5.3	0.90
Medications			
Aspirin, n (%)	40 (100)	38 (95.0)	0.15
Clopidogrel, n (%)	35 (87.5)	33 (82.5)	0.53
ACE inhibitor/ARB, n (%)	35 (87.5)	30 (75.0)	0.15
ARB, n (%)	31 (77.5)	25 (62.5)	0.22
ACE inhibitors, n (%)	4 (10.0)	5 (12.5)	0.99
Perindopril	2 (5.0)	1 (2.5)	0.99
Imidapril	2 (5.0)	4 (10.0)	0.67
Statins, n (%)	36 (90.0)	36 (90.0)	1.00
Atorvastatin	4 (10.0)	7 (17.5)	0.52
Rosuvastatin	18 (45.0)	16 (40.0)	0.82
Pitavastaitn	14 (35.0)	13 (32.5)	0.99
β-blockers, n (%)	21 (52.5)	25(62.5)	0.37

Data are expressed as mean ± SD or number (percentage)
FMD Flow-mediated dilation, *PCI* Percutaneous coronary intervention, *HDL* High-density lipoprotein, *LDL* low-density lipoprotein, *MDA-LDL* Malondialdehyde-modified low-density lipoprotein, *ACE* Angiotensin-converting enzyme, *ARB* Angiotensin II receptor blocker

receptor blockers (ARBs) between the two FMD groups. Additionally, there was no difference in the type of ACE inhibitors between the two groups. There was also no difference in the type of statins between the two groups.

Procedural features of PCI are shown in Table 2. The percentage of the left anterior descending coronary artery as a target vessel artery was greater in the high FMD group than the low FMD group. The use of DES was 68 % in the low FMD group and 78 % in the high FMD group ($p = 0.32$). There were no differences in PCI-related features, such as lesion type, number of stents per lesion, stent diameter, stent length, and stent deployment pressure between the low and high FMD groups.

Patients were retrospectively analyzed for a mean of 21.4 ± 15.9 months after PCI. Table 3 shows the number of cardiovascular disease events when patients were dichotomously categorized as having low FMD or high FMD. During this follow-up period, 34 patients had a cardiovascular event, including cardiac death ($n = 1$), coronary revascularization ($n = 28$), critical limb ischemia ($n = 1$), or ischemic stroke ($n = 4$). Of 19 patients undergoing coronary revascularization due to new lesions, two patients in the low FMD group were hospitalized for unstable angina, but were not diagnosed as having myocardial infarction. PCI for new lesions in the low FMD group was performed significantly more frequently than that in the high FMD group, whereas target lesion revascularization was not different between the groups. FMD in patients with cardiovascular events ($n = 34$) was significantly lower than that in patients without cardiovascular events ($n = 46$) (3.4 ± 1.2 vs 5.1 ± 1.8, $p < 0.01$). There was no difference in the diameter of the brachial artery at baseline and after administration of nitroglycerin between patients with and without cardiovascular disease. The event-free survival curves are shown in Fig. 2. Patients in the low FMD group had significantly more events than those in the high FMD group ($p < 0.01$). In the Cox proportional hazards model including β-blockers and FMD, low FMD (<4.2 %) remained an independent predictor of cardiovascular events (Table 4).

Table 2 Procedural features in patients with FMD <4.2 % and ≥4.2 %

	FMD <4.2 % ($n = 40$)	FMD ≥ 4.2 % ($n = 40$)	p
Target vessel artery	1.08 ± 0.27 (43 lesions)	1.23 ± 0.53 (49 lesions)	0.12
Left mail trunk, n (%)	3 (7.0)	5 (10.2)	0.46
Left anterior descending, n (%)	12 (27.9)	25 (51.0)	<0.01
Left circumflex, n (%)	16 (37.2)	12 (24.5)	0.35
Right coronary disease, n (%)	12 (27.9)	7 (14.3)	0.19
Multivessel coronary disease, n (%)	19 (47.5)	20 (50.0)	0.82
Lesion type B/C2, n (%)	40 (100)	39 (97.5)	0.31
Number of stets per lesion, n (%)	1.3 ± 0.6	1.3 ± 0.7	0.73
Stent diameter (mm)	3.03 ± 0.55	2.85 ± 0.51	0.13
Total stent length (mm)	22.4 ± 14.2	28.3 ± 16.9	0.09
Use of drug eluting stent (%)	27 (67.5)	31 (77.5)	0.32
Stent deployment pressure (atm)	18.3 ± 4.3	18.3 ± 4.5	0.98

Table 3 Cardiovascular events according to FMD

	FMD <4.2 % ($n = 40$)	FMD >4.2 % ($n = 40$)	p
Cardiac death, n (%)	1 (2.5)	0 (0)	0.31
Non-fatal myocardial infarction, n (%)	0 (0)	0 (0)	
Stroke, n (%)	3 (7.5)	1 (2.5)	0.31
Revascularization, n (%)	19 (47.5)	9 (22.5)	0.02
In stent restenosis, n (%)	5 (12.5)	4 (10.0)	0.72
New lesion, n (%)	14 (35.0)	5 (12.5)	0.02
Critical limb ischemia, n (%)	1 (2.5)	0 (0)	0.31
Total, n (%)	24 (60.0)	10 (25.0)	<0.01

Discussion

This study shows that impairment of brachial artery FMD is an independent predictor of cardiovascular events, especially revascularization; however, the brachial artery FMD did not predict in-stent restenosis. Our findings suggest that early evaluation of endothelial function of the brachial artery after PCI can predict cardiovascular events, even in the era of DES.

Our results are in line with previous findings that impaired FMD of the brachial artery is associated with adverse outcomes in patients undergoing coronary stent implantation [8, 11–14, 22], but our study has some differences. In the studies by Patti et al. [14] and Munk et al. [13], the authors reported that impairment of FMD at 30 days after PCI predicted in-stent restenosis in patients with stable CAD at follow-up, while the use of DES was 3 % and 21 %, respectively. However, in our study, almost 70 % of patients were treated with DES. The mechanisms involved in in-stent restenosis include platelet and inflammatory cell activation due to procedural vascular injury, leucocyte adherence, smooth muscle cell proliferation, and extracellular matrix synthesis [23]. Endothelial function affects the association of these factors with in-stent restenosis of bare metal stents. However, in the case of DES, the effect of endothelial function on

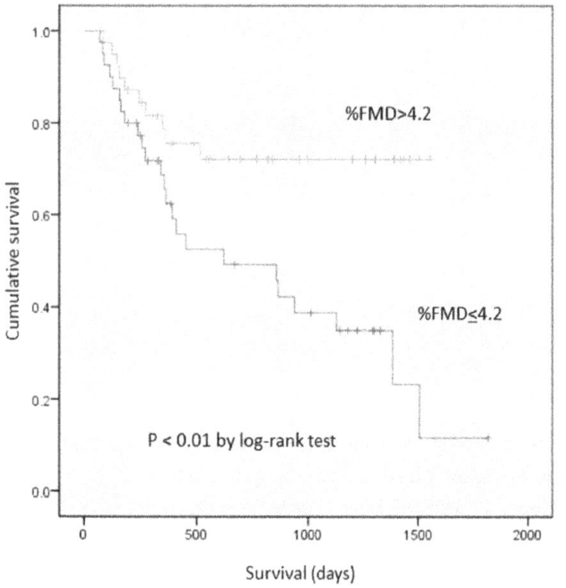

Fig. 2 Kaplan–Meier survival curves for cardiovascular events in patients with FMD <4.2 % and ≥4.2 %

restenosis may be decreased because of strong suppressive effects of coated drugs on the stents.

Endothelial dysfunction has been proposed to be a "barometer" of vascular conditions that integrate the overall effects of risk factors and fundamental defense mechanisms [24]. Therefore, endothelial function determined by FMD in the brachial artery could be associated with the risk of new coronary lesions. In line with this concept, our study showed a significant association of FMD with coronary revascularization in new lesions, but not with in-stent restenosis. Late and very late stent thrombosis is a serious issue associated with DES [25]. Endothelial dysfunction is significantly associated with residual platelet aggregability after dual antiplatelet therapy [26]. The observation period of this study was not sufficient to evaluate late very late stent thrombosis of DES. The association between stent thrombosis and systemic endothelial dysfunction needs to be investigated in a future large study.

Endothelial function reflects the atherosclerotic risk burden at the time of its measurement [27–30]. Our study showed that the low FMD group had lower HDL cholesterol levels and tended to have higher triglyceride levels than the high FMD group, while LDL cholesterol levels were comparable between the two groups. Almost 90 % of our population used statins; therefore, these factors indicated the exact residual risks of CAD. Low HDL

Table 4 Univariate and multivariate Cox proportional hazards analyses of risk factors for cardiovascular events

	Univariate analysis			Multivariate analysis		
	Relative risk	95 % Confidential interval	p	Relative risk	95 % Confidential interval	p
Age >60 years	0.83	0.29–2.39	0.74			
Male	1.07	0.44–2.60	0.88			
Diabetes mellitus	1.53	0.76–3.062	0.23			
Hypertension	0.95	0.45–2.00	0.89			
Dyslipidemia	1.10	0.52–2.31	0.81			
Current smoking	1.32	0.64–2.71	0.45			
Chronic renal insufficiency	0.62	0.31–1.27	0.19			
Previous PCI	0.75	0.290–1.95	0.55			
Previous myocardial infarction	0.04	0.00–11.78	0.27			
LAD vs LCx/RCA	1.03	0.53–2.02	0.93			
Stent diameter <3.0 mm	1.33	0.66–2.67	0.43			
Stented segment length > 15mm	1.00	0.49–2.06	1.00			
Aspirin	21.14	0.00–159472.77	0.50			
Clopidogrel	1.38	0.48–3.93	0.55			
ACE inhibitor / ARB	0.98	0.42–2.26	0.98			
Statins	1.28	0.30–5.37	0.74			
β-blockers	0.50	0.25–1.00	0.05	0.56	0.28–1.13	0.11
FMD <4.2 %	2.60	1.24–5.46	0.01	2.40	1.14–5.06	0.02

PCI Percutaneous coronary intervention, *LAD* Left anterior descending coronary artery, *LCx* Left circumflex coronary artery, *RCA* Right coronary artery, *ACE* Angiotensin-converting enzyme, *ARB* Angiotensin II receptor blocker, *FMD* Flow-mediated dilation cholesterol and high triglyceride levels may contribute to an increase in small dense LDL [31]. Small dense LDL is a highly atherogenic lipoprotein, which affects endothelial function [32, 33]. However, endothelial function is changed by modification of the atherosclerotic risk burden [34, 35]. Our previous study showed that a reduction in triglyceride levels by ezetimibe improved FMD in patients with CAD [36]. In terms of risk factor management, aggressive interventions for residual risks are needed to improve endothelial function, leading to an improvement in the prognosis of patients with CAD.

Endothelial function is affected by several medications. In terms of inhibition of the renin-angiotensin system, a significant difference has been observed between ARBs and ACE inhibitors [37, 38]; some studies have also suggested a difference between different ACE inhibitors [39]. In this study, no difference was observed in the prescription rates of ARBs, ACE inhibitors, or the type of ACE inhibitors between the low and high FMD groups. Statins also improve endothelial function; however, there may be a difference in the effect of different types of statins [40]. We have checked the type of statins used by the study participants, and no difference in the type of statins was observed between the two FMD groups. Thus, the use of these medications is unlikely to have affected the findings of the current study; however, long-term treatment with ACE inhibitors and statins may affect clinical outcome by pleiotropic effects beyond the influence of endothelial function.

Several studies have reported that impairment of endothelial vasomotor function has an adverse effect on clinical outcome in patients with CAD [8, 11–14]. However, there is currently no general agreement on the cut-off value for FMD. Therefore, the application of FMD in clinical practice is difficult. Currently, a large, multicenter prospective study is underway to determine normal values and cut-off values for FMD in the brachial artery, and to assess clinical outcomes [41]. This study will provide important evidence for the usefulness of FMD measurements in the risk stratification for cardiovascular disease.

Recently, use of a bioresorbable vascular scaffold (BVS) has been reported [42, 43]. The implantation of a BVS is a new approach that provides transient vessel mechanical support with drug delivery capability, potentially without permanent metallic implantations. In the process of bioresorption of the polymeric scaffold, endothelial function is important for early and appropriate covering and replacement of the scaffold by endothelial cells and extracellular matrix. Further data relating to the impact of endothelial function on the prognosis of patients with BVS implantation are eagerly awaited.

Limitations

First, this study is preliminary and considerably limited by the small number of study patients. A large prospective trial is required to determine the precise role of systemic endothelial function in the pathogenesis of coronary atherosclerosis. Second, there were relatively few clinical events compared with the numerous variables tested in the multivariate model, resulting in large confidence intervals.

Conclusions

This study shows that impaired brachial artery FMD is an independent determinant of cardiovascular events in the era of DES. In contrast to previous studies, FMD was not a predictor of in-stent restenosis in this study. Our results suggest that early assessment of endothelial function by brachial artery FMD may represent a useful screening tool for risk stratification of future cardiovascular events after PCI using DES. Further large prospective studies are required to evaluate the clinical utility of a brachial artery FMD method in patients with stable angina undergoing PCI.

Abbreviation

ACE inhibitor: Angiotensin-converting enzyme inhibitor; ARB: Angiotensin II receptor blocker; BVS: Bioresorbable vascular scaffold; CAD: Coronary artery disease; DES: Drug-eluting stent; FMD: Flow-mediated dilation; HDL: High-density lipoprotein; LDL: Low-density lipoprotein; PCI: Percutaneous coronary intervention.

Competing interests

The authors declare that they have no competing interests.

Authors' contributions

MK, TM, HO, and YO conceived the study, participated in its design and coordination, and helped to draft the manuscript. KN and HI were involved in drafting the manuscript and critically revising it. All authors read and approved the final manuscript.

Author details

[1]Department of Cardiovascular Medicine, Okayama University Graduate School of Medicine, Dentistry and Pharmaceutical Sciences, Okayama, Japan. [2]Center of Ultrasonography, Okayama University Graduate School of Medicine, Dentistry and Pharmaceutical Sciences, Okayama, Japan.

References

1. Davignon J, Ganz P. Role of endothelial dysfunction in atherosclerosis. Circulation. 2004;109:III27–32.
2. Verma S, Buchanan MR, Anderson TJ. Endothelial function testing as a biomarker of vascular disease. Circulation. 2003;108:2054–9.
3. Charakida M, Masi S, Luscher TF, Kastelein JJ, Deanfield JE. Assessment of atherosclerosis: the role of flow-mediated dilatation. Eur Heart J. 2010;31:2854–61.
4. Corretti MC, Anderson TJ, Benjamin EJ, Celermajer D, Charbonneau F, Creager MA, et al. Guidelines for the ultrasound assessment of endothelial-dependent flow-mediated vasodilation of the brachial artery: a report of the International Brachial Artery Reactivity Task Force. J Am Coll Cardiol. 2002;39:257–65.
5. Donald AE, Halcox JP, Charakida M, Storry C, Wallace SM, Cole TJ, et al. Methodological approaches to optimize reproducibility and power in clinical studies of flow-mediated dilation. J Am Coll Cardiol. 2008;51:1959–64.
6. Muiesan ML, Salvetti M, Paini A, Monteduro C, Galbassini G, Poisa P, et al. Prognostic role of flow-mediated dilatation of the brachial artery in hypertensive patients. J Hypertens. 2008;26:1612–8.

7. Suzuki T, Hirata K, Elkind MS, Jin Z, Rundek T, Miyake Y, et al. Metabolic syndrome, endothelial dysfunction, and risk of cardiovascular events: the Northern Manhattan Study (NOMAS). Am Heart J. 2008;156:405–10.
8. Kitta Y, Obata JE, Nakamura T, Hirano M, Kodama Y, Fujioka D, et al. Persistent impairment of endothelial vasomotor function has a negative impact on outcome in patients with coronary artery disease. J Am Coll Cardiol. 2009;53:323–30.
9. Suwaidi JA, Hamasaki S, Higano ST, Nishimura RA, Holmes Jr DR, Lerman A. Long-term follow-up of patients with mild coronary artery disease and endothelial dysfunction. Circulation. 2000;101:948–54.
10. Kastrati A, Mehilli J, Pache J, Kaiser C, Valgimigli M, Kelbaek H, et al. Analysis of 14 trials comparing sirolimus-eluting stents with bare-metal stents. N Engl J Med. 2007;356:1030–9.
11. Akcakoyun M, Kargin R, Tanalp AC, Pala S, Ozveren O, Akcay M, et al. Predictive value of noninvasively determined endothelial dysfunction for long-term cardiovascular events and restenosis in patients undergoing coronary stent implantation: a prospective study. Coron Artery Dis. 2008;19:337–43.
12. Kitta Y, Nakamura T, Kodama Y, Takano H, Umetani K, Fujioka D, et al. Endothelial vasomotor dysfunction in the brachial artery is associated with late in-stent coronary restenosis. J Am Coll Cardiol. 2005;46:648–55.
13. Munk PS, Butt N, Larsen AI. Endothelial dysfunction predicts clinical restenosis after percutaneous coronary intervention. Scand Cardiovasc J. 2011;45:139–45.
14. Patti G, Pasceri V, Melfi R, Goffredo C, Chello M, D'Ambrosio A, et al. Impaired flow-mediated dilation and risk of restenosis in patients undergoing coronary stent implantation. Circulation. 2005;111:70–5.
15. Serruys PW, Degertekin M, Tanabe K, Abizaid A, Sousa JE, Colombo A, et al. Intravascular ultrasound findings in the multicenter, randomized, double-blind RAVEL (RAndomized study with the sirolimus-eluting VElocity balloon-expandable stent in the treatment of patients with de novo native coronary artery Lesions) trial. Circulation. 2002;106:798–803.
16. Fraker Jr TD, Fihn SD, Gibbons RJ, Abrams J, Chatterjee K, Daley J, et al. 2007 chronic angina focused update of the ACC/AHA 2002 Guidelines for the management of patients with chronic stable angina: a report of the American college of cardiology/American heart association task force on practice guidelines writing group to develop the focused update of the 2002 Guidelines for the management of patients with chronic stable angina. Circulation. 2007;116:2762–72.
17. Yunoki K, Nakamura K, Miyoshi T, Enko K, Kohno K, Morita H, et al. Ezetimibe improves postprandial hyperlipemia and its induced endothelial dysfunction. Atherosclerosis. 2011;217:486–91.
18. Miyoshi T, Noda Y, Ohno Y, Sugiyama H, Oe H, Nakamura K, et al. Omega-3 fatty acids improve postprandial lipemia and associated endothelial dysfunction in healthy individuals - a randomized cross-over trial. Biomed Pharmacother. 2014;68:1071–7.
19. Hicks KA, Tcheng JE, Bozkurt B, Chaitman BR, Cutlip DE, Farb A, et al. 2014 ACC/AHA Key data elements and definitions for cardiovascular endpoint events in clinical trials: a report of the american college of cardiology/ american heart association task force on clinical data standards (Writing Committee to Develop Cardiovascular Endpoints Data Standards). Circulation. 2015;132:302–61.
20. Thygesen K, Alpert JS, Jaffe AS, Simoons ML, Chaitman BR, White HD, et al. Third universal definition of myocardial infarction. Circulation. 2012;126:2020–35.
21. Tonino PA, De Bruyne B, Pijls NH, Siebert U, Ikeno F, Van' t Veer M, et al. Fractional flow reserve versus angiography for guiding percutaneous coronary intervention. N Engl J Med. 2009;360:213–24.
22. Huang PH, Chen JW, Lu TM, Yu-An Ding P, Lin SJ. Combined use of endothelial function assessed by brachial ultrasound and high-sensitive C-reactive protein in predicting cardiovascular events. Clin Cardiol. 2007;30:135–40.
23. Ferns GA, Avades TY. The mechanisms of coronary restenosis: insights from experimental models. Int J Exp Pathol. 2000;81:63–88.
24. Vita JA, Keaney Jr JF. Endothelial function: a barometer for cardiovascular risk? Circulation. 2002;106:640–2.
25. Windecker S, Meier B. Late coronary stent thrombosis. Circulation. 2007;116:1952–65.
26. Fujisue K, Sugiyama S, Ono T, Matsuzawa Y, Akiyama E, Sugamura K, et al. Effects of endothelial dysfunction on residual platelet aggregability after dual antiplatelet therapy with aspirin and clopidogrel in patients with stable coronary artery disease. Circ Cardiovasc Interv. 2013;6:452–9.
27. Bonetti PO, Lerman LO, Lerman A. Endothelial dysfunction: a marker of atherosclerotic risk. Arterioscler Thromb Vasc Biol. 2003;23:168–75.
28. Celermajer DS, Sorensen KE, Gooch VM, Spiegelhalter DJ, Miller OI, Sullivan ID, et al. Non-invasive detection of endothelial dysfunction in children and adults at risk of atherosclerosis. Lancet. 1992;340:1111–5.
29. Vita JA, Treasure CB, Nabel EG, McLenachan JM, Fish RD, Yeung AC, et al. Coronary vasomotor response to acetylcholine relates to risk factors for coronary artery disease. Circulation. 1990;81:491–7.
30. Widlansky ME, Gokce N, Keaney Jr JF, Vita JA. The clinical implications of endothelial dysfunction. J Am Coll Cardiol. 2003;42:1149–60.
31. Querton L, Buysschaert M, Hermans MP. Hypertriglyceridemia and residual dyslipidemia in statin-treated, patients with diabetes at the highest risk for cardiovascular disease and achieving very-low low-density lipoprotein-cholesterol levels. J Clin Lipidol. 2012;6:434–42.
32. Wakatsuki A, Ikenoue N, Shinohara K, Watanabe K, Fukaya T. Small low-density lipoprotein particles and endothelium-dependent vasodilation in postmenopausal women. Atherosclerosis. 2004;177:329–36.
33. Woodman RJ, Watts GF, Playford DA, Best JD, Chan DC. Oxidized LDL and small LDL particle size are independently predictive of a selective defect in microcirculatory endothelial function in type 2 diabetes. Diabetes Obes Metab. 2005;7:612–7.
34. Anderson TJ, Meredith IT, Yeung AC, Frei B, Selwyn AP, Ganz P. The effect of cholesterol-lowering and antioxidant therapy on endothelium-dependent coronary vasomotion. N Engl J Med. 1995;332:488–93.
35. Mancini GB, Henry GC, Macaya C, O'Neill BJ, Pucillo AL, Carere RG, et al. Angiotensin-converting enzyme inhibition with quinapril improves endothelial vasomotor dysfunction in patients with coronary artery disease. The TREND (Trial on Reversing ENdothelial Dysfunction) Study. Circulation. 1996;94:258–65.
36. Yunoki K, Nakamura K, Miyoshi T, Enko K, Kubo M, Murakami M, et al. Impact of hypertriglyceridemia on endothelial dysfunction during statin +/- ezetimibe therapy in patients with coronary heart disease. J Am Coll Cardiol. 2011;108:333–9.
37. Virdis A, Ghiadoni L, Taddei S. Effects of antihypertensive treatment on endothelial function. Curr Hypertens Rep. 2011;13:276–81.
38. Cangiano E, Marchesini J, Campo G, Francolini G, Fortini C, Carra G, et al. ACE inhibition modulates endothelial apoptosis and renewal via endothelial progenitor cells in patients with acute coronary syndromes. Am J Cardiovasc Drugs. 2011;11:189–98.
39. Ceconi C, Francolini G, Bastianon D, Gitti GL, Comini L, Ferrari R. Differences in the effect of angiotensin-converting enzyme inhibitors on the rate of endothelial cell apoptosis: in vitro and in vivo studies. Cardiovasc Drugs Ther. 2007;21:423–9.
40. Reriani MK, Dunlay SM, Gupta B, West CP, Rihal CS, Lerman LO, et al. Effects of statins on coronary and peripheral endothelial function in humans: a systematic review and meta-analysis of randomized controlled trials. Eur J Cardiovasc Prev Rehabil. 2011;18:704–16.
41. Tomiyama H, Kohro T, Higashi Y, Takase B, Suzuki T, Ishizu T, et al. A multicenter study design to assess the clinical usefulness of semi-automatic measurement of flow-mediated vasodilatation of the brachial artery. Int Heart J. 2012;53:170–5.
42. Serruys PW, Chevalier B, Dudek D, Cequier A, Carrie D, Iniguez A, et al. A bioresorbable everolimus-eluting scaffold versus a metallic everolimus-eluting stent for ischaemic heart disease caused by de-novo native coronary artery lesions (ABSORB II): an interim 1-year analysis of clinical and procedural secondary outcomes from a randomised controlled trial. Lancet. 2015;385:43–54.
43. Ormiston JA, Serruys PW, Regar E, Dudek D, Thuesen L, Webster MW, et al. A bioabsorbable everolimus-eluting coronary stent system for patients with single de-novo coronary artery lesions (ABSORB): a prospective open-label trial. Lancet. 2008;371:899–907.

15

Adverse clinical outcomes associated with a low dose and a high dose of aspirin following percutaneous coronary intervention

Pravesh Kumar Bundhun[1], Girish Janoo[2], Abhishek Rishikesh Teeluck[2] and Wei-Qiang Huang[1*]

Abstract

Background: Guidelines from the American Heart Association/American College of Cardiology recommend a higher dosage of aspirin daily following Percutaneous Coronary Intervention (PCI), whereas guidelines from the European Society of Cardiology recommend a lower dosage. This study aimed to compare the adverse clinical outcomes associated with a low dose and a high dose of aspirin following PCI.

Methods: Electronic databases were searched for studies comparing a low dose with a high dose aspirin following PCI. Adverse clinical outcomes were considered as the endpoints in this study. We calculated Odds Ratios (OR) with 95 % Confidence Intervals (CIs) for categorical variables. The pooled analyses were performed with RevMan 5.3 software.

Results: A total number of 25,083 patients were included. Results from this analysis showed that the combination of Cardiovascular (CV) death/Myocardial Infarction (MI) or stroke was not significantly different between a low and high dose of aspirin with OR: 1.08, 95 % CI: 0.98–1.18; $P = 0.11$. Mortality and MI were also not significantly different between these two treatment regimens following PCI with OR: 0.95, 95 % CI: 0.74–1.23; $P = 0.71$ and OR: 1.17, 95 % CI: 0.97–1.41; $P = 0.09$ respectively. However, a high dose of aspirin was associated with a significantly higher rate of Major Adverse Cardiac Events (MACEs) with OR: 1.20, 95 % CI: 1.02–1.41; $P = 0.03$. Thrombolysis In Myocardial Infarction (TIMI) defined minor bleeding was also significantly higher with a high dose aspirin with OR: 1.22, 95 % CI: 1.02–1.47; $P = 0.03$. When Stent thrombosis (ST) was compared, no significant difference was found with OR: 1.28, 95 % CI: 0.59–2.58; $P = 0.53$. Even if TIMI defined major bleeding favored a low dose of aspirin, with OR: 1.42, 95 % CI: 0.95–2.13; $P = 0.09$, or even if major bleeding was insignificantly higher with a high dose aspirin, with OR: 1.78, 95 % CI: 1.01–3.13; $P = 0.05$; $I^2 = 94$ %, higher levels of heterogeneity observed in these subgroups could not be considered significant to any extent.
(Continued on next page)

* Correspondence: huangwq1029@126.com
[1]Institute of Cardiovascular Diseases, the First Affiliated Hospital of Guangxi Medical University, Nanning, Guangxi 530027, People's Republic of China
Full list of author information is available at the end of the article

(Continued from previous page)

Conclusion: According to the results of this analysis, a high dose of aspirin following PCI was not associated with any significantly higher rate of CV death/MI/stroke, mortality or MI. However, MACEs significantly favored a low dose of aspirin. In addition, TIMI defined minor bleeding was significantly higher with a high dose of aspirin whereas the results for the major bleeding outcomes were not statistically significant. However, due to limited data availability and since the subgroups analyzing major bleeding were highly heterogeneous, further studies are recommended to completely solve this issue.

Keywords: Aspirin, Percutaneous coronary intervention, Bleeding, Major adverse cardiac events, Cardiovascular death, Meta-analysis

Abbreviations: ACS, Acute coronary syndrome; MACEs, Major adverse cardiac events; OR, Odds ratio; PCI, Percutaneous coronary intervention; TIMI defined bleeding, Thrombolysis in myocardial infarction defined bleeding

Background

Percutaneous Coronary Intervention (PCI) is considered to be among the most preferred invasive procedures carried out in patients with Acute Coronary Syndrome (ACS). Dual Anti-Platelet Therapy (DAPT) with aspirin and a P2Y12 inhibitor mainly clopidogrel, showed increased benefits in reducing adverse clinical outcomes following PCI with Drug Eluting Stents (DES) or Bare Metal Stents (BMS) [1]. Therefore, the American College of Cardiology/American Heart Association [2] recommends at least one-year treatment with DAPT after PCI with DES whereas the European Society of Cardiology [3] recommends 6 to 12 months DAPT use after intracoronary stenting by DES. For BMS, the duration period for DAPT is even shorter (1 month) compared to DES. However, uncertainty regarding the optimal dosage of aspirin is still a fact which remains to be solved [4]. Guidelines from the American Heart Association/American College of Cardiology recommend higher doses of aspirin (162 to 325 mg) daily following PCI [5], whereas guidelines from the European Society of Cardiology recommend lower doses (75 to 100 mg) [6]. This current analysis aimed to compare the adverse clinical outcomes associated with a low dose and a high dose of aspirin in patients with ACS following PCI with either DES or BMS.

Methods

Data sources and search strategy

The Cochrane Library, PubMed, Medline and EMBASE were searched for studies comparing a low dose with a high dose of aspirin following PCI by typing the words or phrases 'low and high dose aspirin and percutaneous coronary intervention'. Another search was conducted using the words 'aspirin and acute coronary syndrome or drug eluting stents/bare metal stents' [aspirin + acute coronary syndrome/aspirin + percutaneous coronary intervention/aspirin + drug eluting stents/bare metal stents/low and/or high dose aspirin + percutaneous coronary intervention]. In order to enhance this search, abbreviations such as ASA, ACS, DES/BMS and PCI were also used as well as the terms 'coronary angioplasty', 'coronary intervention' and 'single or double dose aspirin' [ASA + PCI/ASA + percutaneous coronary intervention/ASA + acute coronary syndrome/ASA + ACS/ASA + DES/BMS/ASA + coronary angioplasty]. Medical journals which were expected to publish articles related to coronary interventions such as the Journal of Circulation, the Journal of the American College of Cardiology, Euro-intervention, the American Journal of Cardiology and BMC cardiovascular disorders were also searched using the above mentioned terms for relevant articles. Moreover, reference lists of suitable articles were also searched for relevant studies. This search was restricted to articles published in English.

Inclusion and exclusion criteria

Studies were included if:

(a) They were Randomized Controlled Trials (RCTs) or observational studies comparing a low dose with a high dose of aspirin following PCI.
(b) They reported adverse outcomes as their clinical endpoints.
(c) They involved any dosage of aspirin, as far as a low dose was compared with a high dose.

Studies were excluded if:

(a) They were meta-analyses, letter to editors and case studies.
(b) They did not report adverse outcomes as their clinical endpoints.
(c) They were duplicates.

Outcomes, definitions and follow ups

The clinical endpoints analyzed included:

(a) Mortality
(b) Myocardial Infarction (MI)

(c) Cardiovascular (CV) death/MI/stroke
(d) Major adverse cardiac events (MACEs) consisting of death, MI and revascularization
(e) Stent Thrombosis (ST)
(f) Major bleeding which was defined as bleeding that was significantly disabling for example intraocular bleeding that lead to significant vision loss, or bleeding requiring transfusion of 2 units of red blood cells or equivalent whole blood, a drop in hemoglobin concentration of 5 g/L, bleeding causing significant hypotension requiring intravenous inotropes or surgical intervention, symptomatic intracranial hemorrhage or bleeding that was fatal
(g) TIMI defined major bleeding [7]
(h) TIMI defined minor bleeding

The outcomes reported and the dosage of aspirin reported among the cohorts as well as their corresponding follow up periods have been summarized in Table 1.

A low dosage of aspirin was defined as any low dosage in accordance to the high dosage of aspirin reported in the same study. For example, if a dosage of aspirin greater than 200 mg was considered a high dosage, then any dosage below 200 mg in the same study should be considered as a low dosage.

Data extraction and quality assessment

Three authors (PKB, GJ and ART) independently assessed the articles selected for this analysis. Information concerning the type of study reported, the total number of patients treated with a low and high dose of aspirin respectively, data concerning the baseline characteristics of the patients, the reported outcomes and follow up periods were carefully extracted. If any disagreement about including certain data occurred, it was discussed among these three authors and if they could not reach a consensus, a final decision was made by the fourth author (WQH). Bias risk was assessed in accordance to the components recommended by the Cochrane Collaboration [8].

Methodological quality and statistical analysis

Recommendations of the PRISMA (Preferred Reporting Items for Systematic Reviews and Meta-Analyses) statement were followed since this is a meta-analysis involving mostly trials [9]. Heterogeneity across the subgroups was assessed using the Cochrane Q-statistic test (whereby a P value $< 0 \cdot 05$ was considered statistically significant whereas a P value > 0.05 was considered statistically insignificant) and the I^2-statistic test (whereby an I^2 with low percentage represented a lower heterogeneity and an increasing percentage denoted an increasing heterogeneity). If I^2 was less than 50 %, a fixed effect model was used. However, if I^2 was more than 50 %, a random effect model was used. Publication bias was visually estimated by assessing funnel plots. We calculated Odds Ratios (OR) and 95 % Confidence Intervals (CIs) for categorical variables. The pooled analyses were performed with RevMan 5.3 software. Ethical approval was not required for systematic reviews and meta-analyses. All the authors had full access to the data and approved the manuscript as written.

Results

Search results

A total number of 622 articles were obtained from the Cochrane Library, PubMed, Medline and EMBASE and from reference lists of suitable articles. After a careful assessment of titles and abstracts, 584 articles were eliminated since they were not related to our topic. A further 26 articles were eliminated since they were duplicates. 12 full-text articles were assessed for eligibility. Eight more articles were eliminated: one article was a systematic review of the literature, two article did not report adverse clinical outcomes and two articles which could probably satisfy the inclusion and exclusion criteria of our study were not made available by the authors, one article did not include data which could be used in this analysis, and another two trials were the subset of other trials included in this analysis. Finally, four articles (3 trials and 1 observational study) [4, 10–13] were included in this systematic review and meta-analysis. The flow diagram for the study selection has been represented in Fig. 1.

General features of the studies included

The general features of the studies included in this meta-analysis have been listed in Table 2.

A total number of 25,083 patients (14,402 patients were assigned to a low dose of aspirin and 10,681 patients were assigned to a high dose of aspirin) were included in this analysis.

Table 1 Reported outcomes

Studies	Outcomes reported	Dosage of aspirin	Follow up periods
GHOST	MACEs, ST, Death or MI, TIMI bleeding	81 mg vs 160–325 mg	1 year
CURRENT OASIS 7	Death/MI/stroke, death, MI, stroke, TIMI major and minor bleeding	≤100 mg vs ≥ 300 mg	30 days
CURE	CV death/MI/stroke, major bleeding	<200 mg vs ≥ 200 mg	1 year
HORIZONS-AMI	MACEs, mortality, MI, stroke, major bleeding, TIMI major and minor bleeding, ST	≤200 mg vs > 200 mg	3 years

Abbreviations: *MI* myocardial infarction, *TIMI* thrombolysis in myocardial infarction, *MACEs* major adverse cardiac events, *ST* stent thrombosis, *CV* cardiovascular

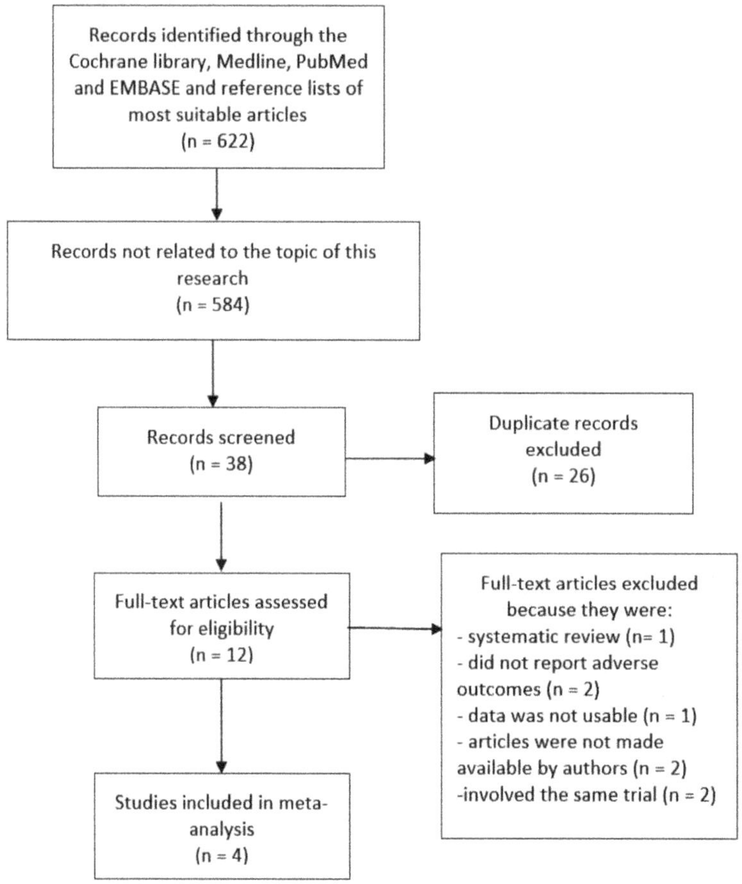

Fig. 1 Flow diagram representing the study selection

Baseline characteristics of the studies included

The baseline features of the patients have been listed in Table 3 whereas Table 4 shows the other antiplatelet/anticoagulants used by the patients during the procedure or following PCI. According to these baseline features, no significant differences were observed between patients assigned to a low dose and a high dose of aspirin respectively.

Clinical outcomes reported

Results from this analysis (Table 5) showed that the combination of CV death/MI or stroke was not significantly different between a low and a high dose of aspirin following PCI with OR: 1.08, 95 % CI: 0.98–1.18; $P = 0.11$, $I^2 = 0$ %. Mortality and MI were also not significantly different between these two treatment regimens after PCI with OR: 0.95, 95 % CI: 0.74–1.23; $P = 0.71$, $I^2 = 7$ % and OR: 1.17, 95 % CI: 0.97–1.41; $P = 0.09$, $I^2 = 33$ % respectively. However, a high dose of aspirin was associated with a significantly higher rate of MACEs with OR: 1.20, 95 % CI: 1.02–1.41; $P = 0.03$, $I^2 = 35$ %. TIMI defined minor bleeding was also significantly higher with a high dose aspirin with OR: 1.22, 95 % CI: 1.02–1.47; $P = 0.03$; $I^2 = 44$ %. These results have been represented in Fig. 2.

Table 2 General features of the studies included

Studies	Type of study	No of patients with low dose ASA (n)	No of patients with high dose ASA (n)	Total no of patients (n)	Type of P2Y12 inhibitor used
GHOST [10]	observational	313	2507	2820	clopidogrel
CURRENT OASIS 7 [11]	RCT	3371	3502	6873	clopidogrel
CURE [4, 12]	RCT	8429	4110	12,539	clopidogrel
HORIZONS-AMI [13]	RCT	2289	562	2851	clopidogrel
Total no of patients (n)		14,402	10,681	25,083	

Only female patients were included from trial CURRENT OASIS 7 in order to avoid the influence of this trial on the results of this analysis
Abbreviations: *ASA* aspirin, *RCT* randomized controlled trials

Table 3 Baseline features of the patients included in this analysis

Studies	Mean age (years)	Males (%)	Ht (%)	Ds (%)	Cs (%)	DM (%)
	L/H	L/H	L/H	L/H	L/H	L/H
GHOST	67.0/64.0	64.0/70.0	73.0/65.0	76.0/72.0	19.0/27.0	12.0/8.0
CURRENT OASIS 7	61.2/61.5	0.00/0.00	60.2/60.4	40.9/41.4	33.6/33.2	23.1/23.8
CURE	-	58.8/65.4	58.8/60.5	-	20.8/25.1	21.0/26.8
HORIZONS-AMI	59.9/58.8	76.3/79.4	50.6/58.2	42.3/47.9	65.0/63.5	16.6/15.8

Abbreviations: *L* low dose, *H* high dose, *Ht* hypertension, *Ds* dyslipidemia, *Cs* current smoker, *DM* diabetes mellitus

When ST was compared between these two groups, no significant difference was found with OR: 1.28, 95 % CI: 0.59–2.58; $P = 0.53$, $I^2 = 65$ %. Even if TIMI defined major bleeding favored a low dose aspirin, with OR: 1.42, 95 % CI: 0.95–2.13; $P = 0.09$; I2 = 59 %, the result was not statistically significant. Moreover, even if major bleeding was higher with a high dose aspirin, with OR: 1.78, 95 % CI: 1.01–3.13; $P = 0.05$; $I^2 = 94$ %, the level of heterogeneity was much higher that it could not be considered significant to any extent. These results have been represented in Fig. 3.

For all of the above analyses, sensitivity analyses yielded consistent results. Based on a visual inspection of the funnel plot obtained, there has been little evidence of publication bias for the included studies that assessed several clinical endpoints. However, a high level of heterogeneity was observed among the subgroups analyzing stent thrombosis and the major bleeding outcomes. The funnel plot showing the sensitivity analysis has been represented in Fig. 4.

Discussion

This study aimed to compare the adverse clinical outcomes associated with a low dose and a high dose of aspirin following PCI. Results of this study showed that a high dose of aspirin was not associated with a significantly higher rate of mortality, CV death/MI/stroke and MI. ST was also not significantly different between these two dosages of aspirin. However, MACEs significantly favored a low dose aspirin. In addition, a high dose of aspirin was associated with a significantly higher rate of TIMI defined minor bleeding, without any significant increase in TIMI defined major bleeding major bleeding after PCI.

The systematic review of literature [14] which was meant to show any association between aspirin dosing and cardiac and bleeding events after treatment of ACS showed no improved clinical outcomes associated with a high dose of aspirin following PCI among the 289,330 patients analyzed. 2.1 % of patients experienced major bleeding when treated with a high dose of aspirin whereas only 1.9 % of patients treated with a low dose of aspirin following stent implantation experienced major bleeding.

Moreover, the investigators of the CURRENT OASIS 7 [11] concluded that in patients with ACS who were referred for an invasive strategy, no significant difference in primary outcome of cardiovascular death, MI or stroke was observed between a low and a high dose of aspirin. However, only a follow up period of 7 days was considered.

Also, the study published by Joyal et al. [15] demonstrating the influence of a low dose (81 mg) versus a high dose (325 mg) of aspirin on the incidence of sirolimus eluting stents showed a similar rate of ST to be associated with either a low or a high dose of aspirin. The

Table 4 Other antiplatelet/anticoagulants used by the patients included in this analysis

Other antiplatelets/ anticoagulants	GHOST	CURRENT OASIS 7	CURE	HORIZONS-AMI
Heparin	+++	–	–	–
GP IIb/IIIa inhibitors	+	+	+++	–
Oral anticoagulants (warfarin/Coumadin)	+	–	+	+
Clopidogrel	++++	++++	++++	++++

Abbreviations: *GP* glycoproteins, "+": less than 25 % of patients, "++": 26 to 50 % of patients, "+++": 51 to 75 % of patients, "++++": 76 to 100 % of patients

Table 5 Results of this analysis

Outcomes analyzed	OR with 95 % CI	*P* value	I^2 (%)
Mortality	0.95 [0.74–1.23]	0.71	7
MI	1.17 [0.97–1.41]	0.09	33
CV death/MI/stroke	1.08 [0.98–1.18]	0.11	0
MACEs	1.20 [1.02–1.41]	0.03	35
ST	1.28 [0.59–2.78]	0.53	65
Major bleeding	1.78 [1.01–3.13]	0.05	94
TIMI major bleeding	1.42 [0.95–2.13]	0.09	59
TIMI minor bleeding	1.22 [1.02–1.47]	0.03	44

Abbreviations: *MI* myocardial infarction, *TIMI* thrombolysis in myocardial infarction, *MACEs* major adverse cardiac events, *ST* stent thrombosis, *CV* cardiovascular, *OR* odds ratio, *CI* confidence intervals

Study or Subgroup	High dose ASA Events	High dose ASA Total	Low dose ASA Events	Low dose ASA Total	Weight	Odds Ratio M-H, Fixed, 95% CI
1.1.1 CV death/MI/stroke						
CURE	715	4110	1355	8429	43.5%	1.10 [1.00, 1.21]
CURRENT OASIS 7	148	3502	147	3371	8.5%	0.97 [0.77, 1.22]
Subtotal (95% CI)		**7612**		**11800**	**52.0%**	**1.08 [0.98, 1.18]**
Total events	863		1502			
Heterogeneity: Chi² = 0.97, df = 1 (P = 0.32); I² = 0%						
Test for overall effect: Z = 1.61 (P = 0.11)						
1.1.2 Mortality						
CURRENT OASIS 7	76	3502	84	3371	5.0%	0.87 [0.63, 1.19]
HORIZONS-AMI	26	562	92	2289	2.1%	1.16 [0.74, 1.81]
Subtotal (95% CI)		**4064**		**5660**	**7.0%**	**0.95 [0.74, 1.23]**
Total events	102		176			
Heterogeneity: Chi² = 1.08, df = 1 (P = 0.30); I² = 7%						
Test for overall effect: Z = 0.37 (P = 0.71)						
1.1.3 Myocardial Infarction (MI)						
CURE	67	1064	77	1594	3.4%	1.32 [0.95, 1.85]
CURRENT OASIS 7	71	3502	70	3371	4.1%	0.98 [0.70, 1.36]
GHOST	153	2507	21	313	2.1%	0.90 [0.56, 1.45]
HORIZONS-AMI	44	562	124	2289	2.7%	1.48 [1.04, 2.12]
Subtotal (95% CI)		**7635**		**7567**	**12.3%**	**1.17 [0.97, 1.41]**
Total events	335		292			
Heterogeneity: Chi² = 4.50, df = 3 (P = 0.21); I² = 33%						
Test for overall effect: Z = 1.67 (P = 0.09)						
1.1.4 Major Adverse Cardiac Events (MACEs)						
CURE	101	1064	147	1594	6.3%	1.03 [0.79, 1.35]
GHOST	231	2507	27	313	2.6%	1.08 [0.71, 1.63]
HORIZONS-AMI	125	562	391	2289	7.1%	1.39 [1.11, 1.74]
Subtotal (95% CI)		**4133**		**4196**	**16.0%**	**1.20 [1.02, 1.41]**
Total events	457		565			
Heterogeneity: Chi² = 3.09, df = 2 (P = 0.21); I² = 35%						
Test for overall effect: Z = 2.20 (P = 0.03)						
1.1.5 TIMI minor bleeding						
CURRENT OASIS 7	173	3502	148	3371	8.5%	1.13 [0.90, 1.42]
GHOST	467	2507	46	313	3.9%	1.33 [0.96, 1.85]
HORIZONS-AMI	6	562	8	2289	0.2%	3.08 [1.06, 8.90]
Subtotal (95% CI)		**6571**		**5973**	**12.6%**	**1.22 [1.02, 1.47]**
Total events	646		202			
Heterogeneity: Chi² = 3.60, df = 2 (P = 0.17); I² = 44%						
Test for overall effect: Z = 2.15 (P = 0.03)						
Total (95% CI)		**30015**		**35196**	**100.0%**	**1.12 [1.05, 1.19]**
Total events	2403		2737			
Heterogeneity: Chi² = 17.34, df = 13 (P = 0.18); I² = 25%						
Test for overall effect: Z = 3.34 (P = 0.0008)						
Test for subgroup differences: Chi² = 3.93, df = 4 (P = 0.42), I² = 0%						

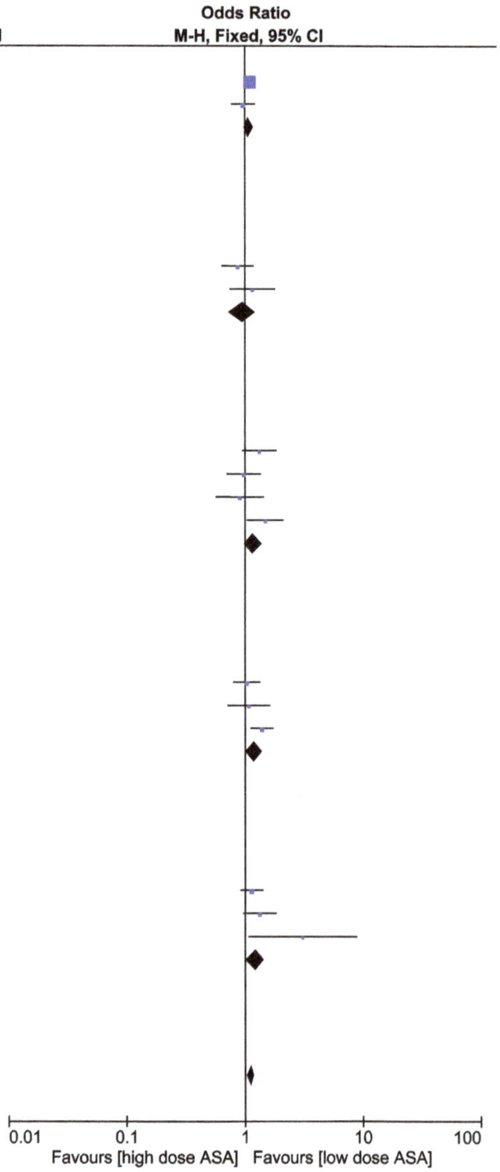

Fig. 2 Adverse clinical outcomes reported between a low and a high dose of aspirin

Ottawa Heart Institute PCI Registry [16] which involved 930 patients discharged on 325 mg aspirin and 910 patients discharged on 81 mg aspirin showed no difference in death or MI at 1 year between these two different dosages of aspirin. In addition, another study investigating the influence of low dose aspirin (81 mg) on the incidence of definite stent thrombosis in patients receiving BMS and DES concluded that a low dose of aspirin following PCI was not associated with any increase in definite stent thrombosis compared to a high dose [17].

However, results from the Dual Antiplatelet Therapy Study [18] showed that a high dose of aspirin might be associated with adverse events and the authors suggested that a low dose of aspirin might be the target to improve clinical outcomes after PCI reflecting the results of this current analysis.

Nevertheless, when prasugrel was compared with clopidogrel, with a high and low dose aspirin respectively, prasugrel was associated with better clinical outcomes irrespective of the dosage of aspirin as demonstrated in the TRITON TIMI 38 trial whereby 12,674 patients were classified into a low and high dose aspirin groups [19]. No meaningful interaction of aspirin with clopidogrel was observed. However, this current analysis was different and was focused mainly on comparing a low with a high dose of aspirin following PCI.

Study or Subgroup	High dose ASA Events	High dose ASA Total	Low dose ASA Events	Low dose ASA Total	Weight	Odds Ratio M-H, Random, 95% CI
1.1.1 Stent thrombosis (ST)						
GHOST	45	2507	7	313	7.7%	0.80 [0.36, 1.79]
HORIZONS-AMI	27	562	63	2289	12.2%	1.78 [1.13, 2.83]
Subtotal (95% CI)		**3069**		**2602**	**19.9%**	**1.28 [0.59, 2.78]**
Total events	72		70			
Heterogeneity: Tau² = 0.21; Chi² = 2.88, df = 1 (P = 0.09); I² = 65%						
Test for overall effect: Z = 0.63 (P = 0.53)						
1.1.2 Major bleeding						
CURE	201	4110	265	8429	16.0%	1.58 [1.31, 1.91]
CURRENT OASIS 7	331	3502	318	3371	16.3%	1.00 [0.85, 1.18]
HORIZONS-AMI	33	562	34	2289	11.8%	4.14 [2.54, 6.74]
Subtotal (95% CI)		**8174**		**14089**	**44.1%**	**1.78 [1.01, 3.13]**
Total events	565		617			
Heterogeneity: Tau² = 0.23; Chi² = 35.87, df = 2 (P < 0.00001); I² = 94%						
Test for overall effect: Z = 1.98 (P = 0.05)						
1.1.3 TIMI major bleeding						
CURRENT OASIS 7	55	3502	49	3371	13.3%	1.08 [0.73, 1.59]
GHOST	467	2507	46	313	14.2%	1.33 [0.96, 1.85]
HORIZONS-AMI	12	562	18	2289	8.5%	2.75 [1.32, 5.75]
Subtotal (95% CI)		**6571**		**5973**	**36.0%**	**1.42 [0.95, 2.13]**
Total events	534		113			
Heterogeneity: Tau² = 0.07; Chi² = 4.85, df = 2 (P = 0.09); I² = 59%						
Test for overall effect: Z = 1.70 (P = 0.09)						
Total (95% CI)		**17814**		**22664**	**100.0%**	**1.54 [1.14, 2.08]**
Total events	1171		800			
Heterogeneity: Tau² = 0.14; Chi² = 43.88, df = 7 (P < 0.00001); I² = 84%						
Test for overall effect: Z = 2.80 (P = 0.005)						
Test for subgroup differences: Chi² = 0.57, df = 2 (P = 0.75), I² = 0%						

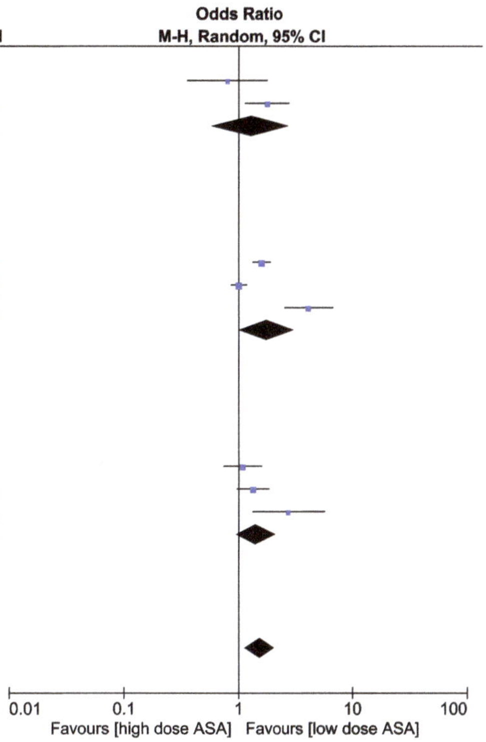

Fig. 3 Stent thrombosis, major bleeding outcomes reported between a low and a high dose of aspirin

Novelty

This study is new in the way that it is among the first systematic review and meta-analyses comparing a low dose with a high dose of aspirin following PCI. Moreover, several adverse outcomes have been analyzed. This study also included a large number of patients from randomized trials compared to patients from observational studies and reported a low or moderate level of heterogeneity among several subgroups assessing these clinical endpoints. Since dosage of aspirin following PCI could

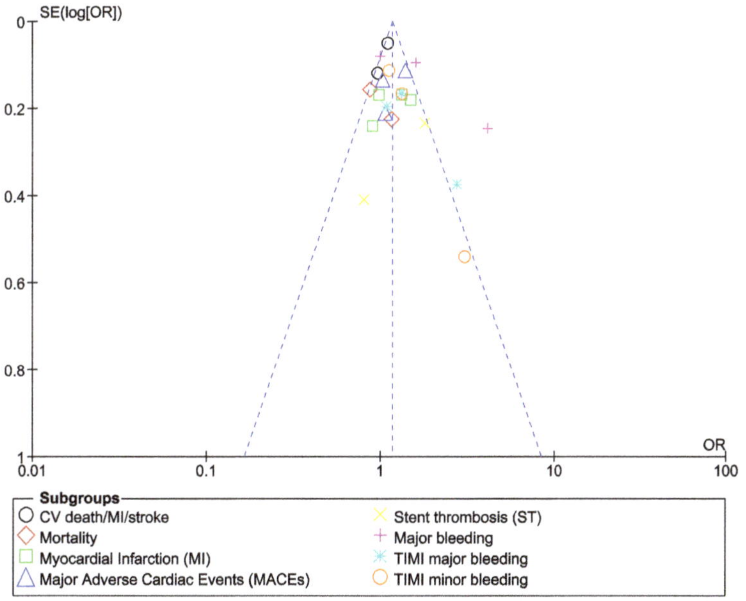

Fig. 4 Funnel plot showing sensitivity analysis

be an important issue in several types of patients, this analysis could inspire other scientists to conduct further research in this particular field.

Limitations

This study also has limitations. First of all, due to the limited number of patients and studies, this analysis might not provide robust results. Secondly, because this analysis also included data obtained from observational studies along with data obtained from randomized trials, selection bias could possibly have been introduced. Moreover, one study had a follow-up period of 3 years and another one had a follow up period of 1 month. They have been included among other studies with a follow-up period of 1 year and analyzed altogether. This could be another limitation. In addition, several subgroups analyzed only compared data from two or three studies which could strictly affect the results and should be considered another limiting factor in this meta-analysis. A high level of heterogeneity observed among the several subgroups analyzing stent thrombosis, and major bleedings could be another limitation in this study. In addition, different studies reported different dosage of aspirin. This could also be a limiting factor in this study. Also, only the percentage of patients representing the female population were included from the trial CURRENT OASIS 7, because its large number of patients could influence the results of this analysis. Therefore, this could also be a limitation in this study. It should also be noted that patients involved in this analysis varied from stable coronary diseases, ST segment elevated MI or non-ST segment elevated MI representing another probable limitation to this study. However, the main focus was on patients who underwent PCI. Also, almost all of the studies were sub-group analysis of trials whereby patients were not randomized specifically to a low and high dosage of aspirin respectively, therefore, the groups might not necessarily be comparable thus rendering the introduction of potentially confounding variables possible, which could have a great impact on the results of this current analysis. Another limitation could be the influence of glycoprotein IIb/IIIa inhibitors used peri-operatively, and other anticoagulants which were used differently following PCI in different studies, possibly affecting the bleeding outcomes.

Conclusion

According to the results of this analysis, a high dose of aspirin following PCI was not associated with any significantly higher rate of CV death/MI/stroke, mortality or MI. However, MACEs significantly favored a low dose of aspirin. In addition, TIMI defined minor bleeding was significantly higher with a high dose of aspirin whereas the results for the major bleeding outcomes were not statistically significant. However, due to limited data availability and since the subgroups analyzing major bleeding were highly heterogeneous, further studies are recommended to completely solve this issue.

Acknowledgements

There was no external source of funding for this research and no writing assistance was required.

Funding

There was no external source of funding for this research.

Authors' contributions

PKB, GJ, ART and WQH were responsible for the conception and design, acquisition of data, analysis and interpretation of data, drafting the initial manuscript and revising it critically for important intellectual content. PKB wrote this manuscript. All authors read and approved the final manuscript.

Competing interests

The authors declare that they have no competing interests.

Author details

[1]Institute of Cardiovascular Diseases, the First Affiliated Hospital of Guangxi Medical University, Nanning, Guangxi 530027, People's Republic of China. [2]Guangxi Medical University, Nanning, Guangxi 530027, People's Republic of China.

References

1. Bhatt DL. Intensifying platelet inhibition–navigating between Scylla and charybdis. N Engl J Med. 2007;357(20):2078–81.
2. Levine GN, Bates ER, Blankenship JC, et al. American college of cardiology foundation; American heart association task force on PracticeGuidelines; society for cardiovascular angiography and interventions. 2011 ACCF/AHA/SCAI guideline for percutaneous coronary intervention. A report of the American college ofCardiology foundation/American heart association task force on practice guidelines and the society for cardiovascular angiography and interventions. J Am Coll Cardiol. 2011;58(24):e44–122. doi:10.1016/j.jacc.2011.08.007.
3. Authors/Task Force members, Windecker S, Kolh P, et al. 2014 ESC/EACTS guidelines on myocardial revascularization: the task force on myocardial revascularizationof the European society of cardiology (ESC) and the European association for cardio-thoracic surgery(EACTS)developed with the special contribution of the European association of percutaneous CardiovascularInterventions (EAPCI). Eur Heart J. 2014;35(37):2541–619. doi:10.1093/eurheartj/ehu278.
4. Peters RJ, Mehta SR, Fox KA, et al. Clopidogrel in unstable angina to preventRecurrent events (CURE) trial investigators. Effects of aspirin dose when used alone or in combination with clopidogrel in patients with acute coronary syndromes: observations from the clopidogrel in unstable angina to prevent recurrent events (CURE) study. Circulation. 2003;108:1682–7.
5. King 3rd SB, Smith Jr SC, Hirshfeld Jr JW, et al. 2007 focused update of the ACC/AHA/SCAI 2005 guideline update for percutaneous coronary intervention: are port of the American college of cardiology/American heart association task force on practice guidelines. J Am Coll Cardiol. 2008;51(2):172–209.
6. Silber S, Albertsson P, Avilés FF, et al. Task force for percutaneous coronary interventions of the European society of cardiology. Guidelines for percutaneous coronary interventions. The task force for percutaneous coronary interventions of the European society of cardiology. Eur Heart J. 2005;26(8):804–47.
7. The Thrombolysis in Myocardial Infarction (TIMI) trial. Phase I findings. TIMI Study Group. N Engl J Med. 1985;312(14):932–6.

8. Higgins JPT, Altman DG. Assessing risk of bias in included studies. In: Higgins JPT, Green S, editors. Cochrane handbook for systematic reviews of interventions. Wiley;2008. p. 187–241.
9. Liberati A, Altman DG, Tetzlaff J, et al. The PRISMA statement for reporting systematic reviews and meta-analyses of studies that evaluate healthcareinterventions: explanation and elaboration. BMJ. 2009;339:b2700.
10. Harjai KJ, Shenoy C, Orshaw P, et al. Low-dose versus high-dose aspirin after percutaneous coronary intervention: analysis from the guthrie health off-label StenT (GHOST) registry. J Interv Cardiol. 2011;24(4):307–14.
11. CURRENT-OASIS 7 Investigators, Mehta SR, Bassand JP, et al. Dose comparisons of clopidogrel and aspirin in acute coronary syndromes. N Engl J Med. 2010;363(10):930–42.
12. Jolly SS, Pogue J, Haladyn K, et al. Effects of aspirin dose on ischaemic events and bleeding after percutaneous coronary intervention: insightsfrom the PCI-CURE study. Eur Heart J. 2009;30(8):900–7. doi:10.1093/eurheartj/ehn417.
13. Yu J, Mehran R, Dangas GD, et al. Safety and efficacy of high- versus low-dose aspirin after primary percutaneous coronary intervention in ST-segment elevation myocardial infarction: the HORIZONS-AMI (Harmonizing Outcomes With Revascularization and Stents in Acute Myocardial Infarction) trial. JACC Cardiovasc Interv. 2012;5(12):1231–8.
14. Berger JS, Sallum RH, Katona B, et al. Is there an association between aspirin dosing and cardiac and bleeding events after treatment of acute coronarysyndrome? A systematic review of the literature. Am Heart J. 2012;164(2):153-162.e5.
15. Joyal D, Freihage JH, Cohoon K, et al. The influence of low (81 mg) versus high (325 mg) doses of ASA on the incidence of sirolimus-eluting stent thrombosis. J Invasive Cardiol. 2007;19(7):291–4.
16. So D, Cook EF, Le May M, et al. Association of aspirin dosage to clinical outcomes after percutaneous coronary intervention: observations from the Ottawa Heart Institute PCI Registry. J Invasive Cardiol. 2009;21(3):121–7.
17. Lotfi A, Cui J, Wartak S, Columbo J, Mulvey S, Davis M, Schweiger M, Giugliano GR. Influence of low-dose aspirin (81 mg) on the incidence of definite stent thrombosis in patients receiving bare-metal and drug-eluting stents. Clin Cardiol. 2011;34(9):567–71.
18. Matteau A, Yeh RW, Kereiakes D, et al. Frequency of the use of low- versus high-dose aspirin in dual antiplatelet therapy after percutaneous coronaryintervention (from the Dual Antiplatelet Therapy study). Am J Cardiol. 2014;113(7):1146–52.
19. Kohli P, Udell JA, Murphy SA, Cannon CP, Antman EM, Braunwald E, Wiviott SD. Discharge aspirin dose and clinical outcomes in patients with acute coronary syndromes treated withprasugrel versus clopidogrel: an analysis from the TRITON-TIMI 38 study (trial to assess improvement in therapeutic outcomes by optimizing platelet inhibition with prasugrel-thrombolysis in myocardial infarction 38). J Am Coll Cardiol. 2014;63(3):225–32.

16

An Australian longitudinal pilot study examining health determinants of cardiac outcomes 12 months post percutaneous coronary intervention

Karen-leigh Edward[1,2*], John Stephenson[1,2], Jo-Ann Giandinoto[1], Andrew Wilson[3], Robert Whitbourn[3], Jack Gutman[3] and Andrew Newcomb[3]

Abstract

Background: Percutaneous coronary intervention (PCI) is a very common revascularisation procedure for coronary artery disease (CAD). The purpose of this study was to evaluate cardiac outcomes, health related quality of life (HRQoL), resilience and adherence behaviours in patients who have undergone a PCI at two time points (6 and 12 months) following their procedure.

Methods: A longitudinal pilot study was conducted to observe the cardiac outcomes across a cohort of patients who had undergone a percutaneous coronary intervention (PCI). Participants who had undergone PCI 6 months prior were invited. Those participants who met the inclusion criteria and provided consent then completed a telephone survey (time point 1). These participants were then contacted 6 months later (i.e. 12 months post-intervention, time point 2) and the measures were repeated.

Results: All patients ($n = 51$) were recorded as being alive at time point 1. The multiple model indicated that controlling for other factors, gender was significantly associated with a linear combination of outcome measures ($p = 0.004$). The effect was moderate in magnitude (partial-$\eta^2 = 0.303$), where males performed significantly better than females 6 months after the PCI procedure physically and with mood. Follow-up univariate ANOVAs indicated that gender differences were grounded in the scale measuring depression (PHQ9) ($p = 0.005$) and the physical component score of the short form measuring HRQoL (SF12-PCS) ($p = 0.003$). Thirteen patients were lost to follow-up between time points 1 and 2. One patient was confirmed to have passed away. The pattern of correlations between outcome measures at time point 2 revealed statistically significant negative correlation between the PHQ instrument and the resilience scale (CD-RISC) ($r = -0.611$; $p < 0.001$); and the physical component score of the SF-12 instrument ($r = -0.437$; $p = 0.054$).

Conclusions: Men were performing better than women in the 6 months post-PCI, particularly in the areas of mood (depression) and physical health. This pilot results indicate gender-sensitive practices are recommended particularly up to 6 months post-PCI. Any gender differences observed at 6 month appear to disappear at 12 months post-PCI. Further research into the management of mood particularly for women post-PCI is warranted. A more detailed inquiry related to access/attendance to secondary prevention is also warranted.

Keywords: Percutaneous coronary intervention, Wellbeing, Quality of life, Depression, Gender, Resilience

* Correspondence: Karen-leigh.edward@acu.edu.au
[1]Australian Catholic University and St Vincent's Private Hospital Melbourne Ltd, Locked Bag 4115 MDC, Fitzroy 3065, Australia
[2]University of Huddersfield, Huddersfield, United Kingdom
Full list of author information is available at the end of the article

Background

Cardiovascular disease (CVD) has over the last decade emerged as the single most important cause for death worldwide [1]. Two recent international studies, the INTERHEART study in 2005 and the INTERSTROKE study in 2010 have confirmed that in both developing and developed countries, the risk factors for CVD include: smoking, hypertension, abdominal obesity, lack of physical activity, abnormal blood lipid profiles, diabetes, alcohol intake, psychosocial factors and a diet deficient in fruits, vegetables and fish [2, 3]. Percutaneous coronary intervention (PCI) is a very common revascularisation procedure for coronary artery disease (CAD), and indications for PCI include myocardial infarction (MI), stable and unstable angina pectoris (SAP and UAP respectively). In 2000, the age-standardised ratio of PCI procedures in males compared to females was around 3.1 to 1; this is despite males experiencing heart attacks at only twice the rate of females [4]. Irrespective of recent advances in surgical technology, PCI is associated with a range of adverse post-procedural complications, including acute bleeding, cardiac events, vascular complications and mortality [5–7].

A significant proportion of PCI patients also experience mental health issues, although the direction of this relationship is unclear. Anxiety and depression are prevalent in 25-50 % of CAD patients [8–10] and are associated with readmission for further cardiovascular morbidity [9, 11, 12], decreased health-related quality of life and mortality [10, 13]. There is evidence to suggest that levels of anxiety and depression in the majority of PCI patients remain relatively stable 12 months post-procedure, and baseline levels of anxiety and depression are associated with either symptom improvement or deterioration among those who experience changes to distress [14].

Research findings are inconclusive as to the impact of PCI on quality of life post-procedure. Some evidence indicates patients over the age of 70 years are more likely to experience deteriorating and poorer mental and physical health-related quality of life than those under 70 years at 36 months post-intervention, irrespective of adverse events during outcomes [15]. The impact of psychopathology such as anxiety and depression is known to increase risk of readmission [11] and mortality [13], but little is known about the efficacy of psychological interventions on long-term outcomes of PCI. The short term impacts (<6 months) of coronary care for patients indicates HRQoL concerns should not drive revascularisation decisions [16], that mood can predict worsening heart health [17, 18] and QoL should be considered in future research in order to inform practice decisions with this group of patients [19]. There appears to be no studies that have examined the notion of personal resilience in this group of patients.

The aim of this longitudinal prognostic study was to evaluate cardiac outcomes, HRQoL, personal resilience, mental health and adherence behaviours in patients who have had undergone a PCI measured at two time points (6 months and 12 months) post-intervention. The objectives of this study were to (1) inform clinical care practice of the care of patients who undergo PCI, and (2) provide pilot information of patients related to QoL, medication adherence behaviours, personal resilience and mental health post a PCI.

Methods

Research design

A longitudinal pilot study design was undertaken. Observational research, such as this study allowed the use of repeated measures of the same cohort over 12 months. The benefit of this type of study is the ability to assess the significance of predictors of outcomes post-PCI.

Participants and recruitment

Sampling

The study aimed to recruit a total of 49 participants. As a pilot, the study was not powered to detect significant effects or was subject to a formal sample size calculation. However, a sample size was desired which would allow the assessment of incidence rates with a 95 % confidence interval with +/- 10 % precision (i.e. to have 95 % confidence that the estimated rate was within 10 % of its true value in the population) assuming a prevalence of hospital readmission of about 15 %. The sample size also provided sufficient power to show that the correlation between continuously distributed variables (adherence, QOL etc.) and was statistically significant if the correlation coefficient was ≥ 0.39 and provided sufficient power to test 3-4 variables in multiple regression models without compromising stability of estimates.

Exclusion criteria

Participants were excluded from the study if they were under the age of 18 years, were unable to give informed consent or English was not their first language.

Ethics, consent and permissions

Ethical clearance was obtained from both the hospital (St Vincent's Hospital Melbourne) and university (Australian Catholic University) Human Research Ethical Committees (protocol numbers LRR 020/13 and 2014 75 V respectively). Informed verbal consent was obtained before data collection was undertaken. Consent to publish findings in aggregated formats was obtained in the consent process for all participants.

Recruitment

Participants were identified via a database. This database is called The Victorian Cardiac Outcomes Registry (VCOR) and became operational in December 2012 as a tool to help improve safety and quality of healthcare provided to cardiovascular patients in the state of Victoria. The collection of data, coordinated by the Victorian Cardiac Clinical Network, and jointly funded by Victorian Department of Health and Medibank Private, invited all public and private health services that perform PCI to join VCOR. St Vincent's Private Hospital Melbourne was the participating site in the original VCOR collection and ethics approval was obtained for the use of this database as a source of recruitment for our study. Participants were invited to participate consecutively using the database contact details and after providing informed consent by the research interviewer completing the questionnaire with participants, they were enrolled in the study. Recruitment took place between 1/2014 and 11/2014.

Data collection

Data was collected via a telephone interview at both time points (6 months and 12 months post-PCI). To evaluate lifestyle cardiac risk factors, patients were asked about their tobacco use, physical activity, diet, cholesterol/lipids (total cholesterol above 5.5 mmol/L is considered high), and about any weight gain. Patients were also asked about their adherence to cardiac rehabilitation, and all cause readmissions. Mortality was recorded if this had occurred (see demographic information Table 1).

Adherence was measured using the Brief Medication Questionnaire (BMQ). This self-report tool for monitoring adherence is used to identify patients who need assistance with their medications, assessing patient concerns, and evaluating new programs. The tool includes a 5-item Regimen Screen that asks patients how they took each medication in the past week, a 2-item Belief Screen that asks about drug effects and bothersome features, and a 2-item Recall Screen about potential difficulties remembering. Validity was assessed in 20 patients using the Medication Events Monitoring System (MEMS). Results varied by type of non-adherence, with the Regimen and Belief Screens having 80–100 % sensitivity for "repeat" non-adherence and the Recall Screen having 90 % sensitivity for "sporadic" non-adherence. The BMQ appears more sensitive than existing tools and may be useful in identifying and diagnosing adherence problems [20].

Depression was evaluated using the Patient Health Questionnaire (PHQ9) [21]. The sensitivity and specificity of the PHQ9 is 83 and 92 % respectively if the scaled response is requested as in the current investigation (i.e. not at all = 0, several days = 1, more than half the days = 2 and nearly every day = 3). The PHQ is positive if the participant scores 3 or more points.., Minor depression

Table 1 Demographics and Health Information

1) Are you male or female?
   - Male ☐
   - Female ☐

2) What is your age?

   ____

3) What is the highest level of education you have completed?
   - Primary school ☐
   - High school ☐
   - TAFE qualification ☐
   - Bachelor degree ☐
   - Post graduate degree ☐
   - Master's degree ☐
   - PhD ☐

4) What is your current marital status?
   - Single ☐
   - Married ☐
   - Defacto ☐
   - Separated ☐
   - Divorced ☐
   - Widowed ☐

5) Do you have high blood pressure?
   - Yes ☐
   - No ☐

   If yes, please indicate your highest and lowest blood pressure in the last month (if known)

   Highest: ____________

   Lowest: ____________

6) Do you smoke tobacco?
   - Yes ☐
   - No ☐

   If yes, please indicate how many cigarettes per day you smoke

   ____

7) Do you have high blood glucose levels, or a diagnosis of diabetes I or II?
   - Yes ☐
   - No ☐

8) How many times per week on average do you undertake exercise?
   - None ☐
   - Once a week ☐
   - Twice a week ☐
   - Three times a week ☐
   - Four times a week ☐
   - Five times a week ☐
   - Six times a week ☐
   - Everyday ☐

9) Including snacks, how many times do you usually have something to eat in a day including evenings?

   ____

10) How many days per week do you usually have something to eat for breakfast?

   ____

11) How many serves of vegetables do you usually eat each day? (a serve = 1/2 cup cooked vegetables or 1 cup of salad vegetables)

   ____

12) How many serves of fruit do you usually eat each day? (a serve = 1 medium piece or 2 small pieces of fruit or 1 cup of diced pieces

   ____

13) Do you have high blood cholesterol?
   - Yes ☐
   - No ☐

14) What is your current height and weight?
   - Height: ____________ (in cms)
   - Weight: ____________ (in kgs)

15) Have you adhered to the cardiac rehabilitation program given to you at discharge
   - Not at all ☐
   - Rarely ☐
   - Sometimes ☐
   - Often ☐
   - Always ☐

16) Have you been readmitted to hospital since your admission for cardiac intervention?
   - Yes ☐
   - No ☐

   If yes, how many times and for what reason?

   Amount of readmission/s: ____________________

   Reason/s: ____________________

was defined to be given by a score between 5 and 9, and severe depression was defined to be given by a score of 20 or more.

To measure resilience, the Connor-Davidson resilience scale (CD-RISC) was used. The original CD-RISC is a 25-item scale assessing resilience during the last month, with higher scores indicating higher resilience capacity [22]. Each item is rated on a 5-point range of responses from not true at all (0) to true nearly all time (4). The total score ranges from 0–100. The CD-RISC has been tested in the general population, as well as in clinical samples, and demonstrates excellent psychometric properties, with good internal consistency and test–retest reliability. The scale exhibits validity relative to other measures of resilience. The CD-RISC is a brief, self-rated measure of resilience that can measure resilience in the context of health status.

The SF-12 was used to evaluate health related quality of life. The SF-12 comprises: two questions about physical functioning; two questions on role limitations because of physical health problems; one question about bodily pain; one question related to general health perceptions; one question on vitality, energy/fatigue; one question on social functioning; two questions about role limitations because of emotional problems; and two questions on general mental health. The 12 items on the SF-12 are summarized in two weighted summary scales - mental health score (MCS) and physical health score (PCS) - where lower scores indicate more severe disability [23]. The SF12 - PCS and MCS component summary scales – were scored using a norm-based method. Regression weight for the PCS and the MCS are derived from the United States of America population [24].

Data analysis

The sample was summarised descriptively. The following outcome measures were considered: resilience (as measured by the Connor-Davidson resilience scale (CD-RISC)) [22]; depression (as measured by the Patient Health Questionnaire (PQ-9)) [21]; adherence (as measured by the Brief Medication Questionnaire (BMQ)) [20] and quality of life (as measured by the MCS and PCS sub-scales of the SF-12 questionnaire) [23]. The following variables collected on patients were initially considered for their association with the outcome measures at each time point: gender, age, hypertension, tobacco use, raised blood glucose (diabetes), physical activity, diet, cholesterol/lipid levels, and weight. Additional demographic and health-related variables were collected for descriptive analysis. The survival status of each patient (i.e. alive or dead) was also recorded at each time point.

Exploratory analyses were conducted on the data to assess the extent of missing data, frequencies of groups in categorical variables, possible collinearity between predictor variables and suitability of the outcome measures for a multivariate treatment. Categorical variables with a high number of categories including low-frequency categories were combined appropriately for analysis to ensure that each category had a sufficient number of individuals for analysis. Patterns of correlations between outcome variables were assessed for suitability for multivariate treatment.

Analysis of variance (ANOVA) and multivariate analysis of variance (MANOVA) were conducted on data collected at 6 months after the PCI procedure (time point 1) and 12 months after the PCI procedure (time point 2), with the outcome measures included in the MANOVA procedure being those found to be substantively correlated. To avoid over-fitting the models, a modelling strategy was derived whereby each predictor variable was initially assessed in a series of uni-variable models. Variables appearing to be important at this stage were then carried forward for inclusion in multiple models, with standard statistics reported from these models. In the event of a particular predictor variable being significantly related to the linear combination of outcome measures, follow-up univariate analyses of variance (ANOVAs) were conducted to investigate the sources of such associations.

A series of doubly multivariate repeated measures analyses of variance was also conducted on the data to further investigate the effect of the time component. A similar modelling strategy was implemented as for the ANOVA/MANOVA models; with between-subjects variables initially assessed on a univariable basis within these models; any variables found to be of substantive significance were carried forward for inclusion in a multiple model.

Results

Descriptive and exploratory analysis

Data was collected on 51 patients for this pilot study. Baseline sample characteristics are summarised descriptively in Table 2.

Exploratory analyses identified a small amount of missing data on certain predictor variables. The total amount of missing data was less than 0.5 %. Missing data on predictor variables only was imputed using expectation maximisation.

Only one participant self-reported as a user of tobacco. This variable was not considered further. No evidence for collinearity was observed between the remaining independent variables considered for analysis.

Analysis – time point 1 (6 months post PCI)

All patients were recorded as being alive at time point 1. The pattern of correlations between outcome measures at time point 1 revealed statistically significant moderate

Table 2 summary of baseline sample characteristics

Categorical factors	Frequency (valid %)
Gender	
Male	41 (80.4 %)
Female	10 (19.6 %)
Highest level of qualification	
Primary school	2 (3.9 %)
High school	33 (64.7 %)
TAFE qualification	13 (25.5 %)
Postgraduate degree	3 (5.9 %)
Marital status	
Single	3 (5.9 %)
Married	37 (72.5 %)
De facto	4 (7.8 %)
Separated	1 (2.0 %)
Divorced	1 (2.0 %)
Widowed	5 (9.8 %)
Hypertension	
Yes	30(58.8 %)
No	21 (41.2 %)
Smoking status	
Smoker	1 (2.0 %)
Non-smoker	50 (98.0 %)
Diabetes	
Yes	12 (23.5 %)
No	39 (76.5 %)
Exercise frequency	
None	3 (5.9 %)
1-3 times per week	14 (27.5 %)
4-6 times per week	6 (11.8 %)
Daily	28 (54.9 %)
Cholesterol level (total above 5.5 mmol/L)	
High	35 (70.0 %)
Normal	15 (30.0 %)
Adherence to cardiac rehabilitation	
Not at all	18 (36.7 %)
Sometimes	6 (12.2 %)
Often	8 (16.3 %)
Always	17 (34.7 %)
Readmission post intervention	
Yes	16 (32.0 %)
No	34 (68.0 %)
Numerical covariates	Mean (SD)
Age	72.3 (8.82)
Height (cm)	173.9 (8.34)
Weight (kg)	82.7 (14.0)

negative correlation between the PQ-9 instrument and: the CD-RISC instrument ($r = -0.331$; $p = 0.018$); the mental component summary (MCS) subscale of the SF-12 instrument ($r = -0.517$; $p < 0.001$); and the physical component summary (PCS) subscale of the SF-12 instrument ($r = -0.506$; $p < 0.001$); implying that a multivariate treatment was appropriate for these outcome measures. The correlations are illustrated in Fig. 1 (a)–(c).

No significant or substantive correlation was recorded between the BMQ instrument and the other outcome measures. Hence a separate univariate analysis was conducted on this outcome.

Univariable models indicated that gender, exercise levels, cholesterol/lipid levels and weight exhibited at least some substantively important association with a linear combination of the PQ-9, CD-RISC, SF12-MCS and SF12-PCS scales. These variables were carried forward to a multiple multivariate model including these outcome measures. The variables age, education, hypertension, diabetes status, frequency of eating, and post-intervention readmission did not appear to be important in univariable models and were not considered further with respect to these outcome measures.

The multiple model indicated that controlling for other factors, gender was significantly associated with a linear combination of outcome measures ($\Lambda = 0.697$; $F_{4,40} = 4.45$; $p = 0.004$). The effect was moderate in magnitude (partial-$\eta^2 = 0.303$). Follow-up univariate ANOVAs indicated that gender differences were grounded in the PQ-9 scale ($F_{1,44} = 8.85$; $p = 0.005$) and the SF12-PCS scale ($F_{1,44} = 10.2$; $p = 0.003$). On the PHQ scale, the mean male score was 13.1 (SD 5.21); the mean female score was 17.1 (SD 3.57). On the SF12-PCS scales, the mean male score was 53.1 (SD 9.58); the mean female score was 44.9 (SD 11.8). Hence males performed significantly better than females on both these scales 6 months after the PCI procedure.

No other factor was found to be statistically significant in the multiple model; however, some of the remaining factors indicated a degree of substantive significance.

None of the categorical factors or covariates considered exhibited any statistically significant or substantive association with the BMQ outcome measure.

Analysis – time point 2 (12 months post PCI)

Thirteen patients were lost to follow-up between time points 1 and 2. One patient was confirmed to have passed away. Twelve patients refused to participate further in the study or did not respond to requests; of these, 10 were known to be alive at time point 2, with the status of two patients being uncertain.

The pattern of correlations between outcome measures at time point 2 revealed statistically significant or near-significant negative correlation between the PHQ

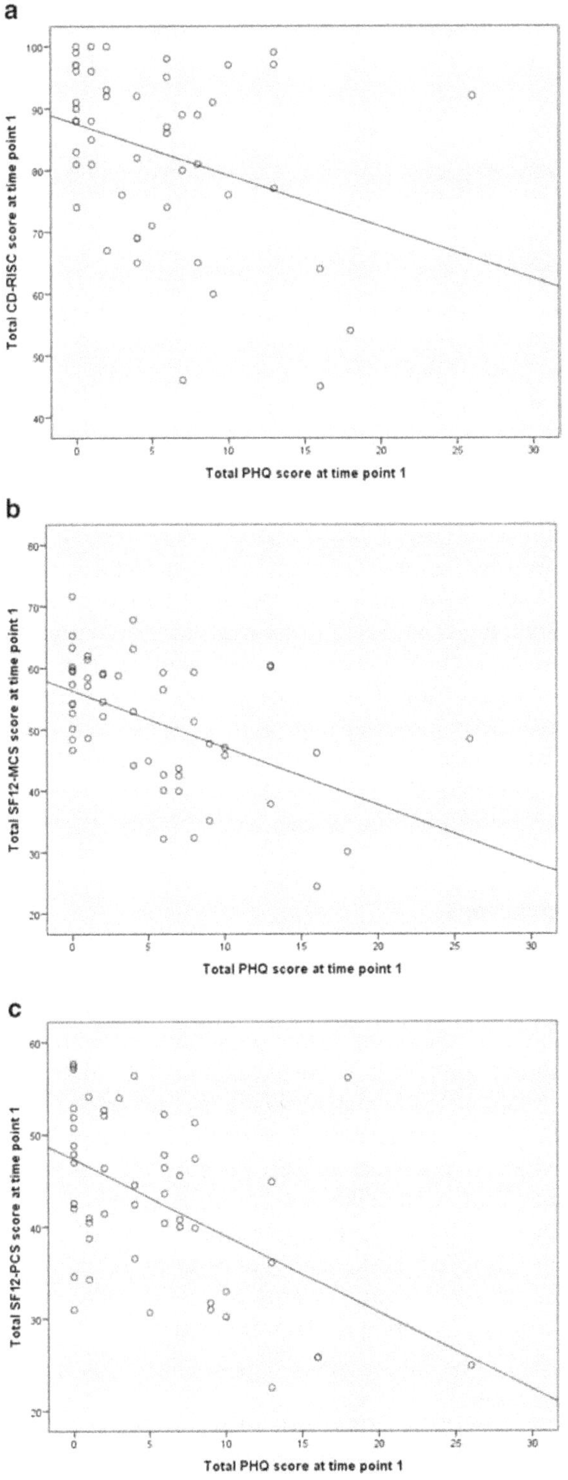

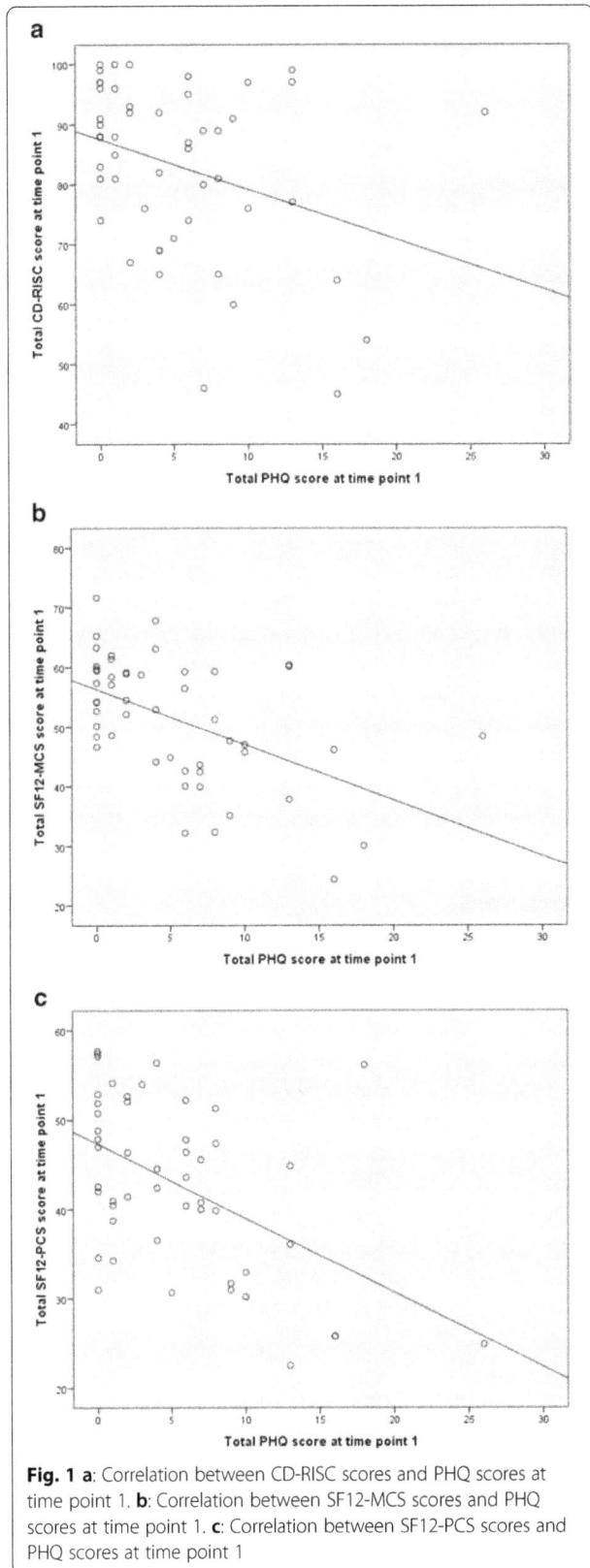

Fig. 1 **a**: Correlation between CD-RISC scores and PHQ scores at time point 1. **b**: Correlation between SF12-MCS scores and PHQ scores at time point 1. **c**: Correlation between SF12-PCS scores and PHQ scores at time point 1

instrument and the CD-RISC instrument ($r = -0.611$; $p < 0.001$); and the PCS subscale of the SF-12 instrument ($r = -0.437$; $p = 0.054$). Most other correlations between outcome measures, were also negative and moderate in magnitude; implying that a multivariate treatment was appropriate for all outcome measures, including the BMQ outcome. Univariable models indicated that education level and hypertension exhibited at least some substantively important association with a linear combination of the PHQ, CD-RISC, BMQ, SF12-MCS and SF12-PCs scales. These variables were carried forward to a multiple model. This model did not indicate either education level or hypertension to be statistically associated with a linear combination of the outcome measures.

Repeated measures analysis

Outcome measured recorded at time points 1 and 2 are summarised in Table 3 below.

Hence a substantive change was recorded in all measures except the CD-RISC measure between the two time points. The reduction in PQ-9 scores, and the increase in SF12-MCS scores represent improvements; the increase in BMQ scores and the reduction in SF12-PCS scores represent deteriorations. A null model with no between-subjects factors or covariates indicated that time point 2 (12-month) scores were significantly different from time point 1 (6-month scores) on the PHQ outcome ($F_{1,18} = 143.7$; $p < 0.001$), the MCS outcome ($F_{1,18} = 24.5$; $p < 0.001$), the PCS outcome ($F_{1,18} = 11.0$; $p = 0.004$) and the BMQ outcome ($F_{1,18} = 6.33$; $p = 0.022$). Scores on the CD-RISC outcome were not significantly different between time points 1 and 2. No between-measures factors or covariates measured in univariable models were statistically significant or exhibited substantive importance.

Discussion

The analysis reveals that men are performing better than women 6 months after the PCI procedure on a range of outcome measures, particularly depression (as measured by the PQ-9 instrument) and physical health (as measured by the SF-12-PCS instrument). Using the PHQ09 improvements in mood particularly depression has been associated with improved adherence in cardiac inpatient cardiac units who were hospitalized for acute coronary syndrome, heart failure, or arrhythmia in the 6 months following hospitalisation [25] however, assessment of gender differences requires further inquiry since the enrolment of women in heart studies remains low. In our study, much of these gender differences have disappeared by 12 months. Furthermore, no other grouping variable discriminates between patients at either 6 or 12 months after PCI. This may be because as a pilot study, the study is underpowered to detect any such

Table 3 summary of outcome measure scores at time points 1 and 2

Measure	Time point 1 (mean (SD)) – all patients	Time point 2 (mean (SD)) – all patients	*p*-value for change (calculated from patients providing values at both time points)
CD-RISC	83.3. (14.0)	80.6 (17.1)	0.083
PQ-9	13.9 (5.16)	4.97 (5.26)	<0.001
BMQ	1.59 (0.876)	2.78 (2.24)	0.022
SF12-MCS	43.0 (9.57)	57.0 (8.28)	<0.001
SF12-PCS	51.4 (10.5)	39.7 (10.8)	0.004

effects that may exist; in particular the analysis of time point 2 data, which was subject to heavy attrition loss.

While significant changes in most outcomes were recorded between the two time points, the overall pattern of improvement is not clear; with the direction of movement being positive for two measures and negative for two measures. Improvement or deterioration is not more noticeable in any sub-group than any other. Again, this may be ascribed to a loss of power as a result of the low sample size. It is also possible that attrition bias was introduced by the loss of 25.5 % of the sample between 6 and 12 months.

Mood and physical health considerations particularly for women patients in the first 6 months post-PCI appears an area for further investigation. It is known that within Australia, data that specifically addresses women and CHD is limited [26–28], even in the knowledge that the traditional risk factors for CVD in women is increasing. Clinically women can present with a wider range of symptoms, which can lead to delayed diagnosis should problems arise post-intervention. In addition, psychosocial factors and conventional CVD risk factors often coexist (i.e. depression and heart disease). Mental health problems such as depression give rise to perceived reduced social support, and can negatively impact of recovery post PCI. Depression can also become chronic over time. Care planning related to prodromal symptoms and devising a plan of action in collaboration with patients post PCI is recommended. In addition, assessment of existing and/or required social supports and pre-existing mental health problems is recommended to ensure access to required supports post-PCI for patients in a timely manner.

Limitations of the study

The longitudinal nature of this study, whilst having an advantage of observing and controlling for differences in the same cohort of people over a period of time when compared to cross-sectional study, does have some limitations. Data collection in this study was time-consuming and resulted in a reduced number of participants completing surveys at the 12-month time point of the study, with the resulting smaller sample size at this time point leading to a reduction in power of analyses conducted at this time point. The sample size was small, with a small number of women being represented in the cohort; therefore interpretations of the findings are to be considered conservatively in the context of the pilot study setting. Another limitation of this study was the use of self-report for smoking status and in surveys: although each of the measures used have been tested for reliability and validity, the nature of surveys relies on participants' ability to recall information, answer truthfully, understand the questions and scales used; and the surveys must have the ability to remove potential for response bias (i.e. participants will answer questions in a certain way regardless of the question being asked). In this study questionnaires were completed over the telephone with a researcher. Future research may consider providing participants with a paper/online copy of the questionnaire where they would be able to answer the questions anonymously.

Conclusions

This pilot study has provided insight into the potential social and physical impacts post-PCI, particularly for women patients with regard to mood and physical health with men performing better physically and with mood 6 months post PCI. In consideration of the differences in symptom presentation between men and women undergoing cardiac care, interventions need to be tailored in an individual and gender sensitive manner following PCI. Given the paucity of research related to women following PCI further research into the management of mood particularly for women is warranted. More detailed inquiry related to access/attendance to secondary prevention is also warranted.

Abbreviations

ANOVA: analysis of variance; BMQ: brief medication questionnaire; CAD: coronary artery disease; CD-RISC: Connor-Davidson resilience scale; CVD: cardiovascular disease; HRQoL: health related quality of life; MANOVA: multivariate analysis of variance; MCS: mental component summary; MI: myocardial infarction; PCI: percutaneous coronary intervention; PCS: physical component summary; PHQ: patient health questionnaire; QOL: quality of life; SF12: short form 12; STEMI: ST-elevation myocardial infarction; VCOR: Victorian Cardiac Outcomes Registry.

Competing interests

The authors declare that they have no competing interests.

Authors' contributions

KLE conception and design, data interpretation, manuscript development. JS statistical methods and manuscript development. J-AG literature review, data collection, manuscript development. AW concept development and design. RW concept development and recruitment. AN recruitment. JG access to database for recruitment, manuscript development. All authors have read and approved the final manuscript.

Acknowledgments

Funded with donations from the community made to St Vincent's Private Hospital Melbourne Ltd.

We wish to also acknowledge Lisa Thompson and Christine Wright for their contribution to data collection for this study.

Author details

[1]Australian Catholic University and St Vincent's Private Hospital Melbourne Ltd, Locked Bag 4115 MDC, Fitzroy 3065, Australia. [2]University of Huddersfield, Huddersfield, United Kingdom. [3]University of Melbourne and St Vincent's Hospital Melbourne, Melbourne, Australia.

References

1. Mann DL, Zipes DP, Libby P, Bonow RO. Braunwald's heart disease: a textbook of cardiovascular medicine. Philadelphia, USA: Elsevier Health Sciences; 2014.
2. Yusuf S, Hawken S, Ounpuu S, Dans T, Avezum A, Lanas F, et al. Effect of potentially modifiable risk factors associated with myocardial infarction in 52 countries (the INTERHEART study): case-control study. Lancet. 2004; 364(9438):937–52.
3. O'Donnell MJ, Xavier D, Liu L, Zhang H, Chin SL, Rao-Melacini P, et al. Risk factors for ischaemic and intracerebral haemorrhagic stroke in 22 countries (the INTERSTROKE study): a case-control study. Lancet. 2010; The Lancet, Early Online Publication, 18 June 2010(doi:10.1016/S0140-6736(10)60834-3).
4. Davies J. Coronary revascularisation in Australia, 2000. Bulletin no. 7. Canberra: Australian Institute of Health and Welfare; 2003.
5. Ajani AE, Reid CM, Duffy SJ, Andrianopoulos N, Lefkovits J, Black A, et al. Outcomes after percutaneous coronary intervention in contemporary Australian practice: insights from a large multicentre registry. Med J Aust. 2008;189(8):423–8.
6. Mehran R, Pocock S, Nikolsky E, Dangas GD, Clayton T, Claessen BE, et al. Impact of bleeding on mortality after percutaneous coronary intervention results from a patient-level pooled analysis of the REPLACE-2 (randomized evaluation of PCI linking angiomax to reduced clinical events), ACUITY (acute catheterization and urgent intervention triage strategy), and HORIZONS-AMI (harmonizing outcomes with revascularization and stents in acute myocardial infarction) trials. JACC Cardiovasc Interv. 2011;4(6):654–64.
7. Aggarwal B, Ellis SG, Lincoff AM, Kapadia SR, Cacchione J, Raymond RE, et al. Cause of death within 30 days of percutaneous coronary intervention in an era of mandatory outcome reporting. J Am Coll Cardiol. 2013;62(5):409–15.
8. Connerney I, Sloan RP, Shapiro PA, Bagiella E, Seckman C. Depression is associated with increased mortality 10 years after coronary artery bypass surgery. Psychosom Med. 2010;72(9):874–81.
9. Strik JJ, Denollet J, Lousberg R, Honig A. Comparing symptoms of depression and anxiety as predictors of cardiac events and increased health care consumption after myocardial infarction. J Am Coll Cardiol. 2003;42(10):1801–7.
10. Lane D, Carroll D, Ring C, Beevers DG, Lip GY. Mortality and quality of life 12 months after myocardial infarction: effects of depression and anxiety. Psychosom Med. 2001;63(2):221–30.
11. Iles-Smith H, McGowan L, Campbell M, Mercer C, Deaton C. A prospective cohort study investigating readmission, symptom attribution and psychological health within six months of primary percutaneous coronary intervention. Eur J Cardiovasc Nurs. 2014.
12. Wang ZJ, Guo M, Si TM, Jiang MM, Liu SM, Liu YY, et al. Association of depression with adverse cardiovascular events after percutaneous coronary intervention. Coron Artery Dis. 2013;24(7):589–95.
13. Damen NL, Pelle AJ, Boersma E, Serruys PW, van Domburg RT, Pedersen SS. Reduced positive affect (anhedonia) is independently associated with 7-year mortality in patients treated with percutaneous coronary intervention: results from the RESEARCH registry. Eur J Prev Cardiol. 2013;20(1):127–34.
14. Damen NL, Pelle AJ, van Geuns R-JM, van Domburg RT, Boersma E, Pedersen SS. Intra-individual changes in anxiety and depression during 12-month follow-up in percutaneous coronary intervention patients. J Affect Disord. 2011;134(1–3):464–7.
15. Panasewicz A, Pedersen SS, Veenhuis SJG, Oemrawsingh RM, van der Giessen WJ, van Geuns R-J, et al. Health-related quality of life in the elderly three years after percutaneous coronary intervention. EuroIntervention. 2013;9(3):373–81.
16. Rumsfeld JS, Magid DJ, Plomondon ME, Sacks J, Henderson W, Hlatky M, et al. Health-related quality of life after percutaneous coronary intervention versus coronary bypass surgery in high-risk patients with medically refractory ischemia. J Am Coll Cardiol. 2003;41(10):1732–8.
17. Rumsfeld JS, Havranek E, Masoudi FA, Peterson ED, Jones P, Tooley JF, et al. Depressive symptoms are the strongest predictors of short-term declines in health status in patients with heart failure. J Am Coll Cardiol. 2003;42(10): 1811–7.
18. van Dijk MR, Utens EM, Dulfer K, Al-Qezweny MN, van Geuns R-J, Daemen J, et al. Depression and anxiety symptoms as predictors of mortality in PCI patients at 10 years of follow-up. Eur J Prev Cardiol. 2015; 2047487315571889.
19. Blankenship JC, Marshall JJ, Pinto DS, Lange RA, Bates ER, Holper EM, et al. Effect of percutaneous coronary intervention on quality of life: a consensus statement from the Society for Cardiovascular Angiography and Interventions. Catheter Cardiovasc Interv. 2013;81(2):243–59.
20. Svarstad BL, Chewning BA, Sleath BL, Claesson C. The brief medication questionnaire: a tool for screening patient adherence and barriers to adherence. Patient Educ Couns. 1999;37(2):113–24.
21. Martin A, Rief W, Klaiberg A, Braehler E. Validity of the brief patient health questionnaire mood scale (PHQ-9) in the general population. Gen Hosp Psychiatry. 2006;28(1):71–7.
22. Connor KM, Davidson JRT. Development of a new resilience scale: the Connor-Davidson Resilience Scale (CD-RISC). Depress Anxiety. 2003;18(2):76–82.
23. Jenkinson C, Layte R, Jenkinson D, Lawrence K, Petersen S, Paice C, et al. A shorter form health survey: can the SF-12 replicate results from the SF-36 in longitudinal studies? J Public Health. 1997;19(2):179–86.
24. Ware J, Kosinski M, Keller S. SF-12: how to score the SF-12 physical and mental health summary scales. 3rd ed. Boston: Quality Metric Inc. and The Health Assessment Lab; 1998.
25. Bauer LK, Caro MA, Beach SR, Mastromauro CA, Lenihan E, Januzzi JL, et al. Effects of depression and anxiety improvement on adherence to medication and health behaviors in recently hospitalized cardiac patients. Am J Cardiol. 2012;109(9):1266–71.
26. Stramba-Badiale M, Fox KM, Priori SG, Collins P, Daly C, Graham I, et al. Cardiovascular diseases in women: a statement from the policy conference of the European Society of Cardiology. Eur Heart J. 2006;27(8):994–1005.
27. Lerman A, Sopko G. Women and cardiovascular heart disease: clinical implications from the Women's Ischemia Syndrome Evaluation (WISE) study. Are we smarter? J Am Coll Cardiol. 2006;47(3 Suppl):S59–62.
28. Worrall-Carter L, Edward K-l, Page K. Women and cardiovascular disease: at a social disadvantage? Collegian. 2012;19(1):33–7.

Does infection with human immunodeficiency virus have any impact on the cardiovascular outcomes following percutaneous coronary intervention?

Pravesh Kumar Bundhun[1], Manish Pursun[2] and Wei-Qiang Huang[1,3*]

Abstract

Background: A direct link between human immunodeficiency virus (HIV)-infected patients and the risk of cardiovascular diseases (CVD) has been shown in recent scientific research. However, this issue is controversial since other previous reports showed no apparent impact of HIV or its anti-retroviral drugs on the cardiovascular system. We aimed to systematically compare the postinterventional adverse cardiovascular outcomes which were observed in patients with and without HIV infection during a mean follow up period ranging from 1 year to 3 years.

Methods: Common electronic databases were searched for studies which compared postinterventional adverse cardiovascular outcomes [mortality, myocardial infarction (MI), cardiac death, target vessel revascularization (TVR), target lesion revascularization (TLR), stroke and major adverse cardiac events (MACEs)] in patients with and without HIV infection. Statistical analysis was carried out by the RevMan 5.3 software whereby Odds Ratios (OR) and 95% Confidence Intervals (CIs) were generated.

Results: Two thousand two hundred and sixty-eight (2268) patients (821 patients were HIV positive and 1147 patients were HIV negative) were analyzed. The current results showed that mortality was not significantly increased among patients who were HIV positive with OR: 1.13, 95% CI: 0.65–1.96; $P = 0.66$. Cardiac death was also similarly reported with OR: 1.16, 95% CI: 0.50–2.68; $P = 0.74$. However, even if recurrent MI, TVR, TLR, MACEs and stroke were higher in patients who were HIV positive, with OR: 1.32, 95% CI: 0.88–2.12; $P = 0.18$, OR: 1.36, 95% CI: 0.88–2.12; $P = 0.17$, OR: 1.22, 95% CI: 0.72–2.06; $P = 0.46$, OR: 1.29, 95% CI: 0.89–1.85; $P = 0.17$ and OR: 1.47, 95% CI: 0.44–4.89; $P = 0.53$ respectively, these results were not statistically significant.

Conclusion: Patients who were infected with HIV had similar mortality post coronary intervention compared to patients who were not infected by the virus, during a mean follow-up period of 1–3 years. In addition, no significant increase in MI, TVR, TLR, MACEs and stroke were observed during this follow up period. Therefore, it might be concluded that no apparent impact of HIV on the cardiovascular outcomes was observed post coronary intervention.

Keywords: Human immunodeficiency virus, Percutaneous coronary intervention, Cardiovascular outcomes, Acquired immune deficiency syndrome, Coronary artery disease, Highly active antiretroviral therapy

* Correspondence: huangwq1029@126.com
[1]Institute of Cardiovascular Diseases, the First Affiliated Hospital of Guangxi Medical University, Nanning, Guangxi 530027, People's Republic of China
[3]Institute of Cardiovascular Diseases, the First Affiliated Hospital of Guangxi Medical University, Nanning, Guangxi 530021, People's Republic of China
Full list of author information is available at the end of the article

Background

In its earlier stage known as Human Immunodeficiency Virus (HIV) infection and later manifesting as Acquired Immune Deficiency Syndrome (AIDS), HIV/AIDS has been in the headlines since the year 1981. For many years, Highly Active Anti-Retroviral Therapy (HAART) has been the main treatment expected to have prolonged survival and improved quality of life in these HIV infected patients [1].

A clear link between HIV-infected patients and the risk of cardiovascular diseases (CVD) has been shown in recent scientific research [2]. The PREmature VAscular LEsions and Antiretroviral Therapy (PREVALEAT II) Cohort further supported this point [3].

However, the use of HAART and cardiovascular manifestations in HIV infected patients has mainly been reported in case studies [4] and compared to infected patients who were not treated by HAART therapy, an increase in the yearly incidence of Myocardial Infarction (MI) was observed among patients who were treated with HAART [5].

Nevertheless, this issue is still controversial. Even if only a minority of research has been carried out on this particular topic, a few studies showed no impact of HIV or its anti-retroviral therapy on the cardiovascular system [6].

Percutaneous Coronary Intervention (PCI) is the most common invasive procedure which is being carried out in this new Era. Any factor which affects the cardiovascular system should probably influence cardiovascular outcomes following PCI. Therefore, this study aimed to systematically compare the postinterventional adverse cardiovascular outcomes which were observed in patients with and without HIV infection during a mean follow up period of 1 to 3 years.

Methods

Data sources and search strategy

Online electronic databases [PubMed/Medline, EMBASE (www.sciencedirect.com) and the Cochrane databases] were searched for Randomized Controlled Trials (RCTs) and Observational studies (which were published in English language) comparing postinterventional adverse cardiovascular outcomes which were reported in patients with and without HIV infection.

The following searched terms were used:

1. Human Immunodeficiency Virus and Percutaneous Coronary Intervention;
2. HIV and PCI;
3. Acquired Immune Deficiency Syndrome/AIDS and PCI;
4. Coronary angioplasty and Human Immunodeficiency Virus;
5. Acute coronary syndrome and Human Immunodeficiency Virus;
6. Coronary revascularization and Human Immunodeficiency Virus;
7. Percutaneous revascularization and Human Immunodeficiency Virus;
8. Coronary stenting and Human Immunodeficiency Virus.

Inclusion and exclusion criteria

Studies were included if:

(a) They were RCTs or observational studies which compared post-interventional adverse cardiovascular outcomes [mortality, myocardial infarction (MI), cardiac death, target vessel revascularization (TVR), target lesion revascularization (TLR), stroke and major adverse cardiac events (MACEs)] in patients with and without HIV infections.

Studies were excluded if:

(a) They were meta-analyses, or case studies.
(b) They did not report the above-mentioned adverse cardiovascular outcomes as their clinical endpoints.
(c) They did not involve patients with HIV infections and their respective controls.
(d) They did not involve patients who underwent PCI.

Definitions, outcomes and follow up periods

The endpoints which were considered relevant in this analysis included:

(a) All-cause mortality
(b) Cardiac mortality
(c) Recurrent MI
(d) TVR
(e) TLR
(f) Stroke
(g) MACEs (death, MI and revascularization). One study reported major adverse cardiovascular and cerebrovascular events (MACCEs). Therefore, we combined MACEs and MACCEs together during the analysis.

This analysis had a follow up period of 1 to 3 years. The outcomes which were reported and their corresponding follow up periods were summarized in Table 1.

Data extraction and review

Two authors (PKB and MP) carefully reviewed the studies and the data which were reported. Information concerning the author names, the year of patients' enrollment, the total number of HIV positive and HIV negative patients

Table 1 Reported Outcomes

Study	Reported outcomes	Follow up periods
Badr 2015 [10]	Death, cardiac death, TLR, TVR, MI, stroke, MACEs	24 months
Boccara 2006 [11]	TVR, MACEs	20 months
Boccara 2011 [12]	MACCEs, cardiac death, stroke, TLR, TVR	12 months
Lorgis 2013 [13]	MI, stroke, death	12 months
Matetzky 2003 [14]	MI, death, cardiac death	14 months
Ren 2009 [15]	MACEs, death, cardiac death, MI, TVR, TLR	37 months

Abbreviations: *MI* myocardial infarction, *TLR* target lesion revascularization, *TVR* target vessel revascularization, *MACEs* major adverse cardiac events, *MACCEs* major adverse cardiac and cerebrovascular events

respectively, the outcomes and follow up periods which were reported as well as the baseline features were carefully extracted from the selected studies. During this data extraction process, any disagreement which was encountered by any of these two authors was discussed and resolved by the third author (WQH)).

Statistical analysis

Reporting guideline which was used: The Preferred Reporting Items for Systematic Reviews and Meta-Analyses [7].

Since this is a meta-analysis of several studies, inconsistency across these studies were possible [8]. Therefore, assessment of heterogeneity was carried out to provide relevant results. Heterogeneity across the studies were assessed by first of all, the Cochrane Q statistic test (*P* value less or equal to 0.05 was considered statistically significant) and secondly the I^2 statistic test (high I^2 value = increased heterogeneity, lower I^2 value = low heterogeneity).

If I^2 was greater than 50%, a random effects model was used during the analysis, whereas if I^2 was less than 50%, a fixed effects model was used.

The latest version of RevMan (version 5.3) was used to carry out this analysis [9], whereby odds ratios (OR) with 95% confidence intervals (CI) were used as the statistical parameters.

Funnel plot was visually assessed for evidence of publication bias.

Ethical committee or medical institutional board approval was not required.

Results

Search result

One hundred and six (106) articles were searched from the electronic databases. After a careful screening of the abstracts and titles, eighty-one (81) articles were eliminated since they were not relevant.

Among the remaining twenty-five (25) articles, eight (8) articles were duplicates and were spontaneously eliminated.

Seventeen (17) full-text articles were assessed for eligibility.

Eleven (11) full text articles were eliminated since:

- four (4) publications were case studies,
- two (2) publications were meta-analyses,
- two (2) articles did not report the relevant adverse cardiovascular outcomes,
- three (3) articles did not involve any control group. Finally, six (6) articles [10–15] were selected and included in this systematic review and meta-analysis (Fig. 1).

General features of the studies which were included

Table 2 represents the general features of the studies which were included in this systematic review and meta-analysis.

Two thousand two hundred and sixty-eight (2268) patients were analyzed. Eight hundred and twenty-one (821) patients were HIV positive whereas 1147 patients were HIV negative. According to Table 2, patients' enrollment period ranged from the year 1998 to the year 2011. Study Lorgis2013 consisted of the highest number of patients among all the other studies which were included in this analysis.

The quality assessment of the studies was carried out by the Newcastle Ottawa Scale (NOS) [16] whereby grades were allotted according to a star system in order to rate the methodological qualities of these studies. NOS consisted of eight items, which were classified in three different groups namely selection, comparability, and outcome or exposure. A maximum total number of nine stars (*********) were possible.

The methodological quality of each study was assessed and graded as followed:

Badr2015: ******* (7 stars).
Boccara2006: ****** (6 stars).
Boccara2011: ******** (8 stars).
Lorgis2013: ******** (8 stars).
Matetzky2003: ***** (5 stars).
Ren2009: ******* (7 stars).

Baseline features of the participants

The baseline characteristics of the participants were represented in Table 3.

According to Table 3, (43.3–68.3 years) was the mean age of the participants. Three studies, namely studies Boccara 2006, Matetzky 2003 and Boccara 2011 consisted of younger patients in comparison to the other studies. Study Ren 2009 consisted only of male patients. Study Badr 2015 consisted of a larger number of patients with hypertension. Only a small percentage of patients suffered

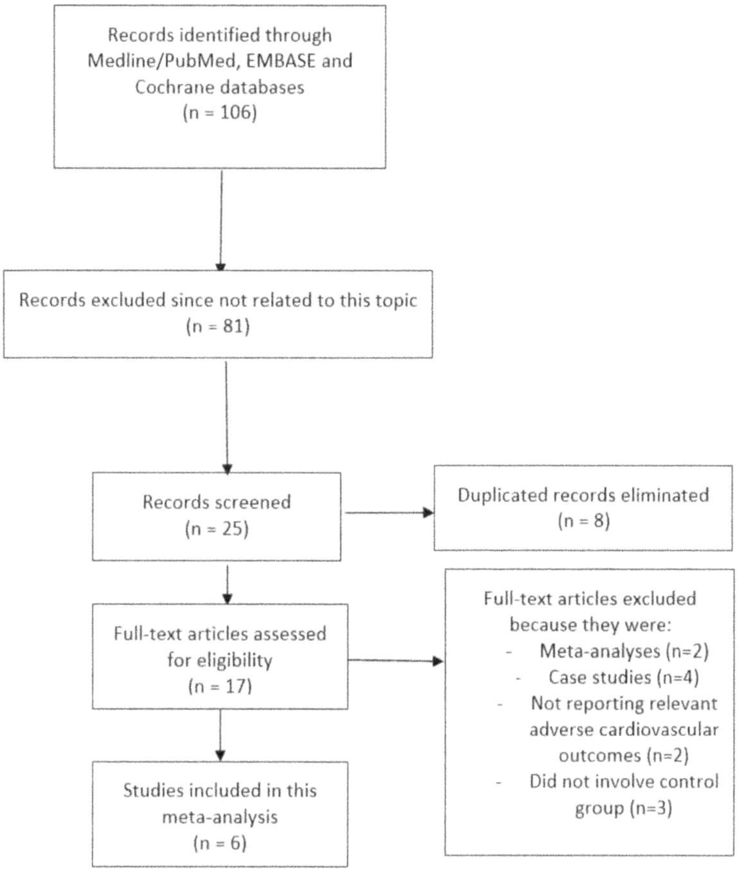

Fig. 1 Flow diagram representing the study selection

from diabetes mellitus. According to Table 3, almost no significant difference was observed in the baseline characteristics of the participants within the two groups.

Analysis of the adverse cardiovascular outcomes

The postinterventional adverse cardiovascular outcomes which were observed in patients with and without HIV infection were represented in Table 4.

Table 2 General features of the studies which were included

Studies	Patients' enrollment	No of HIV positive patients (*n*)	No of HIV negative patients (*n*)	Total no of patients (*n*)
Badr 2015 [10]	2003–2011	112	112	244
Boccara 2006 [11]	2001–2003	50	50	100
Boccara 2011 [12]	2003–2006	103	195	298
Lorgis 2013 [13]	2005–2009	435	945	1380
Matetzky 2003[14]	1998–2000	24	48	72
Ren2009 [15]	2000–2007	97	97	194
Total (*n*)		821	1447	2268

Abbreviations: *HIV* human immunodeficiency virus

Current results showed that, during a mean follow up period of 1–3.1 years, mortality was not significantly increased in the HIV positive group with OR: 1.13, 95% CI: 0.65–1.96; P = 0.66. Cardiac death was also noted to be similar with OR: 1.16, 95% CI: 0.50–2.68; P = 0.74.

However, even if the other adverse cardiovascular outcomes including recurrent MI, TVR, TLR, MACEs and stroke favored HIV negative patients with OR: 1.32, 95% CI: 0.88–2.12; P = 0.18, OR: 1.36, 95% CI: 0.88–2.12; P = 0.17, OR: 1.22, 95% CI: 0.72–2.06; P = 0.46, OR: 1.29, 95% CI: 0.89–1.85; P = 0.17 and OR: 1.47, 95% CI: 0.44–4.89; P = 0.53 respectively, the results were not statistically significant in this analysis. These results have been summarized in Table 4 and illustrated in Fig. 2.

Sensitivity analysis

Six observational studies were included in this analysis. Therefore, to make sure that the result of this analysis was not influenced by any of the studies, we carried out a sensitivity analysis (one by one exclusion of studies with re-assessment of the results). Excluding study Badr2015 did not affect the main result of this analysis

Table 3 Baseline features of the participants

Study	Mean age (yrs)	Males (%)	HT (%)	CS (%)	DM (%)
	HIV/Non-HIV	HIV/Non-HIV	HIV/Non-HIV	HIV/Non-HIV	HIV/Non-HIV
Badr 2015 [10]	58.0/58.0	64.3/64.3	84.8/83.0	30.4/26.8	12.7/12.7
Boccara 2006 [11]	43.3/44.0	90.0/88.0	-	-	-
Boccara 2011 [12]	48.0/50.0	93.0/94.0	18.0/24.0	59.0/64.0	9.0/12.0
Lorgis 2013 [13]	50.0/68.3	88.6/66.3	17.4/35.9	29.6/14.2	9.1/18.2
Matetzky 2003 [14]	47.0/48.0	88.0/88.0	29.0/44.0	58.0/48.0	12.0/19.0
Ren 2009 [15]	53.0/54.0	100/100	46.0/67.0	24.0/26.0	10.0/26.0

Abbreviations: *yrs.* years, *HIV* human immunodeficiency virus, *HT* hypertension, *CS* current smoker, *DM* diabetes mellitus

with OR: 0.86, 95% CI: 0.39–1.90; $P = 0.71$ for mortality, OR: 0.61, 95% CI: 0.11–3.32; $P = 0.57$ for cardiac death, OR: 1.20, 95% CI: 0.79–1.83; $P = 0.39$ for recurrent MI, OR: 1.31, 95% CI: 0.79–2.16; $P = 0.29$ for TVR, OR: 1.31, 95% CI: 0.71–2.42; $P = 0.38$ for TLR and OR: 1.15, 95% CI: 0.74–1.79; $P = 0.53$ for MACEs. There was no significant difference in outcomes.

When study Matetzky2003 was excluded and a new analysis was carried out, still no significant difference in results were obtained with OR: 1.19, 95% CI: 0.68–2.08; $P = 0.55$ for mortality, OR: 1.21, 95% CI: 0.50–2.91; $P = 0.67$ for cardiac death and OR: 1.22, 95% CI: 0.81–1.85; $P = 0.34$ for recurrent MI.

When study Ren2009 was excluded, still no significant difference was observed in the results with OR: 1.10, 95% CI: 0.62–1.96; $P = 0.75$ for mortality, OR: 1.17, 95% CI: 0.49–2.83; $P = 0.72$ for cardiac death, OR: 1.35, 95% CI: 0.89–2.05; $P = 0.16$ for recurrent MI, OR: 1.56, 95% CI: 0.87–2.79; $P = 0.13$ for TVR, OR: 1.11, 95% CI: 0.55–2.25; $P = 0.78$ for TLR and OR: 1.37, 95% CI: 0.87–2.15; $P = 0.18$ for MACEs.

When the remaining studies were excluded and a new analysis was carried out, still no significant difference in results was obtained as shown in Table 5, implying that for all of the above analyses, sensitivity analyses yielded consistent results.

Also, almost no evidence of publication bias was observed (Fig. 3).

Discussion

This study aimed to compare the postinterventional adverse cardiovascular outcomes which were observed in patients with and without HIV infection.

Current results showed no significant difference in cardiovascular outcomes among patients who were or were not infected by HIV during a follow up period of 1 to 3 years post- PCI.

Previous studies showed a moderate contribution of HIV virus and HAART therapy in the pathogenesis and development of atherosclerosis in infected patients further accelerating coronary artery disease (CAD). Recent observational studies involving larger number of HIV-infected patients showed an increase incidence of MI in association with a longer exposure to antiretroviral therapies [17]. Dysfunction of the endothelium, and premature atherosclerosis have been observed among HIV positive patients who were treated by HAART whose mechanism is considered to affect lipid alteration and inflammatory mechanisms contributing to premature atherosclerosis [18]. Studies have also shown AIDS virus to contribute to these effects by inducing inflammatory reactions intracellularly. HIV virus is able to penetrate coronary artery endothelial cell membrane and induce inflammatory and intracellular responses and reactions further activating endothelial cells [19].

A study carried out by Boccara et al. consisted of data that suggested the presence of an accelerated process of

Table 4 Results of this meta-analysis

Outcomes analyzed	OR with 95% CI	*P* value	I^2 (%)	Fixed or random effects model used
Mortality	1.13 [0.65–1.96]	0.66	0	Fixed
Cardiac death	1.16 [0.50–2.68]	0.74	0	Fixed
Recurrent MI	1.32 [0.88–2.12]	0.18	28	Fixed
TVR	1.36 [0.88–2.12]	0.17	0	Fixed
TLR	1.22 [0.72–2.06]	0.46	0	Fixed
MACEs	1.29 [0.89–1.85]	0.17	0	Fixed
Stroke	1.47 [0.44–4.89]	0.53	0	Fixed

Abbreviations: *MI* myocardial infarction, *TVR* target vessel revascularization, *TLR* target lesion revascularization, *MACEs* major adverse cardiac events, *OR* odds ratios, *CI* confidence intervals

Study or Subgroup	HIV positive Events	HIV positive Total	HIV negative Events	HIV negative Total	Weight	Odds Ratio M-H, Fixed, 95% CI
1.1.1 Mortality						
Badr2015	17	112	12	112	5.4%	1.49 [0.68, 3.29]
Lorgis2013	6	435	16	945	5.3%	0.81 [0.32, 2.09]
Matetzky2003	0	24	2	48	0.9%	0.38 [0.02, 8.22]
Ren2009	3	97	2	97	1.0%	1.52 [0.25, 9.28]
Subtotal (95% CI)		**668**		**1202**	**12.6%**	**1.13 [0.65, 1.96]**
Total events	26		32			
Heterogeneity: Chi² = 1.53, df = 3 (P = 0.68); I² = 0%						
Test for overall effect: Z = 0.44 (P = 0.66)						
1.1.2 Cardiac death						
Badr2015	10	112	7	112	3.4%	1.47 [0.54, 4.01]
Boccara2011	0	103	2	195	0.9%	0.37 [0.02, 7.86]
Matetzky2003	0	24	1	48	0.5%	0.65 [0.03, 16.46]
Ren2009	1	97	1	97	0.5%	1.00 [0.06, 16.22]
Subtotal (95% CI)		**336**		**452**	**5.3%**	**1.16 [0.50, 2.68]**
Total events	11		11			
Heterogeneity: Chi² = 0.88, df = 3 (P = 0.83); I² = 0%						
Test for overall effect: Z = 0.34 (P = 0.74)						
1.1.3 Recurrent myocardial infarction						
Badr2015	7	112	2	112	1.0%	3.67 [0.74, 18.05]
Lorgis2013	29	435	57	945	17.8%	1.11 [0.70, 1.77]
Matetzky2003	4	24	2	48	0.6%	4.60 [0.78, 27.19]
Ren2009	4	97	4	97	2.0%	1.00 [0.24, 4.12]
Subtotal (95% CI)		**668**		**1202**	**21.4%**	**1.32 [0.88, 1.97]**
Total events	44		65			
Heterogeneity: Chi² = 4.14, df = 3 (P = 0.25); I² = 28%						
Test for overall effect: Z = 1.34 (P = 0.18)						
1.1.4 Target vessel revascularization						
Badr2015	12	112	8	112	3.8%	1.56 [0.61, 3.98]
Boccara2006	8	50	4	50	1.8%	2.19 [0.61, 7.81]
Boccara2011	8	103	12	195	4.1%	1.28 [0.51, 3.25]
Ren2009	22	97	20	97	8.2%	1.13 [0.57, 2.24]
Subtotal (95% CI)		**362**		**454**	**17.8%**	**1.36 [0.88, 2.12]**
Total events	50		44			
Heterogeneity: Chi² = 0.92, df = 3 (P = 0.82); I² = 0%						
Test for overall effect: Z = 1.37 (P = 0.17)						
1.1.5 Target lesion revascularization						
Badr2015	8	112	8	112	3.9%	1.00 [0.36, 2.76]
Boccara2011	7	103	11	195	3.8%	1.22 [0.46, 3.25]
Ren2009	17	97	13	97	5.7%	1.37 [0.63, 3.01]
Subtotal (95% CI)		**312**		**404**	**13.4%**	**1.22 [0.72, 2.06]**
Total events	32		32			
Heterogeneity: Chi² = 0.23, df = 2 (P = 0.89); I² = 0%						
Test for overall effect: Z = 0.74 (P = 0.46)						
1.1.6 Major Adverse Cardiac Events						
Badr2015	28	112	19	112	7.6%	1.63 [0.85, 3.13]
Boccara2006	10	50	8	50	3.4%	1.31 [0.47, 3.66]
Boccara2011	10	103	18	195	6.0%	1.06 [0.47, 2.38]
Ren2009	32	97	29	97	10.3%	1.15 [0.63, 2.12]
Subtotal (95% CI)		**362**		**454**	**27.2%**	**1.29 [0.89, 1.85]**
Total events	80		74			
Heterogeneity: Chi² = 0.86, df = 3 (P = 0.84); I² = 0%						
Test for overall effect: Z = 1.36 (P = 0.17)						
1.1.7 Stroke						
Boccara2011	0	103	1	195	0.5%	0.63 [0.03, 15.51]
Lorgis2013	4	435	5	945	1.7%	1.74 [0.47, 6.53]
Subtotal (95% CI)		**538**		**1140**	**2.2%**	**1.47 [0.44, 4.89]**
Total events	4		6			
Heterogeneity: Chi² = 0.34, df = 1 (P = 0.56); I² = 0%						
Test for overall effect: Z = 0.62 (P = 0.53)						
Total (95% CI)		**3246**		**5308**	**100.0%**	**1.27 [1.06, 1.54]**
Total events	247		264			
Heterogeneity: Chi² = 9.21, df = 24 (P = 1.00); I² = 0%						
Test for overall effect: Z = 2.52 (P = 0.01)						
Test for subgroup differences: Chi² = 0.43, df = 6 (P = 1.00), I² = 0%						

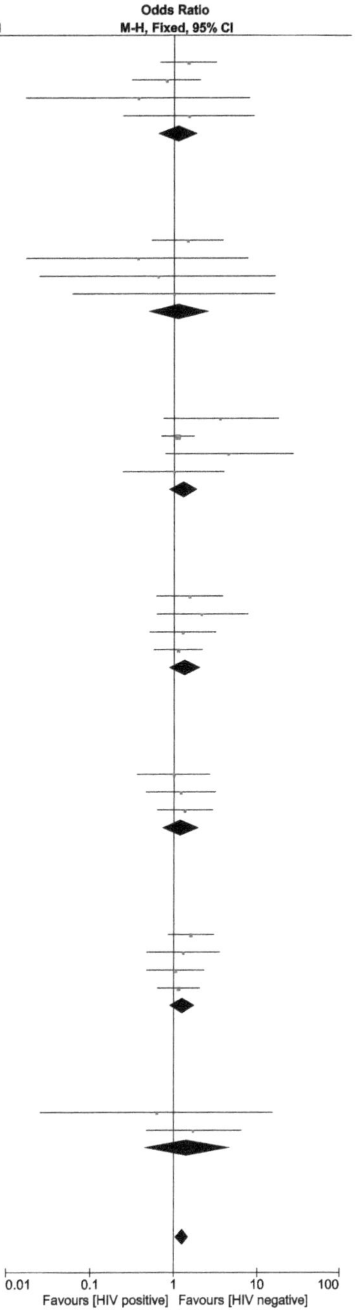

Fig. 2 Postinterventional Adverse Cardiovascular Outcomes which were observed between HIV positive and HIV negative patients

coronary atherosclerosis in HIV positive due to factors including a higher prevalence of conventional and emerging risk factors such as chronic inflammation and immune activation and the role of antiretroviral therapy [20].

Similar to the current analysis, the single-centered study involving patients from MedStar Washington Hospital showed similar short and long-term outcomes reported between HIV positive and HIV negative patients who underwent PCI with drug eluting stents. Moreover, the retrospective study of prospectively collected cohorts investigating the clinical presentation of ACS in HIV infected adults showed a similar prognosis between HIV positive and HIV negative patients [21]. Another study showing the outcomes of patients with HIV undergoing cardiac surgery in the United States showed no increase in mortality among patients with HIV infection compared to those patients not infected by the virus [22].

Table 5 Sensitivity analysis showing odds ratios, with 95% confidence interval, the *P* value and the I^2 value

Study which was excluded	Mortality	Cardiac death	Recurrent MI	TVR	TLR	MACEs
Badr 2015 [10]	0.86 [0.39–1.90], $P = 0.71$, $I^2 = 0\%$	0.61 [0.11–3.32], $P = 0.57$, $I^2 = 0\%$	1.20 [0.79–1.83], $P = 0.39$, $I^2 = 15\%$	1.31 [0.79–2.16], $P = 0.29$, $I^2 = 0\%$	1.31 [0.71–2.42], $P = 0.38$, $I^2 = 0\%$	1.15 [0.74–1.79], $P = 0.53$, $I^2 = 0\%$
Boccara 2006 [11]	-	-	-	1.27 [0.79–2.04], $P = 0.32$, $I^2 = 0\%$	-	1.28 [0.87–1.89], $P = 0.21$, $I^2 = 0\%$
Boccara 2011 [12]	-	1.32 [0.54–3.23], $P = 0.55$, $I^2 = 0\%$	-	1.39 [0.84–2.29], $P = 0.20$, $I^2 = 0\%$	1.22 [0.66–2.27], $P = 0.53$, $I^2 = 0\%$	1.35 [0.90–2.03], $P = 0.15$, $I^2 = 0\%$
Lorgis 2013 [13]	1.36 [0.68–2.72], $P = 0.38$, $I^2 = 0\%$	-	2.32 [0.96–5.58], $P = 0.06$, $I^2 = 11\%$	-	-	-
Matetzky 2003 [14]	1.19 [0.68–2.08], $P = 0.55$, $I^2 = 0\%$	1.21 [0.50–2.91], $P = 0.67$, $I^2 = 0\%$	1.22 [0.81–1.85], $P = 0.34$, $I^2 = 3\%$	-	-	-
Ren 2009 [15]	1.10 [0.62–1.96], $P = 0.75$, $I^2 = 0\%$	1.17 [0.49–2.83], $P = 0.72$, $I^2 = 0\%$	1.35 [0.89–2.05], $P = 0.16$, $I^2 = 50\%$	1.56 [0.87–2.79], $P = 0.13$, $I^2 = 0\%$	1.11 [0.55–2.25], $P = 0.78$, I2 = 0%	1.37 [0.87–2.15], $P = 0.18$, $I^2 = 0\%$

Abbreviations: *MI* myocardial infarction, *TVR* target vessel revascularization, *TLR* target lesion revascularization, *MACEs* major adverse cardiac events

However, results from the study by Hsue et al. involving data from San Francisco General Hospital unexpectedly showed a higher rate of restenosis after PCI in patients who were positive for HIV virus [23], which was completely different from the current results. But their study involved HIV positive patients with a low level of high density lipoproteins.

A systematic review and meta-analysis investigating acute coronary syndrome (ACS) in HIV positive patients showed HIV infected patients who were admitted due to ACS faced a substantial risk of short term death, and a significant long term risk of MI and revascularization, especially in those patients receiving protease inhibitors [24]. However, our analysis, which involved a larger number of patients, showed a completely different result from that study.

In addition, registry data involving twelve sites in Europe, South Africa and the United States also showed HIV patients suffering from ACS to have a significantly increased risk for cardiovascular death if specific treatments with nucleoside-reverse transcriptase inhibitors were not started [25]. The study also showed a significantly higher risk of MI with a low CD4 cell count (<200 cells/mm^3) indicating that HIV/AIDS with lower CD4 cell counts might further contribute to cardiovascular complications.

This analysis satisfied almost all the criteria to be considered solid enough for a meta-analysis. Despite the inclusion of observational studies, a very low level of heterogeneity was surprisingly reported among all the subgroups assessing the different clinical outcomes which should be considered a strong point of this analysis.

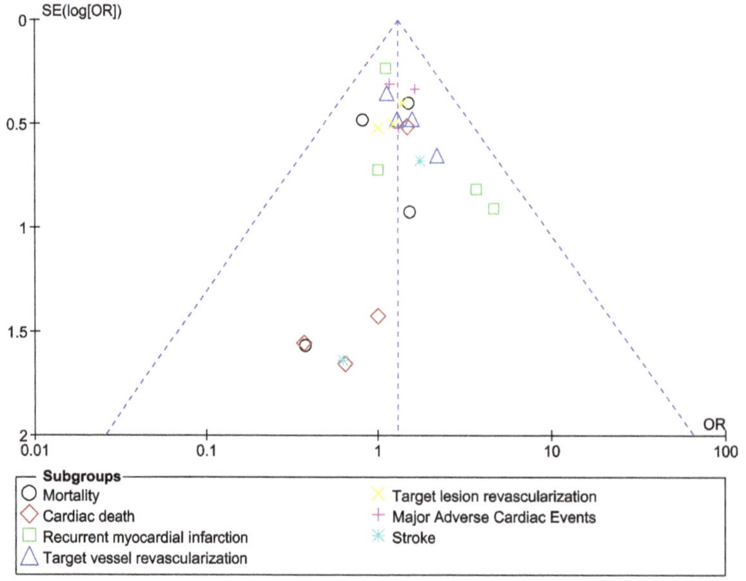

Fig. 3 Funnel plot showing publication bias

This analysis is also among the first meta-analyses comparing postinterventional adverse cardiovascular outcomes in patients with and without HIV infection. Moreover, it consisted of a larger number of patients (both HIV positive and HIV negative). The low level of heterogeneity reported among all the subgroups should further add up to its novelty.

However, due to a limited number of HIV positive patients, the analysis might not generate robust results. In addition, this analysis only involved data which were obtained from observational studies which are not considered as good as data which are found in RCTs. Moreover, all the studies did not report similar cardiovascular outcomes. Therefore, when the outcomes were analyzed, not all of the studies were involved each time.

Conclusion

Patients who were infected with HIV had similar mortality post coronary intervention compared to patients who were not infected by the virus, during a mean follow-up period of 1–3 years. In addition, no significant increase in MI, TVR, TLR, MACEs and stroke were observed during this follow up period. Therefore, it might be concluded that no apparent impact of HIV on the cardiovascular outcomes was observed post coronary intervention.

Abbreviations

AIDS: acquired immune deficiency syndrome; CAD: coronary artery disease; HAART: highly active antiretroviral therapy; HIV: human immunodeficiency virus; MACEs: major adverse cardiac events; PCI: percutaneous coronary intervention

Acknowledgements

Not applicable.

Funding

This research was supported by the Promotional Project of Guangxi Medical and Health Appropriate Technology (No. S201518).

Authors' contributions

PKB, MP and WQH were responsible for the conception and design, acquisition of data, analysis and interpretation of data, drafting the initial manuscript and revising it critically for important intellectual content. PKB wrote this manuscript. All authors read and approved the final manuscript.

Authors' information

Dr. Pravesh Kumar Bundhun (M.D) is the first author. From the Department of Cardiovascular Diseases, the First Affiliated Hospital of Guangxi Medical University, Nanning, Guangxi, China.

Competing interests

The authors declare that they have no competing interests.

Author details

[1]Institute of Cardiovascular Diseases, the First Affiliated Hospital of Guangxi Medical University, Nanning, Guangxi 530027, People's Republic of China. [2]Guangxi Medical University, Nanning, Guangxi 530027, People's Republic of China. [3]Institute of Cardiovascular Diseases, the First Affiliated Hospital of Guangxi Medical University, Nanning, Guangxi 530021, People's Republic of China.

References

1. Palella FJ Jr, Delaney KM, Moorman AC, et al. Declining morbidity and mortality among patients with advanced human immunodeficiency virus infection. HIVOutpatient study investigators. N Engl J Med. 1998;338(13):853–60.
2. Guo F, Hsieh E, Lv W, Han Y, Xie J, Li Y, Song X, Li T. Cardiovascular disease risk among Chinese antiretroviral-naïve adults with advanced HIV disease. BMC Infect Dis. 2017;17(1):287.
3. Maggi P, Bellacosa C, Leone A, et al. Cardiovascular risk in advanced naïve HIV-infected patients starting antiretroviral therapy: Comparison of three different regimens - PREVALEAT II cohort. Atherosclerosis. 2017;
4. Henry K, Melrow H, Huebsch J, et al. Severe coronary heart disease with protease inhibitors. Lancet. 1998;351:1328.
5. Rickerts V, Brodt H, Staszewski S, et al. Incidence of myocardial infarctions in HIV-infected patients between 1983 and 1998: the Frankfurt HIV-cohort study. Eur J Med Res. 2000;5:329–33.
6. Baker JV, Sharma S, Achhra AC, et al. Changes in cardiovascular disease risk factors with immediate versus deferred antiretroviral therapy initiation among HIV-positive participants in the START (strategic timing of antiretroviral treatment) trial. J Am Heart Assoc. 2017;6(5)
7. Liberati A, Altman DG, Tetzlaff J, et al. The PRISMA statement for reporting systematic reviews and meta-analyses of studies that evaluate healthcareinterventions: explanation and elaboration. BMJ. 2009;339:b2700.
8. Higgins JP, Altman DG, Gøtzsche PC, Jüni P, Moher D, et al. The Cochrane Collaboration's tool for assessing risk of bias in randomised trials. BMJ. 2011;343:d5928.
9. HigginsJPT, Green S. Cochrane Handbook for Systematic Reviews of Interventions Version 5.1.0. Cochrane Library, 2011.
10. Badr S, Minha S, Kitabata H, et al. Safety and long-term outcomes after percutaneous coronary intervention in patients with human immunodeficiency virus. Catheter Cardiovasc Interv. 2015;85(2):192–8.
11. Boccara F, Teiger E, Cohen A, et al. Percutaneous coronary intervention in HIV infected patients: immediate results and long term prognosis. Heart. 2006 Apr;92(4):543–4.
12. Boccara F, Mary-Krause M, Teiger E, et al. Prognosis of Acute Coronary Syndrome in HIV-infected patients (PACS) Investigators. Acute coronary syndrome in human immunodeficiency virus-infected patients: characteristics and 1 year prognosis. Eur Heart J. 2011;32(1):41–50.
13. Lorgis L, Cottenet J, Molins G, et al. Outcomes after acute myocardial infarction in HIV-infected patients: analysis of data from a French nationwide hospital medical information database. Circulation. 2013;127(17):1767–74.
14. Matetzky S, Domingo M, Kar S, et al. Acute myocardial infarction in human immunodeficiency virus-infected patients. Arch Intern Med. 2003;163(4):457–60.
15. Ren X, Trilesskaya M, Kwan DM, Nguyen K, Shaw RE, Hui PY. Comparison of outcomes using bare metal versus drug-eluting stents in coronary artery disease patients with and without human immunodeficiency virus infection. Am J Cardiol. 2009;104(2):216–22.
16. Wells GA, Shea B, O'Connell D, Peterson J, Welch V, Losos M, et al. The Newcastle-Ottawa Scale (NOS) for assessing the quality if nonrandomized studies in meta-analyses. http://www.ohri.ca/programs/clinical_epidemiology/oxford.htm 2009 [cited 2009 19]; Available from: URL: http://www.ohri.ca/programs/clinical_epidemiology/oxford.htm
17. Calza L, Manfredi R, Pocaterra D, Chiodo F. Risk of premature atherosclerosis and ischemic heart disease associated with HIV infection and antiretroviral therapy. J Infect. 2008;57(1):16–32.
18. Hwang SJ, Ballantyne CM, Sharrett AR, et al. Circulating adhesion molecules VCAM-1, ICAM-1, and E-selectin in carotid atherosclerosis and incident coronaryheart disease cases: the Atherosclerosis Risk In Communities (ARIC) study. Circulation. 1997;96(12):4219–25.
19. Ren Z, Yao Q, Chen C. HIV-1 envelope glycoprotein 120 increases intercellular adhesion molecule-1 expression by human endothelial cells. Lab Invest. 2002;82(3):245–55.
20. Boccara F, Lang S, Meuleman C, et al. HIV and coronary heart disease: time for a better understanding. J Am Coll Cardiol. 2013;61(5):511–23.
21. Perelló R, Calvo M, Miró O, et al. Clinical presentation of acute coronary syndrome in HIV infected adults: a retrospective analysis of a prospectively collected cohort. Eur J Intern Med. 2011;22(5):485–8.
22. Robich MP, Schiltz N, Johnston DR, et al. Outcomes of patients with human immunodeficiency virus infection undergoing cardiovascular surgery in the United States. J Thorac Cardiovasc Surg. 2014;148(6):3066–73.

18

Impact of hyperuricemia on clinical outcomes after percutaneous coronary intervention for in-stent restenosis

Hyung Joon Joo, Han Saem Jeong, Hyungdon Kook, Seung Hun Lee, Jae Hyoung Park, Soon Jun Hong, Cheol Woong Yu and Do-Sum Lim*

Abstract

Background: There have been limited data on the impact of hyperuricemia on long-term clinical outcomes after percutaneous coronary intervention (PCI) for in-stent restenosis (ISR).

Methods: From January 2009 to July 2015, 317 patients who underwent repeat PCI for ISR were divided into two groups: patients with normal serum uric acid (UA) levels (normal UA group) and patients with higher serum UA levels (higher UA group). The higher UA group included patients with serum UA levels > 6.8 mg/dL or patients who were taking anti-hyperuricemic medication.

Results: During a median follow-up period of 1088 days, the cumulative incidence rates of major adverse event (MAE), including a composite of all-cause death, non-fatal myocardial infarction, and any revascularization, were similar between the two groups (higher UA 36.4% vs. normal UA 29.9%, $p = 0.389$, log-rank $p = 0.367$). Follow-up angiographic data showed similar outcomes of late lumen loss (0.8 ± 0.9 mm vs. 0.8 ± 1.1 mm, $p = 0.895$) and binary restenosis rate (28.1% vs. 34.7%, $p = 0.622$). Multivariate Cox regression analysis indicated higher levels of low-density lipoprotein cholesterol (hazard ratio [HR] 1.011, 95% confidence interval [CI] 1.003–1.019, $p = 0.006$) and lower left ventricular ejection fraction (HR 0.972, 95% CI 0.948–0.996, $p = 0.022$), but not UA levels, to be the independent risk predictors of MAE.

Conclusion: Hyperuricemia is not associated with poor clinical outcomes after repeat PCI for ISR lesions.

Keywords: Uric acid, Major adverse event, In-stent restenosis, Percutaneous coronary intervention

Background

Drug-eluting stent (DES) implantation has remarkably decreased the in-stent restenosis (ISR) rate compared with bare metal stent (BMS) implantation [1]. Long-term follow-ups of previous large clinical trials on first-generation DES showed an annual ISR rate of approximately 6–8% [2–4]. Many clinical studies reflecting real-world situations, such as complex lesion interventions and high-risk patient populations, reported higher rates of ISR [5, 6]. Although the appropriate treatment for ISR lesions, especially after DES implantation, still remains debatable, repeat percutaneous coronary intervention (PCI) for ISR lesions is becoming more frequently used, and an overall increase of ISR can be expected in the coming years. In addition, recent studies showed an extremely high rate of ISR (between 20 and 40%) at the 6–9 months angiographic follow-up after repeat PCI [7, 8].

Many clinical, lesional, and procedural risk factors for ISR have been reported, including diabetes mellitus, chronic kidney disease, complex lesion, balloon injury, and stent underexpansion [9–12]. Pathophysiologically, ISR is considered to be an intrinsic cellular and biological response after stent implantation. Inflammation has been considered to be involved in this process. A recent study showed that high-sensitivity C-reactive protein (hsCRP) was associated with ISR and poor clinical outcomes after DES implantation [13]. Other studies also suggested different circulating inflammatory biomarkers as risk predictors

* Correspondence: dslmd@kumc.or.kr
Department of Cardiology, Cardiovascular Center, Korea University Anam Hospital, 126-1, 5ka, Anam-dong, Sungbuk-ku, Seoul 136-705, Republic of Korea

of ISR [14–16]. However, prognostic biomarkers after repeat PCI for ISR have not been well studied.

Uric acid (UA) is the main metabolite of purines in the human body [17]. A hyperuricemic state could inhibit endothelial nitric oxide synthesis, promote vascular smooth muscle cell proliferation, induce microvascular injury, and trigger metabolic dysregulation [18]. Therefore, hyperuricemia is associated with other cardiovascular risk factors such as hypertension, diabetes mellitus, and chronic kidney disease [19, 20]. Previous studies have shown that hyperuricemia is a significant risk factor for cardiovascular disease and mortality in the general population [21]. In addition, it was reported as an independent risk predictor of ISR after BMS implantation [22]. It was associated with poor clinical outcomes after DES implantation [23]. The aim of this study was to determine whether a high serum UA level is associated with poor clinical outcomes in patients undergoing repeat PCI for ISR lesions.

Methods

Study design

We screened all consecutive patients who underwent PCI at Korea University Anam Hospital between January 2009 and July 2015. Among them, 353 patients had ISR lesions (> 50% restenosis in the stent or within 5 mm of the stent edges) and underwent repeat PCI for ISR lesions. Thirty-six patients had missing data on serum UA level and were excluded. Finally, 317 patients (328 lesions) were analyzed in this study. Clinical events were monitored until June 2016 through medical record reviews and telephone calls. The present study was approved by the hospital's institutional review board (IRB no. AN16238-002) and performed in accordance with the Declaration of Helsinki. The need for written informed consent was waived owing to the retrospective nature of the study.

Definitions

A serum UA level of > 6.8 mg/dL was defined as hyperuricemia for both sexes [24]. This cutoff is the limit of urate solubility in the serum, and supersaturation of urate in extracellular fluid has been known to predispose a person to various pathologic conditions, including gout and cardiovascular diseases. Thus, the higher UA group included patients with hyperuricemia (serum UA level ≥6.8 mg/dL) or patients treated with anti-hyperuricemic agents such as allopurinol and febuxostat.

The primary end point, major adverse event (MAE), was defined as a composite of all-cause death; non-fatal myocardial infarction; any revascularization, including target-vessel revascularization (TVR) and non-TVR; and coronary artery bypass graft surgery. Myocardial infarction was defined as present when patients had elevated cardiac enzymes with compatible symptoms or electrocardiographic findings. Stent thrombosis was defined as definite stent thrombosis based on Academic Research Consortium Criteria [25].

Procedures

Interventional procedures were performed according the standard clinical guidelines. Interventional strategies, including drug-coated balloon (DCB) angioplasty, DES implantation, and use of adjunctive devices and pharmacotherapy, were decided according to the operators' discretion. Balloon pre-dilatation was performed for all ISR lesions. The first-generation DES included CYPHER® (Cordis, Johnson & Johnson, Miami Lake, FL, USA) and TAXUS™ (Boston Scientific Corp., Marlborough, MA, USA). The second-generation DES included XIENCE™ series (Abbott Vascular Devices, Temecula, CA, USA) and Endeavor® series (Medtronic Cardiovascular, Santa Rosa, CA, USA). The third-generation DES included BioMatrix (Biosensors, Singapore, Singapore) and Nobori (Terumo Corporation, Tokyo, Japan). The DCB (SeQent® Please balloon catheter; B.Braun, Melsungen, Germany) became available and was used from July 2010.

Laboratory measurements

Laboratory profiles, including lipid panel, creatinine, glucose, hsCRP, and UA levels, were obtained within 4 weeks before the index PCI or at the index admission date. Serum UA level was measured by using an enzymatic method with an automatic biochemistry analyzer (Beckman Coulter AU 5800; Beckman Coulter Inc., Brea, CA, USA). Creatinine clearance was calculated using the Cockcroft and Gault formula [26].

Angiographic analysis

Three radiologic technologists blinded to the patients' treatment performed analyses with a quantitative coronary angiographic system (CASS system; Pie Medical Instruments, Maastricht, the Netherlands). By using the guiding catheter for magnification-calibration, the diameter of the reference vessel, minimal luminal diameter, and percent diameter stenosis were measured from diastolic frames in a single, matched view showing the smallest minimal luminal diameter. ISR lesions were classified according to the Mehran classification [27]. Multifocal, diffuse, proliferative, and occlusive ISR lesions were classified as non-focal-type restenosis lesions. Acute gain was calculated as the increase in minimal lumen diameter of the treated lesion immediately after the index procedure compared with that before the procedure. Late lumen loss was defined as a decrease in minimal lumen diameter of the treated lesion at the follow-up coronary angiography compared with that immediately after the index procedure. All quantitative angiographic measurements were obtained before and after PCI, and at the follow-up coronary angiography.

Statistics

Categorical variables are reported as count (percentage), and continuous variables are reported as mean ± standard deviation. To compare the baseline clinical characteristics, angiographic features, procedural details, and the cumulative incidence of clinical events between the higher UA and normal UA groups, the chi-square test for categorical variables and Student's *t* test (or Wilcox test) for continuous variables were performed. Kaplan–Meier survival curves with a log-rank test were generated to compare the long-term incidence of MAE between the two groups. In order to identify the risk predictors of MAE, the multivariate Cox proportional hazard model was used to evaluate the possible contributing factors. The following variables were included in the Cox regression model: age, sex, body mass index, current smoking, hypertension, diabetes mellitus, acute myocardial infarction at the index PCI, low-density lipoprotein (LDL)-cholesterol level, triglyceride level, UA level, creatinine clearance, left ventricular ejection fraction (LVEF), previous first-generation DES implantation, multivessel involvement, chronic total occlusion lesion, ISR type (III, IV), and PCI type (DES or DCB). Hazard ratios with 95% confidence intervals and *p*-values were reported. All tests were two-tailed, and p-values < 0.05 were considered statistically significant. All statistical analyses were performed using SPSS software (v20; IBM SPSS Corp., Armonk, NY, USA).

Results

The baseline characteristics of 317 patients who underwent PCI for ISR lesions are presented in Table 1. Eighteen patients (27.3%) already treated with anti-hyperuricemic agents before UA measurement were categorized into the higher UA group. No additional patient was started on anti-hyperuricemic agents during follow-up. Among the total 317 patients, 285 had follow-up data on serum UA levels (Additional File 1:Table S1). The normal UA group showed increased UA levels at the follow-up measurement (4.8 ± 1.1 mg/dL vs. 5.2 ± 1.3 mg/dL, $p = 0.002$). There was no significant difference between the baseline and follow-up UA levels in the higher UA group (7.3 ± 1.5 mg/dL vs. 6.7 ± 2.0 mg/dL, $p = 0.092$). The significant difference in serum UA levels between the normal UA group and the higher UA group was maintained at the follow-up measurement (5.2 ± 1.3 mg/dL vs. 6.7 ± 2.0 mg/dL, $p < 0.001$).

The serum UA level was 7.4 ± 1.6 mg/dL in the higher UA group and 4.9 ± 1.1 mg/dL in the normal UA group ($p < 0.001$). The higher UA group had more men (86.4% vs. 72.5%, $p = 0.03$) and lower creatinine clearance (63.3 ± 26.2 mL/min vs. 72.3 ± 22.5 mL/min, $p = 0.006$). The higher UA group showed a trend of higher body mass index than the normal UA group (25.6 ± 2.9 vs. 24.8 ± 3.0, $p = 0.056$).

The significant PCI characteristics of 328 ISR lesions are shown in Table 2. The diffuse type of ISR (II, III, IV) was more frequent in the higher UA group than in the normal UA group (53.5% vs. 37.0%, $p = 0.017$; Additional File 1: Table S2,). The higher UA group showed a longer interval between the previous PCI and the index PCI (1669 days vs. 990 days, $p = 0.045$). The stent diameter was statistically larger in the higher UA group than in the normal UA group (3.0 ± 0.5 mm vs. 2.9 ± 0.4 mm, p = 0.01). Qualitative comparative analysis data also showed a trend of larger target lesion reference vessel diameter in the higher UA group than in the normal UA group (3.0 ± 0.5 mm vs. 2.9 ± 0.4 mm, $p = 0.055$; Table 3). Angiographic follow-up was performed in 150 (45.7%) lesions. There were no significant differences in late lumen loss and binary restenosis rate between the two groups.

Table 1 Baseline clinical characteristics

	Normal UA (*n* = 251)	Higher UA (*n* = 66)	*p*-value
Age (year)	64.6 ± 9.9	65.3 ± 10.3	0.609
Men, *n* (%)	182 (72.5)	57 (86.4)	0.030
Body mass index	24.8 ± 3.0	25.6 ± 2.9	0.056
Current smoker, *n* (%)	61 (24.3)	16 (24.2)	1.000
Hypertension, *n* (%)	175 (69.7)	53 (80.3)	0.122
Diabetes, *n* (%)	91 (36.3)	25 (37.9)	0.920
Prior MI, *n* (%)	69 (27.5)	23 (34.8)	0.308
Diagnosis at the index PCI			
SA/UA, *n* (%)	210 (83.7)	54 (81.8)	0.863
NSTEMI/STEMI, *n* (%)	41 (16.3)	12 (18.2)	
Laboratory findings			
Uric acid (mg/dL)	4.9 ± 1.1	7.4 ± 1.6	<.001
Total cholesterol (mg/dL)	150.1 ± 37.3	148.8 ± 43.8	0.817
LDL-C (mg/dL)	85.9 ± 29.5	90.6 ± 36.4	0.345
HDL-C (mg/dL)	43.6 ± 11.0	42.0 ± 12.7	0.333
Triglyceride (mg/dL)	127.5 ± 75.6	147.2 ± 78.1	0.064
Glucose (mg/dL)	122.5 ± 42.0	121.8 ± 42.9	0.900
Creatinine Clearance (mL/min)	72.3 ± 22.5	63.3 ± 26.2	0.006
hsCRP (mg/L)	4.3 ± 10.6	5.8 ± 12.9	0.407
LVEF (%)	56.2 ± 7.9	53.5 ± 11.4	0.095
Medications			
DAPT	248 (98.8)	64 (97.0)	0.610
Anti-hyperuricemic agent	–	18 (27.3)	–

Data were presented as *n* (%) or mean ± SD. DES, drug-eluting stent; DCB, drug-coated balloon; MI, myocardial infarction; PCI, percutaneous coronary intervention; SA, stable angina; UA, unstable angina; NSTEMI, non-ST segment elevation myocardial infarction; STEMI, ST segment elevation myocardial infarction; LDL-C, low density lipoprotein cholesterol; HDL-C, high density lipoprotein cholesterol; hsCRP, high sensitivity C-reactive protein; LVEF, left ventricular ejection fraction; DAPT, dual anti-platelet treatment

Table 2 Angiographic features and procedural details

	Normal UA (n = 257)	Higher UA (n = 71)	p-value
Previous PCI characteristics			
Stent type			
BMS, n (%)	21 (8.3)	5 (7.5)	
1st generation DES, n (%)	88 (34.9)	35 (52.2)	0.075
2nd generation DES, n (%)	108 (42.9)	21 (31.3)	
3rd generation DES, n (%)	35 (13.9)	6 (9.0)	
Stent diameter (mm)	2.9 ± 0.3	2.9 ± 0.3	0.900
Stent length (mm)	22.7 ± 7.2	22.0 ± 7.5	0.504
Median duration between previous PCI to the index procedure (day)	990	1669	0.045
Lesion characteristics at the index PCI			
Target vessel, n (%)			
LAD	166 (64.6)	49 (69.0)	0.478
LCX	40 (15.6)	7 (9.9)	
RCA	51 (19.8)	15 (21.1)	
Multivessel involvement, n (%)	166 (64.6)	53 (74.6)	0.147
CTO, n (%)	17 (6.6)	7 (9.9)	0.502
ISR type (II, III, IV), n (%)	95 (37.0)	38 (53.5)	0.017
Procedures of the index PCI			
PCI type			
DES	174 (67.7)	52 (73.2)	0.455
DCB	83 (32.3)	19 (26.8)	
DES type			
1st generation DES, n (%)	17 (9.8)	7 (13.5)	0.354
2nd generation DES, n (%)	116 (66.7)	29 (55.8)	
3rd generation DES, n (%)	41 (23.6)	16 (30.8)	
DES diameter (mm)	2.9 ± 0.4	3.0 ± 0.5	0.010
DES length (mm)	23.1 ± 11.5	23.8 ± 10.3	0.685
DCB diameter (mm)	2.8 ± 0.3	2.9 ± 0.3	0.344
DCB length (mm)	20.2 ± 5.2	20.0 ± 5.1	0.875

Data were presented as n (%) or mean ± SD. PCI, percutaneous coronary intervention; BMS, bare metal stent; DES, drug-eluting stent; LAD, left anterior descending artery; LCX, left circumflex artery; RCA right coronary artery; CTO, chronic total occlusion; ISR, in-stent restenosis; DCB, drug-coated balloon

During the follow-up period (median: 748 days for the total population, 676 days for the higher UA group, and 755 days for the normal UA group; p = 702), the cumulative incidence rates of MAE were similar between the two groups (36.4% in the higher UA group vs. 29.9% in the normal UA group, p = 0.389; Fig. 1a). There were also no significant differences in other clinical events between the two groups even at different time points (Additional File 1: Table S3). Kaplan–Meier analysis indicated that the long-term incidences of MAE were similar between the two groups (log-rank test, p = 0.367; Fig. 1b).

Table 3 Quantitative coronary angiography analysis

	Normal UA	Higher UA	p-value
Index PCI			
n	257	71	
Pre-procedural RVD (mm)	2.9 ± 0.4	3.0 ± 0.5	0.055
Pre-procedural MLD (mm)	0.6 ± 0.4	0.6 ± 0.4	0.396
Pre-procedural DS (mm)	79.0 ± 12.6	78.5 ± 12.4	0.749
Pre-procedural lesion length (mm)	20.1 ± 11.0	20.2 ± 10.2	0.959
Post-procedural MLD (mm)	2.7 ± 0.4	2.8 ± 0.6	0.105
Post-procedural DS (%)	8.6 ± 6.8	8.5 ± 11.9	0.925
Acute gain (mm)	2.1 ± 0.5	2.2 ± 0.6	0.293
Follow-up CAG			
n	118	32	
Median follow-up period (day)	462	527	0.559
Target lesion RVD (mm)	2.9 ± 0.5	2.9 ± 0.5	0.888
Target lesion MLD (mm)	1.9 ± 1.1	2.0 ± 1.1	0.590
Target lesion DS (%)	36.2 ± 34.2	33.4 ± 33.0	0.686
Late lumen loss (mm)	0.8 ± 1.1	0.8 ± 0.9	0.895
Binary restenosis, n (%)	41 (34.7)	9 (28.1)	0.622

Data were presented as n (%) or mean ± SD. PCI, percutaneous coronary intervention; UA, uric acid; CAG, coronary angiography; RVD, reference vessel diameter; MLD, minimal lumen diameter; DS, diameter stenosis

Univariate Cox regression analysis suggested that serum UA level was unable to predict MAE (hazard ratio 1.110, 95% confidence interval 0.980–1.257, p = 0.100). Multivariate Cox regression analysis revealed that high LDL-cholesterol level and low LVEF were independent predictors of MAE (Table 4).

Discussion

The present study is the first to investigate the association between serum UA level and cardiovascular prognosis, especially in patients who underwent repeat PCI for ISR lesions. Hyperuricemia was present in 20.8% of patients with ISR lesions. The diffuse type of ISR was more frequent in patients with hyperuricemia. However, hyperuricemia was not associated with the incidence of MAE and angiographic ISR after re-intervention. Interestingly, high LDL-cholesterol level and low LVEF were associated with poor clinical outcomes.

Definition of hyperuricemia

Many studies have reported that hyperuricemia is associated with cardiovascular disease. A recent meta-analysis including 29 prospective cohort studies also showed that hyperuricemia is an independent risk factor for cardiovascular morbidity and mortality [28]. Biologically, UA exerts pro-oxidant or nitric-oxide-reducing effects depending on its concentration and chemical microenvironment [29]. When the urate concentration exceeds 6 mg/dL, the risk of urate crystal formation and

a

	Normal UA (n = 251)	Higher UA (n = 66)	*p*-value
Major adverse event, n (%)	75 (29.9)	24 (36.4)	0.389
All-cause death, n (%)	8 (3.2)	3 (4.5)	0.874
Non-fatal MI, n (%)	10 (4)	0 (0)	0.211
TVR, n (%)	56 (22.3)	14 (21.2)	0.980
Non-TVR, n(%)	15 (6)	7 (10.6)	0.296
CABG, n (%)	4 (1.6)	2 (3.0)	0.799
Stent thrombosis, n (%)	6 (2.4)	0 (0)	0.447

b

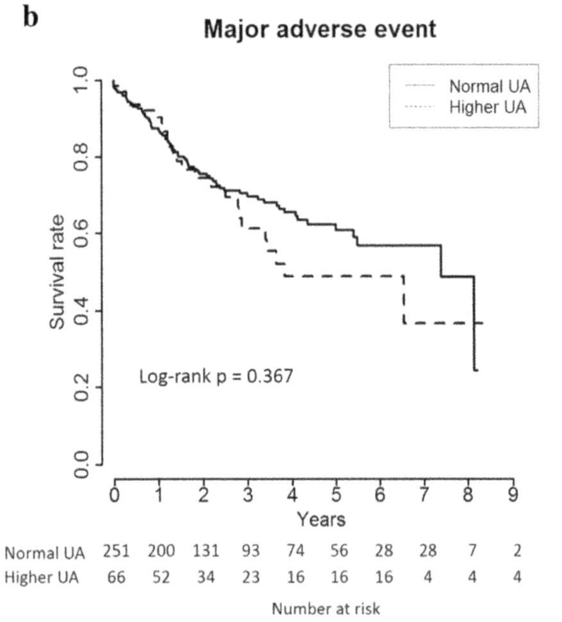

Fig. 1 Clinical outcome. **a** Cumulative incidence of clinical events. **b** Kaplan–Meier curve for major adverse event. Data are presented as n (%). MI, myocardial infarction; TVR, target vessel revascularization; CABG, coronary artery bypass graft. Major adverse event was defined as a composite event of all-cause death, non-fatal myocardial infarction, and any revascularization, including TVR, non-TVR, and CABG

Table 4 Cox-proportional hazard models for major adverse event

	HR	95% CI	*p*-value
Univariate			
Age	1.000	0.981 – 1.019	0.992
Men	1.015	0.654 – 1.577	0.947
Body mass index	0.971	0.909 – 1.039	0.401
Current smoking	1.587	1.067 – 2.359	0.022
Hypertension	1.435	0.917 – 2.246	0.114
Diabetes mellitus	0.929	0.629 – 1.372	0.712
NSTEMI/STEMI at index PCI	1.170	0.727 – 1.884	0.518
LDL-C	1.009	1.002 – 1.015	0.008
Triglyceride	1.001	0.999 – 1.004	0.312
Uric acid	1.110	0.980 – 1.257	0.100
Creatinine clearance	0.997	0.989 – 1.006	0.494
LVEF	0.976	0.955 – 0.998	0.031
Previous 1st generation DES	1.204	0.824 – 1.758	0.338
Multivessel involvement	1.225	0.819 – 1.833	0.324
CTO lesion	0.784	0.364 – 1.689	0.534
ISR type (II, III, IV)	0.951	0.647 – 1.400	0.800
DCB (vs DES)	1.487	0.974 – 2.271	0.066
Multivariate			
Current smoking	1.521	0.957 - 2.416	0.076
Hypertension	1.469	0.870 - 2.481	0.150
LDL-C	1.011	1.003 - 1.019	0.006
LVEF	0.972	0.948 - 0.996	0.022
DCB (vs DES)	1.475	0.912 - 2.386	0.113

HR, hazard ratio; 95% CI, 95% confidence interval; NSTEMI, non-ST segment elevation myocardial infarction; STEMI, ST segment elevation myocardial infarction; LDL-C, low density lipoprotein cholesterol; LVEF, left ventricular ejection fraction; DES, drug-eluting stent; CTO, chronic total occlusion; ISR, in-stent restenosis; DCB, drug-coated balloon

precipitation increases. Therefore, hyperuricemia is generally defined as a serum UA level of > 6.8 mg/dL [30]. The present study adopted this cutoff value. However, the optimal threshold for serum UA level remains debatable. Some studies used different cutoff values based on sex, considering the significant difference in reference ranges of serum UA levels between men and women. Recently, the clinically detrimental effect of serum UA seems to be evident even below its saturation limit, likely independent of urate crystal formation in cardiovascular diseases. Receiver-operating characteristic curve analysis of serum UA level for MAE in the present study showed an area under the curve of 0.544 (95% confidence interval 0.474–0.615, data not shown). In addition, when we further analyzed the clinical outcomes between two groups determined using the median UA level (5.3 mg/dL), the results also showed similar clinical outcomes between patients with lower UA level (≤5.3 mg/dL) and patients with higher UA level (> 5.3 mg/dL) (Additional File 1: Table S4 and Additional File 1: Figure S1). These data suggested that the association between serum UA level and poor clinical outcomes was very weak, and the optimal cutoff value of hyperuricemia might be obscure in those high-risk patients who underwent repeat PCI for ISR lesions.

Clinical and angiographic characteristics of hyperuricemic patients

In the present study, patients with hyperuricemia were predominantly male and somewhat obese. Additionally, they had lower creatinine clearance and showed a trend of higher serum triglyceride levels. Interestingly, patients with hyperuricemia had a higher frequency of non-focal-type restenosis lesions than normouricemic patients. Previously, elevated serum hsCRP level was reported as a risk predictor of non-focal-type ISR after DES implantation, suggesting that inflammatory activity might contribute to aggressive restenosis [31]. In addition, old age, hypertension, diabetes mellitus, and paclitaxel-eluting stent implantation were also reported to be associated with the non-focal type of ISR [32–34]. Thus, considering that hyperuricemia is associated with elevated hsCRP level and other inflammatory markers, it could also be another possible biomarker for non-focal-type ISR. In addition, the present study showed a significant difference in the interval between previous PCI and index PCI between the low UA group and the high UA group. The high UA group took a longer time to develop ISR than the lower UA group. A previous study using an intravascular imaging modality demonstrated that neointimal hyperplasia is associated with earlier ISR, whereas neoatherosclerosis is associated with later ISR [35]. It also suggested the potential role of a high serum UA level in the development of neoatherosclerosis and ISR.

Risk predictors for poor prognosis after repeat PCI for ISR

The present study did not show an association between hyperuricemia and clinical outcomes after repeat PCI for ISR lesions. Previous stent type, stent number, bifurcation lesion, ISR type, and repeat first-generation DES implantation were suggested as risk predictors of poor prognosis [36–39]. Conventional demographic risk factors, such as diabetes mellitus, failed to reach clinical significance after repeat PCI for ISR [40]. These findings suggested that the pathologic mechanisms of recurrent ISR are rather different from those of de novo coronary atherosclerosis, and implied that lesional, technical, and mechanical factors might play important roles in recurrent ISR development after repeat PCI for ISR. A recent study even suggested DCB angioplasty as a predictor of target lesion failure in the second-generation DES era [41]. When we analyzed the impact of hyperuricemia in patients treated with DES or in patients treated with DCB separately, there were no significant differences in clinical outcomes between the low UA group and the high UA group in both the DES- and DCB-treated patients (Additional File 1: Table S5).

In addition, it was previously demonstrated that serum LDL-cholesterol level was significantly associated with the development of neoatherosclerosis, which has been studied as an important pathologic process related to poor clinical outcome after PCI in the DES era [42]. There was also a case of recurrent neoatherosclerosis after repeat PCI for ISR [43]. These data suggested that the residual risk of altered lipid metabolism should be considered after repeat PCI for ISR lesions. The present study indicated LDL-cholesterol level and LVEF as important risk predictors of MAEs (Table 4). However, the Cox proportional hazard model for TVR failed to suggest any independent risk factor from the 17 potential risk factors including age, sex, body mass index, current smoking, hypertension, diabetes mellitus, presentation of acute myocardial infarction, LDL-C, triglyceride, UA, creatinine clearance, LVEF, prior first-generation DES use, multivessel involvement, chronic total occlusion, ISR type, and PCI strategy (data not shown). The Cox proportional hazard model for non-TVR proposed LDL-C and LVEF as the independent risk factors for non-TVR in patients after repeat PCI for ISR (Additional File 1: Table S6). These results suggested that LDL-C and LVEF contribute to MAE development mainly driven by non-TVR rather than TVR. Management of lipid profile and heart failure could be emphasized as a fundamental strategy to prevent adverse clinical outcomes in patients after repeat PCI for ISR, although their association with TVR is obscure. However, the present study showed that TVR rather than non-TVR formed a majority of MAEs (70.7%, 70 of 99). Thus, although the present study failed to suggest the important risk predictor for repeat target vessel failure, further studies should resolve this issue.

Study limitations

The present study has several limitations. First, this is a single-center, retrospective study. The study population was enrolled for a long duration and the baseline characteristics were heterogeneous. Moreover, the PCI strategy was dependent on the discretion of the operators, and a selection bias should be considered in the interpretation of our results. Second, the sample size was too small to discriminate the clinical impact of hyperuricemia, although the patients were followed-up for a long duration. Third, the present study did not analyze intravascular imaging data (intravascular ultrasound or optical coherence tomography) because of their limited usage (36.9%). Considering that mechanical and technical factors may contribute to ISR, detailed lesional information could provide an insight into the clinical relevance of hyperuricemia. Therefore, our findings should be extended and validated further by other studies.

Conclusions

The non-focal-type ISR lesion was more frequent in patients with hyperuricemia. However, hyperuricemia was not associated with poor clinical outcomes after repeat PCI for ISR lesions. Serum LDL-cholesterol level and LVEF were independent risk predictors of poor clinical outcomes.

Additional file

Additional file 1: Table S1. Changes in serum uric acid level, **Table S2.** In-stent restenosis patterns at the index procedure, **Table S3.** Cumulative incidence of clinical events between patients with lower uric acid level (≤6.8 mg/dL) and those with higher uric acid level (> 6.8 mg/dL), **Table S4.** Cumulative incidence of clinical events between patients with lower uric acid level (≤5.3 mg/dL) and those with higher uric acid level (> 5.3 mg/dL), **Table S5.** Subgroup analyses of the cumulative incidence of clinical events between the low uric acid group and the high uric acid group, **Table S6.** Cox-proportional hazard models for non-target vessel revascularization, **Figure S1.** Kaplan-Meier curve for major adverse event between patients with lower uric acid level (≤5.3 mg/dL) and those with higher uric acid level (> 5.3 mg/dL). UA, uric acid.

Abbreviations

BMS: Bare metal stent; DCB: Drug-coated balloon; DES: Drug-eluting stent; hsCRP: High-sensitivity C-reactive protein; ISR: In-stent restenosis; LDL: Low-density lipoprotein; LVEF: Left ventricular ejection fraction; MAE: Major adverse event; PCI: Percutaneous coronary intervention; TVR: Target-vessel revascularization; UA: Uric acid.

Acknowledgements

The authors thank Joon Won Kang and Yon Won Lee of the cardiac catheterization laboratory for their skilled technical assistance.

Authors' contributions

HJJ designed the study, planned and performed statistical analyses, and wrote the first draft. HJJ, HSJ, HK, SHL, JHP, SJH, CWY and DSL contributed to the collection of data, discussions, and interpretation of data. The decision to submit this manuscript for publication was made by HJJ, HSJ, HK, SHL, JHP, SJH, CWY and DSL. All authors read and approved the final manuscript.

Competing interests

The authors declare that they have no competing interests.

References

1. Stone GW, Moses JW, Ellis SG, Schofer J, Dawkins KD, Morice MC, Colombo A, Schampaert E, Grube E, Kirtane AJ, et al. Safety and efficacy of sirolimus- and paclitaxel-eluting coronary stents. N Engl J Med. 2007;356(10):998–1008.
2. Moses JW, Leon MB, Popma JJ, Fitzgerald PJ, Holmes DR, O'Shaughnessy C, Caputo RP, Kereiakes DJ, Williams DO, Teirstein PS, et al. Sirolimus-eluting stents versus standard stents in patients with stenosis in a native coronary artery. N Engl J Med. 2003;349(14):1315–23.
3. Weisz G, Leon MB, Holmes DR Jr, Kereiakes DJ, Clark MR, Cohen BM, Ellis SG, Coleman P, Hill C, Shi C, et al. Two-year outcomes after sirolimus-eluting stent implantation: results from the Sirolimus-eluting stent in de novo native coronary lesions (SIRIUS) trial. J Am Coll Cardiol. 2006;47(7):1350–5.
4. Stone GW, Ellis SG, Cox DA, Hermiller J, O'Shaughnessy C, Mann JT, Turco M, Caputo R, Bergin P, Greenberg J, et al. One-year clinical results with the slow-release, polymer-based, paclitaxel-eluting TAXUS stent: the TAXUS-IV trial. Circulation. 2004;109(16):1942–7.
5. Turco MA, Ormiston JA, Popma JJ, Hall JJ, Mann T, Cannon LA, Webster MW, Mishkel GJ, O'Shaughnessy CD, McGarry TF, et al. Reduced risk of restenosis in small vessels and reduced risk of myocardial infarction in long lesions with the new thin-strut TAXUS Liberte stent: 1-year results from the TAXUS ATLAS program. JACC Cardiovasc Interv. 2008;1(6):699–709.
6. Schofer J, Schluter M, Gershlick AH, Wijns W, Garcia E, Schampaert E, Breithardt G, Investigators ES. Sirolimus-eluting stents for treatment of patients with long atherosclerotic lesions in small coronary arteries: double-blind, randomised controlled trial (E-SIRIUS). Lancet. 2003;362(9390):1093–9.
7. Alfonso F, Perez-Vizcayno MJ, Dutary J, Zueco J, Cequier A, Garcia-Touchard A, Marti V, Lozano I, Angel J, Hernandez JM, et al. Implantation of a drug-eluting stent with a different drug (switch strategy) in patients with drug-eluting stent restenosis. Results from a prospective multicenter study (RIBS III [restenosis intra-stent: balloon angioplasty versus drug-eluting stent]). JACC Cardiovasc Interv. 2012;5(7):728–37.
8. Mehilli J, Byrne RA, Tiroch K, Pinieck S, Schulz S, Kufner S, Massberg S, Laugwitz KL, Schomig A, Kastrati A, et al. Randomized trial of paclitaxel- versus sirolimus-eluting stents for treatment of coronary restenosis in sirolimus-eluting stents: the ISAR-DESIRE 2 (intracoronary stenting and angiographic results: drug eluting stents for in-stent restenosis 2) study. J Am Coll Cardiol. 2010;55(24):2710–6.
9. Alfonso F, Cequier A, Angel J, Marti V, Zueco J, Bethencourt A, Mantilla R, Lopez-Minguez JR, Gomez-Recio M, Moris C, et al. Value of the American College of Cardiology/American Heart Association angiographic classification of coronary lesion morphology in patients with in-stent restenosis. Insights from the restenosis intra-stent balloon angioplasty versus elective stenting (RIBS) randomized trial. Am Heart J. 2006;151(3):681. e681-681 e689
10. Zahn R, Hamm CW, Schneider S, Richardt G, Kelm M, Levenson B, Bonzel T, Tebbe U, Sabin G, Nienaber CA, et al. Coronary stenting with the sirolimus-eluting stent in clinical practice: final results from the prospective multicenter German Cypher stent registry. J Interv Cardiol. 2010;23(1):18–25.
11. Kastrati A, Dibra A, Mehilli J, Mayer S, Pinieck S, Pache J, Dirschinger J, Schomig A. Predictive factors of restenosis after coronary implantation of sirolimus- or paclitaxel-eluting stents. Circulation. 2006;113(19):2293–300.
12. Dangas GD, Claessen BE, Caixeta A, Sanidas EA, Mintz GS, Mehran R. In-stent restenosis in the drug-eluting stent era. J Am Coll Cardiol. 2010;56(23):1897–907.
13. Hsieh IC, Chen CC, Hsieh MJ, Yang CH, Chen DY, Chang SH, Wang CY, Lee CH, Tsai ML. Prognostic impact of 9-month high-sensitivity C-reactive protein levels on long-term clinical outcomes and in-stent restenosis in patients at 9 months after drug-eluting stent implantation. PLoS One. 2015;10(9):e0138512.
14. Jiang H, Liu W, Liu Y, Cao F. High levels of HB-EGF and interleukin-18 are associated with a high risk of in-stent restenosis. Anatol J Cardiol. 2015; 15(11):907–12.
15. Jing XD, Wei XM, Deng SB, Du JL, Liu YJ, She Q. The relationship between the high-density lipoprotein (HDL)-associated sphingosine-1-phosphate (S1P) and coronary in-stent restenosis. Clin Chim Acta. 2015;446:248–52.
16. Liang S, Aiqun M, Jiwu L, Ping Z. TLR3 and TLR4 as potential clinical biomarkers for in-stent restenosis in drug-eluting stents patients. Immunol Res. 2016;64(2):424–30.
17. Mene P, Punzo G. Uric acid: bystander or culprit in hypertension and progressive renal disease? J Hypertens. 2008;26(11):2085–92.
18. Battelli MG, Polito L, Bolognesi A. Xanthine oxidoreductase in atherosclerosis pathogenesis: not only oxidative stress. Atherosclerosis. 2014;237(2):562–7.
19. Jalal DI, Chonchol M, Chen W, Targher G. Uric acid as a target of therapy in CKD. Am J Kidney Dis. 2013;61(1):134–46.
20. Zoppini G, Targher G, Chonchol M, Ortalda V, Abaterusso C, Pichiri I, Negri C, Bonora E. Serum uric acid levels and incident chronic kidney disease in patients with type 2 diabetes and preserved kidney function. Diabetes Care. 2012;35(1):99–104.
21. Fang J, Alderman MH. Serum uric acid and cardiovascular mortality the NHANES I epidemiologic follow-up study, 1971-1992. National Health and nutrition examination survey. JAMA. 2000;283(18):2404–10.
22. Turak O, Canpolat U, Ozcan F, Mendi MA, Oksuz F, Isleyen A, Gurel OM, Cay S, Aras D, Aydogdu S. Usefulness of preprocedural serum uric acid level to predict restenosis of bare metal stents. Am J Cardiol. 2014;113(2):197–202.
23. Yin Z, Fang Z, Yang M, Du X, Nie B, Gao K. Predictive value of serum uric acid levels on mortality in acute coronary syndrome patients with chronic kidney disease after drug-eluting stent implantation. Cardiology. 2013; 125(4):204–12.
24. Wilcox WR, Khalaf A, Weinberger A, Kippen I, Klinenberg JR. Solubility of uric acid and monosodium urate. Med Biol Eng. 1972;10(4):522–31.
25. Cutlip DE, Windecker S, Mehran R, Boam A, Cohen DJ, van Es GA, Steg PG, Morel MA, Mauri L, Vranckx P, et al. Clinical end points in coronary stent trials: a case for standardized definitions. Circulation. 2007;115(17):2344–51.
26. Cockcroft DW, Gault MH. Prediction of creatinine clearance from serum creatinine. Nephron. 1976;16(1):31–41.
27. Mehran R, Dangas G, Abizaid AS, Mintz GS, Lansky AJ, Satler LF, Pichard AD, Kent KM, Stone GW, Leon MB. Angiographic patterns of in-stent restenosis: classification and implications for long-term outcome. Circulation. 1999; 100(18):1872–8.

28. Li M, Hu X, Fan Y, Li K, Zhang X, Hou W, Tang Z. Hyperuricemia and the risk for coronary heart disease morbidity and mortality a systematic review and dose-response meta-analysis. Sci Rep. 2016;6:19520.
29. Kanellis J, Kang DH. Uric acid as a mediator of endothelial dysfunction, inflammation and vascular disease. *Semin Nephrol*. 2005;25(1):39–42.
30. Becker MA, Schumacher HR Jr, Wortmann RL, MacDonald PA, Eustace D, Palo WA, Streit J, Joseph-Ridge N. Febuxostat compared with allopurinol in patients with hyperuricemia and gout. N Engl J Med. 2005;353(23):2450–61.
31. Niccoli G, Conte M, Cosentino N, Todaro D, Brugaletta S, Montone RA, Minelli S, Fracassi F, Galiffa V, Leone AM, et al. Baseline C-reactive protein serum levels and in-stent restenosis pattern after m-TOR inhibitors drug-eluting stent implantation. J Invasive Cardiol. 2011;23(1):16–20.
32. Lee S, Yoon CH, Oh IY, Suh JW, Cho YS, Cho GY, Chae IH, Choi DJ, Youn TJ. Angiographic patterns of restenosis with 2nd generation drug-eluting stent: comparative analysis from a 10-year single-center experience. Int Heart J. 2015;56(1):6–12.
33. Kitahara H, Kobayashi Y, Takebayashi H, Nakamura Y, Kuroda N, Miyazaki A, Haruta S, Komuro I. Angiographic patterns of restenosis after sirolimus-eluting stent implantation. Circ J. 2009;73(3):508–11.
34. Corbett SJ, Cosgrave J, Melzi G, Babic R, Biondi-Zoccai GG, Godino C, Morici N, Airoldi F, Michev I, Montorfano M, et al. Patterns of restenosis after drug-eluting stent implantation: insights from a contemporary and comparative analysis of sirolimus- and paclitaxel-eluting stents. Eur Heart J. 2006;27(19):2330–7.
35. Jinnouchi H, Kuramitsu S, Shinozaki T, Tomoi Y, Hiromasa T, Kobayashi Y, Domei T, Soga Y, Hyodo M, Shirai S, et al. Difference of tissue characteristics between early and late restenosis after second-generation drug-eluting stents implantation- an optical coherence tomography study. Circ J. 2017; 81(4):450–7.
36. Yamashita K, Ochiai M, Yakushiji T, Ebara S, Okabe T, Yamamoto MH, Saito S, Hoshimoto K, Isomura N, Araki H, et al. Repeat drug-eluting stent implantation for in-stent restenosis: first- or second-generation stent. J Invasive Cardiol. 2012;24(11):574–8.
37. Almalla M, Pross V, Marx N, Hoffmann R. Effectiveness of everolimus-eluting stents in the treatment of drug-eluting stent versus bare-metal stent restenosis. Coron Artery Dis. 2012;23(7):492–6.
38. Zhu W, Li J, Luo H, Wang G, Hua Q. Comparison of 2-year outcomes of repeated second-generation drug-eluting stent implantation for focal-type versus nonfocal-type in-stent restenosis. Coron Artery Dis. 2015;26(7):587–91.
39. Naganuma T, Latib A, Costopoulos C, Oreglia J, Testa L, De Marco F, Candreva A, Chieffo A, Naim C, Montorfano M, et al. Drug-eluting balloon versus second-generation drug-eluting stent for the treatment of restenotic lesions involving coronary bifurcations. EuroIntervention. 2016;11(9):989–95.
40. Zhao L, Zhu W, Zhang X, He D, Guo C. Effect of diabetes mellitus on long-term outcomes after repeat drug-eluting stent implantation for in-stent restenosis. BMC Cardiovasc Disord. 2017;17(1):16.
41. Lee JM, Rhee TM, Hahn JY, Hwang D, Park J, Park KW, Kim HL, Kim SH, Chae IH, Doh JH, et al. Comparison of outcomes after treatment of in-stent restenosis using newer generation drug-eluting stents versus drug-eluting balloon: patient-level pooled analysis of Korean multicenter in-stent restenosis registry. Int J Cardiol. 2017;230:181–90.
42. Kuroda M, Otake H, Shinke T, Takaya T, Nakagawa M, Osue T, Taniguchi Y, Iwasaki M, Nishio R, Kinutani H, et al. The impact of in-stent neoatherosclerosis on long-term clinical outcomes: an observational study from the Kobe University Hospital optical coherence tomography registry. EuroIntervention. 2016;12(11):e1366–74.
43. Bastante T, Rivero F, Benedicto A, Cuesta J, Alfonso F. Recurrent Neoatherosclerosis after Bioresorbable vascular scaffold treatment of in-stent restenosis. JACC Cardiovasc Interv. 2015;8(9):1264–5.

19

Successful percutaneous coronary intervention for an in-stent chronic total occlusion in a patient with dextrocardia

Johannes Wild[1*], Tommaso Gori[1,2], Thomas Münzel[1,2,3] and Philip Wenzel[1,2,3]

Abstract

Background: Percutaneous coronary interventions of chronic total occlusion represent one of the most challenging issues in interventional cardiology. A Caucasian patient with dextrocardia presented with an in-stent chronic total occluded right coronary artery, a constellation which has not been described previously in the literature.

Case presentation: A 69-year-old man with pre-known situs inversus totalis and a long history of coronary artery disease with multiple interventions and stent-implantations presented to our department suffering from episodes of chest pain under exercise. A coronary angiogram showed a completely occluded right coronary artery in the area of a drug-eluting stent which had been implanted eight years before. We found collaterals from the left coronary artery system and signs of calcification, so the lesion was classified as chronic total occlusion and the recanalization using an antegrade wire escalation technique successfully performed.

Conclusion: This is the first reported case of an in-stent chronic total occlusion in situs inversus with dextrocardia. Our experience in this case demonstrates the feasibility of recanalization of in-stent chronic total occlusions even in the rare setting of this congenital cardiac malposition combined with severe coronary artery disease.

Keywords: Dextrocardia, Coronary artery disease, Chronic total occlusion

Background

Dextrocardia is a congenital malposition which occurs in only 1 of 10,000 humans [1]. Atherosclerosis in general occurs as often in patients with dextrocardia as in the general population, so, given the rarity of the malposition, chronic total coronary occlusions (CTO) seen in this special population are extremely rare. We now report the case of a patient with dextrocardia and coronary three-vessel disease with the successful ad-hoc recanalization of an in-stent chronic total occluded right coronary artery.

Case presentation

A 69-year-old man with known situs inversus totalis and dextrocardia presented to our department due to frequent episodes of chest pain under minimal exercise (Canadian Cardiovascular Society grading of angina pectoris Class III). The patient presented with arterial hypertension, hypolipoproteinemia and nicotine abuse (45 pack years) as cardiovascular risk factors and a known history of a complex coronary three-vessel disease. About eight years ago, the patient was admitted to a hospital abroad with an acute coronary syndrome and the right coronary artery (RCA) was treated with a drug-eluting stent. Four years ago the patient had reported typical chest pain and the left main was treated with an everolimus-eluting stent as well as the proximal left anterior descending artery (LAD) and left circumflex artery (RCX) dilated in kissing balloon technique. At this previous coronary angiography, the RCA had not shown any de-novo stenosis or in-stent restenosis.

Now, the patient presented with typical chest pain and dyspnea under minimal exercise which had increased

* Correspondence: johannes.wild@unimedizin-mainz.de
[1]Center for Cardiology – Cardiology I, University Medical Center Mainz, Langenbeckstrasse 1, 55131 Mainz, Germany

during the previous months. The patient denies palpitations or other symptoms. In the physical examination, he did not show any pathologies. The heart sounds could be auscultated on the right side of his chest without any murmurs, no peripheral edema could be seen. An ECG with the usual placement of the electrodes showed typical signs of dextrocardia: right axis deviation, positive QRS complexes (with upright P and T waves) in aVR, 'global negativity' (inverted P wave, negative QRS, inverted T wave) in I and absent R-wave progression in the chest leads (Fig. 1a). As recommended in the literature, an additional electrocardiogram was recorded after placing the precordial leads in a mirror-image position on the right side of the chest and reversing the left and right arm leads. As sign of the known former myocardial infarction Q-waves in II/III/aVF were present (Fig. 1b).

The laboratory findings did not show any pathologic results, especially the cardiac markers troponin and creatine kinase were normal. A transthoracic echocardiography at rest revealed a regular left ventricular function with apical hypokinesia which had already been described in the previous echocardiography. No abnormalities of the valves were seen. A stress echocardiogram by treadmill could not be performed due to severe arthralgia and significant dyspnea. Because of the typical symptoms and the complicated coronary three vessel-disease with a history of percutaneous coronary interventions and stent-implantations, the indication for a coronary angiography was given.

The vascular access was established by the right femoral artery and a 6French Terumo® sheath inserted. Due to known dextrocardia, we exceptionally preferred the femoral access over the radial access route in this specific case. The coronary angiography showed a good result after the previous left main stenting and RCX/LAD percutaneous coronary intervention (Fig. 2a). In contrast, the RCA was completely occluded in segment two right in the area of the stent that was implanted ten years before (Fig. 2b). We found collaterals from the left coronary artery system and signs of calcification (Fig. 2a), so the diagnostically criteria of a CTO were fulfilled. Collaterals were grade I – II according to Rentrop classification. The Japanese-CTO-score (J-CTO-score) [2] which describes the complexity of the lesion was 3 (due to the occlusion length of more than 20 mm, bending and the present calcification), indicating a very difficult lesion. Ventriculography showed a regular-sized left ventricle with good systolic function. Because of the present symptoms of the patient and evidence for vital myocardium by echocardiography, an ad-hoc revascularization of the CTO was attempted.

A Cordis 6F SRC® no-torque guidance catheter was used and the standard antegrade wire escalation technique attempted. A buddy-wire (Abbott® BMW-CW) was inserted in a right-ventricular branch of the RCA. A Terumo Finecross® microcatheter was inserted with the help of a BMW-wire which was exchanged to an Abbott Hi-Torque Progress 200 T® which allowed the successful recanalization (Fig. 3a/b). Due to rapid guidewire success and clear demarcation of the CTO segment, we refrained form using a second arterial access to visualize collaterals. Balloon angioplasty was performed with Terumo Tazuna® 1.25/10 mm, Boston Scientific Maverick® 1.5/20 mm and Abbott NC Trek® 2.5/20 mm (eight insufflations with 16 bar maximum, Fig. 3c). Two everolimus eluting stents (Abbott Xience Pro® 2.5/23 mm with 18.0 bar and Xience Pro 2.75/23 mm with 14 bar) were successfully implanted with very good angiographic result (Fig. 3d).

The patient was loaded with clopidogrel for dual platelet aggregation inhibition in addition to his premedication with aspirin. Overall, 254 ml of contrast agent were used during this procedure. Even though the J-CTO-score

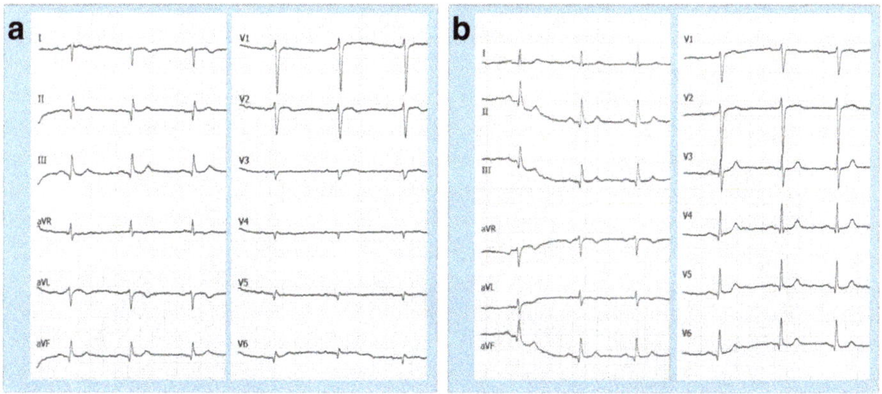

Fig. 1 Electrocardiogram in dextrocardia (25 mm/s, 10 mm/mV). **a** Conventional placement of the ECG leads with the typical findings of dextrocardia: right axis deviation, positive QRS complexes (with upright P and T waves) in aVR, 'global negativity' (inverted P wave, negative QRS, inverted T wave) in I and absent R-wave progression in the chest wall leads. **b** Mirror inverted placement of the ECG leads on the right side of the chest and reversing the left and right arm leads

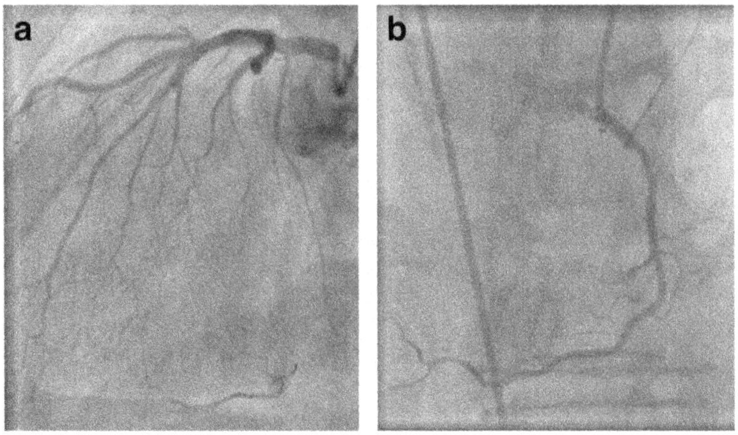

Fig. 2 Coronary angiogram of RCA-in-stent CTO in dextrocardia. **a** In-stent RCA-CTO (angulation RAO 2.1°, CRAN 28.1°). **b** Left coronary artery with collaterals to the right coronary artery (angulation LAO 30°, CRAN 0°)

(indicating the complexity of the lesion) was 3 and thus higher than the average at our department (which is 2,46), the lesion could be treated faster (116 min vs 126 min) and with lower fluoroscopy time (23 min vs 28,3 min) than the average at our department.

After the procedure, there was no clinical sign for pericardial effusion and no significant elevation of cardiac markers. The patient reported no symptoms and was discharged the next day after the procedure.

Discussion and conclusions

According to the current guidelines of the European Society of Cardiology, a CTO lesion is defined as a coronary TIMI flow of zero for at least three months [3]. Since the time of occlusion is – as in the presented case - not always known, the EuroCTO club published different levels of certainty if an occlusion can be classified as CTO. Due to this classification [3], the presented case would be judged with the level of certainty as possible

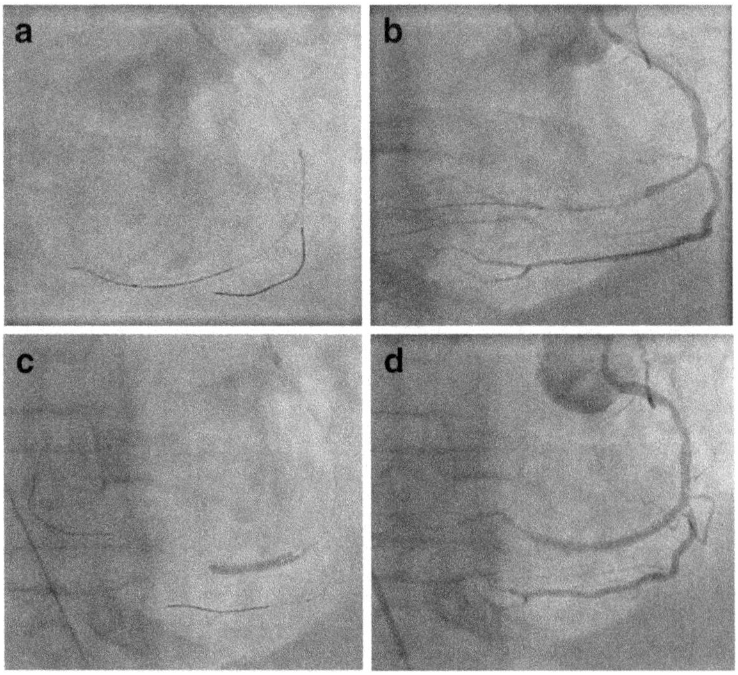

Fig. 3 Coronary angiogram of in-stent CTO-PCI in dextrocardia. **a** Placement of a buddy wire (Abbott® BMW-CW) in a right-ventricular branch and an Abbott Hi-Torque Progress wire for recanalization (angulation RAO 29.30° CAUD 0.2°). **b** Successful recanalization of the RCA-CTO. **c** PTCA with an Abbott NC Trek® 2.5/20 mm balloon. **d** Final result with complete recanalization and TIMI III flow after implantation of two everolimus eluting stents (Abbott Xience Pro® 2.5/23 mm and Xience Pro 2.75/23 mm)

or undetermined. The occlusion showed a TIMI 0 flow and the angiographic anatomy was suggestive of long-standing occlusion with collateral development and no contrast staining. The Japanese CTO register [2] suggests for patients who did not undergo previous catheterization the definition as a CTO based on the patient's clinical history and the angiogram, especially the presence of severe calcification as diagnosed in this patient is seen as a diagnostic criteria for CTO.

Due to growing experience with the percutaneous interventional approach for this kind of lesions and new technical features, the procedural success rates for CTO-revascularizations have significantly improved within the last years and is now considered within the 90% range [4]. In experienced centers, it can nowadays routinely be performed by radial approach [5]. Despite these improvements, the lesion subset of in-stent CTOs has always been associated with lower procedural success rates (63% to 71%) [6] and still remains challenging for interventional cardiologists. In general, coronary chronic total occlusions due to in-stent restenosis are quite common, representing 5% to 25% of all CTO percutaneous coronary interventions. Regarding the presented case, given the rarity of dextrocardia, this is only the third report of a successful percutaneous CTO treatment in a patient with dextrocardia [7, 8] and the first report of the diagnosis and successful treatment of an in-stent CTO in this rare congenital condition.

The risk for structural heart disease is elevated in patients with situs inversus and dextrocardia, anomalies which are diagnosed more frequently in these patients are ventricular septal defect, transposition of the great arteries, double outlet right ventricle and atrial appendage juxtaposition [9]. On the contrary, the risk for atherosclerosis is as high in patients with dextrocardia as in the general population [10].

Our experience in this case demonstrates the feasibility of recanalization of an in-stent CTO even in the rare setting of this congenital cardiac malposition.

Abbreviations

CTO: Chronic total occlusion; LAD: Left anterior descending artery; RCA: Right coronary artery; RCX: Left circumflex artery

Acknowledgements

None

Funding

There was no funding received for this manuscript.

Authors' contributions

JW performed data analyses and wrote the manuscript. PW conducted the percutaneous coronary intervention. JW, PW, TG, and TM conducted the clinical diagnosis and data collection. All authors read and approved the final manuscript.

Competing interests

The authors declare that they have no competing interests.

Author details

[1]Center for Cardiology – Cardiology I, University Medical Center Mainz, Langenbeckstrasse 1, 55131 Mainz, Germany. [2]German Center for Cardiovascular Research (DZHK) – Partner site Rhine-Main, University Medical Center Mainz, Langenbeckstrasse 1, 55131 Mainz, Germany. [3]Center for Thrombosis and Hemostasis, University Medical Center Mainz, Langenbeckstrasse 1, 55131 Mainz, Germany.

References

1. Bohun CM, Potts JE, Casey BM, Sandor GG. A population-based study of cardiac malformations and outcomes associated with dextrocardia. Am J Cardiol. 2007;100(2):305–9.
2. Morino Y, Abe M, Morimoto T, Kimura T, Hayashi Y, Muramatsu T, Ochiai M, Noguchi Y, Kato K, Shibata Y, et al. Predicting successful guidewire crossing through chronic total occlusion of native coronary lesions within 30 minutes: the J-CTO (multicenter CTO registry in Japan) score as a difficulty grading and time assessment tool. JACC Cardiovasc Interv. 2011;4(2):213–21.
3. Di Mario C, Werner GS, Sianos G, Galassi AR, Buttner J, Dudek D, Chevalier B, Lefevre T, Schofer J, Koolen J, et al. European perspective in the recanalisation of chronic Total occlusions (CTO): consensus document from the EuroCTO Club. EuroIntervention. 2007;3(1):30–43.
4. Azzalini L, Vo M, Dens J, Agostoni P. Myths to debunk to improve management, referral, and outcomes in patients with chronic Total occlusion of an Epicardial coronary artery. Am J Cardiol. 2015;116(11):1774–80.
5. Tumscitz C, Pirani L, Tebaldi M, Campo G, Biscaglia S. Seven french radial artery access for PCI: a prospective single-center experience. Int J Cardiol. 2014;176(3):1074–5.
6. Abdel-karim AR, Lombardi WB, Banerjee S, Brilakis ES. Contemporary outcomes of percutaneous intervention in chronic total coronary occlusions due to in-stent restenosis. Cardiovasc Revasc Med. 2011;12(3):170–6.
7. Munawar M, Hartono B, Iskandarsyah K, Nguyen TN. Successful percutaneous coronary intervention for chronic total occlusion of right coronary artery in patient with dextrocardia. Cardiovasc Interv Ther. 2013;28(3):303–6.
8. Celebi OO, Deveci B, Ilkay E. Successful percutaneous coronary intervention for chronic Total occlusion of left anterior descending coronary artery in a patient with Dextrocardia. Int J Angiol. 2016;25(5):e70–2.
9. Maldjian PD, Saric M: Approach to dextrocardia in adults: review. *AJR Am J Roentgenol* 2007, 188(6 Suppl):S39–S49; quiz S35–38.
10. Hynes KM, Gau GT, Titus JL. Coronary heart disease in situs inversus totalis. Am J Cardiol. 1973;31(5):666–9.

Double product reflects the association of heart rate with MACEs in acute coronary syndrome patients treated with percutaneous coronary intervention

Tan Xu[1†], Youqin Zhan[1†], Nan Lu[1], Zhuoqiao He[1], Xi Su[2*] and Xuerui Tan[1*]

Abstract

Background: There is little information about the prognostic value of double product (DP) for acute coronary syndrome (ACS) patients treated with percutaneous coronary intervention (PCI). The aim of this study was to investigate whether DP reflects the predictive power of heart rate (HR) or systolic blood pressure (SBP) in ACS patients treated with PCI.

Methods: A total of 7590 ACS patients who had undergone PCI, free from cardiac shock, were included. The follow-up duration was two years. The main adverse cardiovascular events (MACEs) included all-cause death, recurrent myocardial infarction and stroke.

Results: In the unadjusted model, significantly higher rates of MACEs were recorded in the high DP group (relative risk 1.41, 95%CI 1.08 to 1.83, $p = 0.012$). However, in the full adjusted models, after including HR and SBP, the predictive value of DP was not significant (relative risk 0.86, 95%CI 0.55 to1.33, $p = 0.499$). The predictive value of HR for MACEs was statistically significant (relative risk 1.74, 95% CI 1.33–2.28, $p < 0.001$). It was worth noting that the history of hypertension was strongly associated with MACEs (relative risk 1.53, 95% CI 1.11–2.11, $p = 0.009$).

Conclusion: High DP is associated with MACEs for ACS patients treated with PCI. However, the predictive value of DP weakened when adjusted for HR. Therefore, we have shown that DP may reflect the predictive power of HR for ACS patients treated with PCI.

Background

It has been widely recognized that high blood pressure, especially high systolic blood pressure (SBP), is a risk factor for cardiovascular diseases [1]. Some studies have shown that heart rate (HR) is also a risk factor for mortality and cardiovascular morbidity in patients with acute coronary syndrome (ACS) [2]. Recently, our meta-analysis concluded that elevated HR may increase the mortality of ACS patients in the percutaneous coronary intervention era, irrespective of admission, rest or discharge HR [3].

Double product (DP), which includes both the values of SBP and HR, was initially calculated to indirectly assess myocardial oxygen uptake during stress testing [4, 5]. DP has been demonstrated as a predictive parameter to evaluate prognosis in acute myocardial infarction patients treated with thrombolytic agents [6]. However, in the general population, one study found that DP did not have any value in predicting mortality in addition to SBP and HR [7].

To date, there is little information about the prognostic value of DP for ACS patients who were treated with percutaneous coronary intervention (PCI). This study aimed to investigate whether DP reflects the predictive ability of HR or SBP in ACS patients treated with PCI.

* Correspondence: yaxin_suxi@163.com; 15992287952@163.com
†Equal contributors
[2]Department of Cardiology, Wuhan Asian Heart Hospital, Wuhan, Hubei 430022, China
[1]Department of Cardiology, First Affiliated Hospital of Shantou University Medical College, Changping Road NO.57, Shantou, Guangdong 515041, China

Methods

Study population

A total of 7824 ACS patients who had undergone PCI between January 2011 and December 2014 at Wuhan Asian Heart Disease Hospital, Wu Han, China were included. This is a tertiary hospital that has performed over ten thousand coronary intervention procedures.

The diagnosis of ACS, which includes ST elevated myocardial infarction and non-ST elevated acute coronary syndrome, was based on the standard guidelines [8, 9]. After admission, patients received reperfusion therapy with PCI. Appropriate medication strategies were used according to the practical guidelines of ACS management [8, 9].

Study design

This is a retrospective study of prospectively collected data. The primary source of data was the hospital electronic medical record database and the follow-up database, which contains doctors' performance records. The electronic medical record database included baseline demographics, clinical manifestation, procedure details and complications. The information in the follow-up database was mainly based on telephone and clinic visits.

Written informed consent was not obtained from participants because the primary source of data was collected for clinical audits and evaluation of our services. However, this study was approved by Wuhan Asian Heart Disease Hospital Ethics Committee for data extraction and acquisition from the hospital databases.

Data collection

Patient characteristics, including gender, age, height, weight and medical history (hypertension, diabetes mellitus and dyslipidaemia) were collected at baseline. Patients were determined to be hypertensive if any one of the following conditions was present: SBP was 140 mmHg or higher, diastolic blood pressure was over 90 mmHg or use of antihypertensive medication [10]. Type 2 diabetes mellitus was diagnosed according to the criteria of the American Diabetes Association as a self-reported diagnosis of diabetes, plasma fasting glucose ≥7.0 mmol/L (or 2-h postprandial glucose ≥11.1 mmol/L), or use of diabetes medication at admission [11]. Dyslipidaemiawas defined according to the guidelines or use of statins [12]. BMI was defined as the body weight divided by the square of the body height.

HR and blood pressure at admission were measured accurately at the first medical contact by physicians using calibrated mercury sphygmomanometers. DP was defined as the product of SBP (mmHg) and HR (beats per minutes).

The follow-up duration was two years, during which the occurrence of main adverse cardiovascular events (MACEs) was recorded. The MACEs included all-cause death, recurrent myocardial infarction and stroke. All outcome analyses only considered the first occurrence of an event. All outcome information was extracted from the follow-up database.

Statistical analysis

Categorical variables are presented as percentages. Chi-square tests were performed for categorical variables. Continuous variables are presented as the mean and standard deviation. The continuous variables, such as age, BMI, SBP, diastolic blood pressure, and HR, were compared using Mann–Whitney tests because they were all not normally distributed.

Because there is no established optimal threshold for DP, receiver operator characteristics (ROC) curve analysis was performed to assess the predictive ability of DP and HR on the MACEs. The point where sensitivity and specificity were maximized was determined as the best cut-off point.

We used Cox proportional hazards regression analysis to estimate the relative risk of two-year MACEs. Models for DP and HR were initially adjusted for fundamental biological characteristics, which were age (quartile), gender and body mass index (BMI) (quartile). The fully adjusted models for DP included age (quartile), gender, BMI (quartile), history of hypertension, dyslipidaemia, diabetes mellitus, HR (quartile) and SBP (quartile). The fully adjusted models for HR included age (quartile), gender, BMI (quartile), history of hypertension, dyslipidaemia, diabetes mellitus and SBP (quartile). Interactions between DP, HR and SBP were tested by adding interaction terms to the model.

A *p*-value of 0.05 was considered statistically significant. All statistical analyses were performed using SPSS version 16.0 (SPSS Inc., Chicago, Illinois, USA).

Results

Baseline characteristics

Of the 7824 patients, 214 patients were excluded because of incomplete data. In addition, 20 patients with cardiogenic shock at admission were excluded because of their labile haemodynamic parameters.

A total of 7590 consecutive ACS patients were included in this study. The mean age was 60.13 ± 9.76 years, and 73.4% of them were males. In this population, 64.43% had hypertension, 26.63% had diabetes mellitus, and 24.63% had known dyslipidaemia. The majority of patients (75.59%) were admitted with a non-ST-elevation acute myocardial infarction.

The ROC analysis showed that a D*P* value of 9657 was the cut-off with highest sensitivity and specificity in terms of prognostic significance. DP > 9657 was considered the high DP group, and DP ≤ 9657 was considered the low DP group. The population clinical characteristics were grouped by dichotomy of DP, which was based on the ROC cut-off (Table 1).

Incidence of MACE events

During the two years of follow-up, 124 (1.56%) patients died, including 103 cardiovascular deaths and 21 from another cause of death. Fifty-four patients experienced non-fatal recurrent myocardial infarctions; and forty-eight had non-fatal strokes. In total, the incidence rate of MACEs was 2.94%. MACEs occurred in 94(2.45%) patients with DP < 9657 and 129(3.43%) patients with DP > 9657.

Double product

In the unadjusted model, the high DP group (DP > 9657) had significantly higher rates of MACEs than the low DP group (DP ≤ 9657) (relative risk (RR) 1.41, 95% confidence interval (CI) 1.08 to 1.83, $p = 0.012$) (Fig. 1a). In multivariate Cox regression models that only adjusted for fundamental biological characteristics, high DP was also a significant predictor for MACEs (RR 1.36, 95%CI 1.04 to 1.78, $p = 0.022$). However, in the full adjusted models, after including HR and SBP, DP was not significant (RR 0.86, 95%CI 0.55 to1.33, $p = 0.499$) (Table 2). Interestingly, HR (treated with quartile) was significantly associated with MACEs (RR 1.75, 95%CI 1.083 to 2.817, $p = 0.022$). Therefore, we analysed heart rate separately in the following. Although the relationship between SBP and MACEs was not statistically significant in the fully adjusted model, it is important to note that history of hypertension was a risk factor for MACEs in this population (RR 1.54, 95% CI 1.118 to 2.115, $p = 0.008$). However, there was no significant association between DP and mortality.

Heart rate

A HR value of 76 was determined as the best cut-off. The population was grouped by dichotomy of HR (threshold as 76 beats per minute) into a high HR group and low HR group. In the unadjusted model, significantly higher rates of MACEs were found in the high HR group than in the low HR group (relative risk 1.71, 95%CI 1.31 to 2.23, $p < 0.001$) (Fig. 2).

Initially, the multivariate Cox model was adjusted by gender, sex, age and BMI. High HR was also a significant predictor for MACEs (RR 1.76, 95%CI 1.35 to 2.28, $p < 0.001$). In the fully adjusted model, history of hypertension, diabetes mellitus and dyslipidaemia, and SBP were included (Table 3). The predictive value of HR for MACEs was statistically significant (relative risk 1.74, 95% CI 1.33–2.28, $p < 0.001$). As in the DP model, there was no significant association between SBP and MACEs. It was worth noting that the history of hypertension was strongly associated with MACEs (relative risk 1.53, 95% CI 1.11–2.11, $p = 0.009$). No significant association was found between HR and mortality.

Discussion

This is the first study investigating the predictive ability of DP for ACS patients. Retrospective evaluation of DP in ACS patients with two years of follow up yielded the following salient findings. The main conclusions were as follows: (i) high DP, which was calculated from the product of admission HR and SBP, is associated with MACEs; (ii) after adjusting for HR and SBP, the predictive ability of DP disappeared. However, HR was strongly associated with MACEs, which suggests that DP reflects the predictive ability of HR in ACS patients over the two years of follow-up. (iii) Additionally, history of hypertension

Table 1 Population clinical characteristics stratified by dichotomy of DP based on ROC cut-off (9657 mmHg* bpm)

Characteristic	All	Dichotomy of double product		*p* value
	n = 7590	Low(*n* = 3830)	High(*n* = 3760)	
Male, n (%)	5559(73.24)	2902(75.77)	2657(70.66)	<0.001
Age (year)	60.13 ± 9.73	59.60 ± 9.73	60.66 ± 9.71	<0.001
BMI (kg/m^2)	24.84 ± 3.20	24.63 ± 3.17	25.05 ± 3.22	<0.001
STEMI, n (%)	1853(24.41)	1012(26.42)	841(22.37)	<0.001
Diabetes mellitus, n (%)	2021(26.63)	866(22.61)	1155(30.72)	<0.001
Hypertension, n (%)	4890(64.43)	2139(55.85)	2751(73.16)	<0.001
Dyslipidemia, n (%)	1958(24.63)	937(24.46)	1021(27.15)	<0.001
Heart rate (bpm)	73.23 ± 11.98	66.58 ± 7.75	80.01 ± 11.72	<0.001
SBP (mmHg)	129.77 ± 18.74	118.89 ± 13.65	140.86 ± 16.60	<0.001
DBP (mmHg)	78.22 ± 11.24	73.37 ± 9.31	83.15 ± 10.90	<0.001
DP (mmHg* bpm)	9525.70 ± 2201.88	7874.43 ± 955.85	11,208.73 ± 1800.17	<0.001

DP double product, *ROC* receiver operator characteristics, *BMI* body mass index, *STEMI* ST-segment elevated myocardial infarction, *SBP* systolic blood pressure, *DBP* diastolic blood pressure, *bpm* beats per minutes
*means multiply by

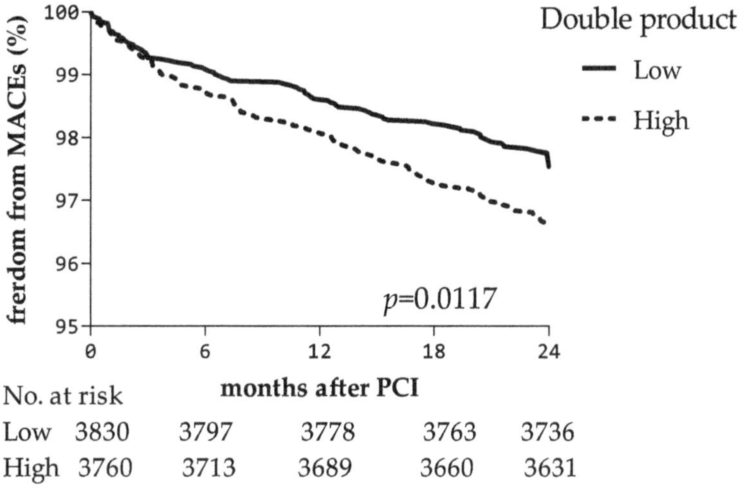

Fig. 1 Kaplan-Meier curve showing the risk of MACEs, stratified by double product ($p = 0.0117$, cut-off9657mmHg*bpm). The number of patients at risk at the beginning of each half year is shown below the horizontal axis

was associated with increased risk of two-year MACEs, but not the level of systolic blood pressure SBP, in both the DP and HR models.

Initially, DP aimed to indirectly estimate myocardial oxygen uptake during exercise stress testing [4, 5]. Villella and colleagues demonstrated that DP was a predictive index to evaluate prognosis in survivors of acute myocardial infarction treated with thrombolytic agents able to perform an exercise test after acute myocardial infarction [6]. Their results showed that low DP was significantly associated with a higher 6-month mortality rate (RR 1.71, $p = 0.020$) [6]. However, in our analysis, low admission DP was a protective factor for two-year MACEs. The DP in our study was derived from the admission HR and SBP in the acute phrase of ACS patients. This may explain the inconsistency between the two studies. Overall, these results show the reliability of DP as a predictor.

Table 2 Full-adjusted multivariate analysis using Cox proportional hazards regression testing the relation between double product and two-year MACEs

Characteristic	Relative risks	95% CI	*P* value
DP	.859	0.554–1.333	0.499
Gender	1.142	.846–1.541	.387
hypertension	1.537	1.118–2.115	.008
Diabetes mellitus	1.308	.981–1.743	0.067
Dyslipidemia	.893	.646–1.233	0.492
SBP			0.605
Q1(<120 mmHg)	reference		
Q4(>140 mmHg)	.786	.498–1.240	.301
Heart rate			0.012
Q1(<66 bpm)	reference		
Q4(>80 bpm)	1.746	1.083–2.817	.022
Age			0.000
Q1(<54 years)	reference		
Q4(>67 years)	3.017	2.017–4.512	.000
Body mass index			0.155
Q1(<23 kg/m^2)	reference		
Q4(>26 kg/m^2)	.647	.438–0.957	.029

MACEs main adverse cardiovascular events, *DP* Double product, *SBP* systolic blood pressure, *Q1* first quartile, *Q4* fourth quartile

In Japanese Ohasama populations, the DP at rest based on home blood pressure measurement was significantly associated with mortality [13]. Notably, the association between the home-measured DP and mortality was stronger than that between mortality and SBP or HR [13]. The results of the Ohasama study were partially consistent with our study. Although both revealed that high DP was associated with adverse events, the predictive value of DP in our study disappeared after adjusting for HR and SBP. This discrepancy may be due to differences in study population, outcomes and measurement methods of biomarkers. All participants in Ohasama study were from a Japanese population without a history of cardiovascular disease, and the DP was evaluated based on the home-measured SBP and HR. Nevertheless, all participants in our study were ACS patients, and the DP was measured based on admission SBP and HR in the acute phrase.

Recently, a study of 9937 participants in the general population demonstrated that DP reflects the predictive power of SBP, as the DP was not associated with mortality after adjusting for SBP [7]. These results were completely opposite from those of the aforementioned

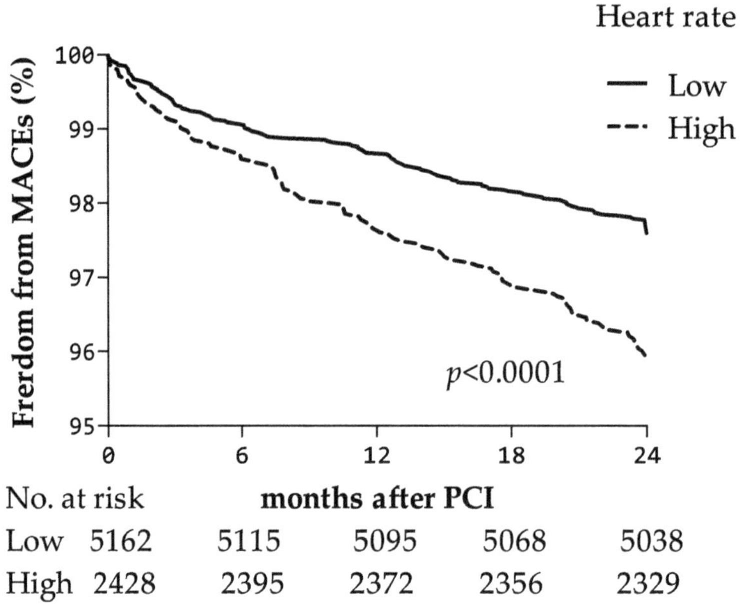

Fig. 2 Kaplan-Meier curve showing the risk of MACEs, stratified by heart rate ($p < 0.0001$, cut-off 76 beats per minute). The number of patients at risk at the beginning of each half year is shown below the horizontal axis

Ohasama study [13] but partially in agreement with ours. Overall, the role of DP has been seriously questioned in previous studies-, especially in different populations.

In addition, the TAIST trial reported that a high DP in the acute phase of stroke can predict poor outcome [14]. However, there is no evidence regarding the predictive value of DP for ACS patients after PCI.

Table 3 Full-adjustedmultivariate analysis using Cox proportional hazards regression testing the relation between heart rate and two-year MACEs

Characteristic	Relative risks	95% CI	*p*value
Heat rate	1.744	1.334–2.279	0.000
Gender	1.138	.843–1.537	0.397
Diabetes mellitus	1.307	.980–1.742	.068
hypertension	1.530	1.112–2.105	.009
Dyslipidemia	.887	.642–1.225	.467
SBP			0.703
Q1(<120 mmHg)	reference		
Q4(>140 mmHg)	.868	.601–1.254	.451
Age			0.000
Q1(<54 years)	reference		
Q4(>67 years)	2.993	2.003–4.474	.000
Body mass index			0.144
Q1(<23 kg/m^2)	reference		
Q4(>26 kg/m^2)	.642	.434–0.950	.027

MACEs main adverse cardiovascular events, *SBP* systolic blood pressure, *Q1* first quartile, *Q4* fourth quartile

As reported, admission SBP and HR have been demonstrated as predictors for in-hospital mortality and long-term mortality [2, 15–17]. Currently, some ACS risk models, such as PURSUIT [18] and GRACE [19], have also included admission HR as a prognostic factor. DP, which takes into account both SBP and HR, was assumed to be a strong predictor for ACS patients in our study. Unfortunately, the results from our study suggest that DP was not useful after HR and SBP were used to predict MACEs in ACS patients because the predictive value of DP was weakened after the model was adjusted for other haemodynamic parameters, such as HR. HR has been demonstrated as an independent risk factor of MACE events in ACS patients, as we have reviewed in a meta-analysis [3].

In our study, there was no significant relationship between SBP and two-year MACEs, which was inconsistent with previous study [15, 16]. This may be due to the exclusion of cardiogenic shock patients and in-hospital MACEs. Our results showed that DP or HR were not associated with mortality, which may be due to the low incidence of mortality in our population. However, our study revealed that history of hypertension is a risk factor of MACE in ACS patients, as reported in previous studies [20, 21].

Study limitations

The present study must be interpreted within the context of its potential limitations. First, this is a retrospective observational analysis with inherent flaws in study design, although the data were prospectively collected and stored. Second, information about medication prior to hospital admission was not available, which may partly influence the HR and SBP. Third, the follow-up was mainly based on telephone interviews, which may bias events.

Conclusion

In conclusion, our data suggest that DP is associated with main adverse cardiovascular events for ACS patients before adjustment for HR. However, the association of DP with MACEs disappeared when adjusted for HR. Therefore, we showed that DP may reflect the predictive ability of HR. Overall, among ACS patients treated with PCI, a history of hypertension is associated with two-year MACEs, not the level of SBP.

Abbreviations

ACS: Acute coronary syndromes; DP: Double product; HR: Heart rate; MACEs: Main adverse cardiovascular events; PCI: Percutaneous coronary intervention; SBP: Stolic blood pressure

Acknowledgements

We gratefully acknowledge the expert Jian Yong as a native English speaker and statistician for revision of the manuscripts. Meanwhile, we sincerely thank Xiaocong Zhang for the assistance of data management.

Funding

The present study was partially supported by grants from National Natural Science Foundation of China (grant number 81473063) to Xuerui Tan.

Authors' contributions

TX and YQZ performed the survey and wrote the draft of manuscript. XRT, NL, ZQH and XS designed the study, helped interpret the analysis results, and assisted inmodifying the manuscript. All authors read and approved the final manuscript.

Competing interests

The authors declare that they have no competing interests.

References

1. Lewington S, Clarke R, Qizilbash N, Peto R, Collins R. Age-specific relevance of usual blood pressure to vascular mortality: a meta-analysis of individual data for one million adults in 61 prospective studies. Lancet. 2002;360(9349):1903–13.
2. Noman A, Balasubramaniam K, Das R, Ang D, Kunadian V, Ivanauskiene T, Zaman AG. Admission heart rate predicts mortality following primary percutaneous coronary intervention for ST-elevation myocardial infarction: an observational study. Cardiovasc Ther. 2013;31(6):363–9.
3. Xu T, Zhan Y, Xiong J, Lu N, He Z, Su X, Tan X. The relationship between heart rate and mortality of patients with acute coronary syndromes in the coronary intervention era: meta-analysis. Medicine. 2016;95(46):e5371.
4. Kitamura K, Jorgensen CR, Gobel FL, Taylor HL, Wang Y. Hemodynamic correlates of myocardial oxygen consumption during upright exercise. J Appl Physiol. 1972;32(4):516–22.
5. Gobel FL, Norstrom LA, Nelson RR, Jorgensen CR, Wang Y. The rate-pressure product as an index of myocardial oxygen consumption during exercise in patients with angina pectoris. Circulation. 1978;57(3):549–56.
6. Villella M, Villella A, Barlera S, Franzosi MG, Maggioni AP. Prognostic significance of double product and inadequate double product response to maximal symptom-limited exercise stress testing after myocardial infarction in 6296 patients treated with thrombolytic agents. GISSI-2 investigators. Grupo Italiano per lo studio della Sopravvivenza nell-Infarto Miocardico. Am Heart J. 1999;137(3):443–52.
7. Schutte R, Thijs L, Asayama K, Boggia J, Li Y, Hansen TW, Liu YP, Kikuya M, Bjorklund-Bodegard K, Ohkubo T, et al. Double product reflects the predictive power of systolic pressure in the general population: evidence from 9,937 participants. Am J Hypertens. 2013;26(5):665–72.
8. Wright RS, Anderson JL, Adams CD, Bridges CR, Casey DE, Jr., Ettinger SM, Fesmire FM, Ganiats TG, Jneid H, Lincoff AM et al: 2011 ACCF/AHA focused update of the guidelines for the Management of Patients with unstable angina/non-ST-elevation myocardial infarction (updating the 2007 guideline): a report of the American College of Cardiology Foundation/ American Heart Association task force on practice guidelines developed in collaboration with the American College of Emergency Physicians, Society for Cardiovascular Angiography and Interventions, and Society of Thoracic Surgeons. J Am Coll Cardiol 2011, 57(19):1920–1959.
9. Kushner FG, Hand M, Smith SC, Jr., King SB, 3rd, Anderson JL, Antman EM, Bailey SR, Bates ER, Blankenship JC, Casey DE, Jr. et al: 2009 Focused updates: ACC/AHA guidelines for the Management of Patients with ST-elevation myocardial infarction (updating the 2004 guideline and 2007 focused update) and ACC/AHA/SCAI guidelines on percutaneous coronary intervention (updating the 2005 guideline and 2007 focused update): a report of the American College of Cardiology Foundation/American Heart Association task force on practice guidelines. Circulation 2009, 120(22):2271–2306.
10. Chobanian AV, Bakris GL, Black HR, Cushman WC, Green LA, Izzo JL, Jr., Jones DW, Materson BJ, Oparil S, Wright JT, Jr. et al: The seventh report of the joint National Committee on prevention, detection, evaluation, and treatment of high blood pressure: the JNC 7 report. JAMA 2003, 289(19): 2560–2572.
11. Report of the expert committee on the diagnosis and classification of diabetes mellitus. Diabetes Care 2003, 26 Suppl 1:S5–20.
12. Catapano AL, Reiner Z, De Backer G, Graham I, Taskinen MR, Wiklund O, Agewall S, Alegria E, Chapman MJ, Durrington P, et al. ESC/EAS guidelines for the management of dyslipidaemias: the task force for the management of dyslipidaemias of the European Society of Cardiology (ESC) and the European atherosclerosis society (EAS). Atherosclerosis. 2011;217(Suppl 1):S1–44.
13. Inoue R, Ohkubo T, Kikuya M, Metoki H, Asayama K, Kanno A, Obara T, Hirose T, Hara A, Hoshi H, et al. Predictive value for mortality of the double product at rest obtained by home blood pressure measurement: the Ohasama study. Am J Hypertens. 2012;25(5):568–75.
14. Sprigg N, Gray LJ, Bath PM, Boysen G, De Deyn PP, Friis P, Leys D, Marttila R, Olsson JE, O'Neill D, et al. Relationship between outcome and baseline blood pressure and other haemodynamic measures in acute ischaemic stroke: data from the TAIST trial. J Hypertens. 2006;24(7):1413–7.
15. Ma WF, Liang Y, Zhu J, Yang YM, Tan HQ, LT Y, Gao X, Feng GX, Li JD. Comparison of 4 admission blood pressure indexes for predicting 30-day mortality in patients with ST-segment elevation myocardial infarction. Am J Hypertens. 2016;29(3):332–9.
16. Bangalore S, Qin J, Sloan S, Murphy SA, Cannon CP. What is the optimal blood pressure in patients after acute coronary syndromes?: relationship of blood pressure and cardiovascular events in the PRavastatin OR atorVastatin evaluation and infection therapy-thrombolysis in myocardial infarction (PROVE IT-TIMI) 22 trial. Circulation. 2010;122(21):2142–51.
17. Antoni ML, Boden H, Delgado V, Boersma E, Fox K, Schalij MJ, Bax JJ. Relationship between discharge heart rate and mortality in patients after acute myocardial infarction treated with primary percutaneous coronary intervention. Eur Heart J. 2012;33(1):96–102.
18. Boersma E, Pieper KS, Steyerberg EW, Wilcox RG, Chang WC, Lee KL, Akkerhuis KM, Harrington RA, Deckers JW, Armstrong PW, et al. Predictors of outcome in patients with acute coronary syndromes without persistent ST-segment elevation. Results from an international trial of 9461 patients. The PURSUIT investigators. Circulation. 2000;101(22):2557–67.
19. Granger CB, Goldberg RJ, Dabbous O, Pieper KS, Eagle KA, Cannon CP, Van De Werf F, Avezum A, Goodman SG, Flather MD, et al. Predictors of hospital mortality in the global registry of acute coronary events. Arch Intern Med. 2003;163(19):2345–53.
20. Majahalme SK, Smith DE, Cooper JV, Kline-Rogers E, Mehta RH, Eagle KA, Bisognano JD. Comparison of patients with acute coronary syndrome with and without systemic hypertension. Am J Cardiol. 2003;92(3):258–63.

Combined value of left ventricular ejection fraction and the Model for End-Stage Liver Disease (MELD) score for predicting mortality in patients with acute coronary syndrome who were undergoing percutaneous coronary intervention

Tuncay Kırıs[1], Eyüp Avcı[2*] and Aykan Çelik[1]

Abstract

Background: The purpose of the study was to investigate whether the addition of left ventricular ejection fraction (LVEF) to the MELD score enhances the prediction of mortality in patients with acute coronary syndrome (ACS) undergoing percutaneous coronary intervention (PCI).

Methods: This retrospective study analyzed 846 consecutive patients with ACS undergoing PCI who were not receiving previous anticoagulant therapy. The patients were grouped as survivors or non-survivors. The MELD score and LVEF were calculated in all patients. The primary end point was all-cause death during the median follow-up of 28 months.

Results: During the follow-up, there were 183 deaths (21.6%). MELD score was significantly higher in non-survivors than survivors (10.1 ± 4.4 vs 7.8 ± 2.4, $p < 0.001$). LVEF was lower in non-survivors compared with survivors (41.3 ± 11.8% vs. 47.5 ± 10.0%, $p < 0.001$). In multivariate analysis, both MELD score and LVEF were independent predictors of total mortality. (HR: 1.116, 95%CI: 1.069–1.164, $p < 0.001$; HR: 0.972, 95%CI: 0.958–0.986, $p < 0.001$, respectively). The addition of LVEF to MELD score was associated with significant improvement in predicting mortality compared with the MELD score alone (AUC:0.733 vs 0.690, $p < 0.05$). Also, the combining LVEF with MELD score improved the reclassification (NRI:24.6%, $p < 0.001$) and integrated discrimination (IDI:0.045, $p < 0.001$) of patients compared with MELD score alone.

Conclusions: Our study demonstrated that the combining LVEF with MELD score may be useful to predict long-term survival in patients with ACS who were undergoing PCI.

Keywords: MELD score, LVEF, Acute coronary syndromes, Mortality

Background

Acute coronary syndromes (ACSs) which encompass unstable angina (UA) together with non-ST-elevation myocardial infarction (NSTEMI) and ST-elevation myocardial infarction (STEMI) are the leading cause of death and high morbidity worldwide [1, 2]. Various biomarkers and risk stratification scores have been developed and used to predict prognosis of these patients [3, 4]. The Model for End-stage Liver Disease (MELD) score including serum creatinine (sCr), total bilirubin (TB), and international normalized ratio (INR) are commonly used to estimate prognosis among patients with chronic liver diseases of different etiologies [5]. In addition, this score can be effective in the prediction of nonoperative outcomes, such as evaluating risk for patients with congestive heart failure [6].

Serum creatinin and total bilirubin levels measured at hospital admission seem to be associated with mortality in patients with ACS [7, 8]. Similarly, it has recently

* Correspondence: dreyupavci@gmail.com
[2]Department of Cardiology, Balikesir University Faculty of Medicine, 10345 Balikesir, Turkey
Full list of author information is available at the end of the article

been shown that an increase INR in the absence of anticoagulant therapy is associated with mortality in patients with both acute pulmonary embolism (PE) and heart failure [9, 10]. Left ventricular systolic dysfunction has been associated with increased mortality after ACSs [11].

As both MELD score include the above-mentioned laboratory parameters and left ventricular ejection fraction (LVEF) related to mortality in cardiovascular diseases, we aimed to investigate whether the addition of LVEF to MELD score creates additional prognostic value for all-cause mortality in patients with ACS treated with percutaneous coronary intervention (PCI) who were not on anticoagulant therapy.

Methods

Study population

We retrospectively evaluated 910 consecutive patients with ACS treated with PCI from april 2008 and July 2015. To be enrolled in the study, patients had to have angiographically proven ACS and baseline INR, sCr, and TB measurements. Nine patients with incomplete data, two with a history of liver cirrhosis, 14 who had received anticoagulant therapy (vitamin-K antagonists, direct thrombin inhibitors, direct factor Xa inhibitors, or enoxaparin), 29 patients with right ventricular dilatation/failure and moderate to severe tricuspid regurgitation were excluded from the analysis. Consequently, the final study population consisted of 846 patients. They were divided into survivors ($n = 663$) and non-survivors ($n = 183$) based on the total mortality at follow-up. The local ethics committee approved the study. The study conforms to the Declaration of Helsinki.

Blood sampling and calculation of MELD score

All measurements of INR, sCr, and TB were performed at the presentation of the patients prior to the initiation of anticoagulant therapy and coronary angiography. The blood-collection tubes contained 3.2% sodium citrate (0.5 ml citrate, 4.5 ml blood) for INR, measurement. Samples were immediately centrifuged for routine testing, and analysis was performed within 1 h after sampling. INR was measured using the reagent HemosIL RecombiPlasTin 2G (Instrumentation Laboratory, Bedford, MA, USA). Complete blood count was determined via an Abbott Cell-Dyn 3700 autoanalyzer using commercial assay kits (Abbott Diagnostic, CA, US). Biochemical measurements were performed using Siemens Healthcare Diagnostic Products kits and calibrators (Marburg, Germany).

The standard MELD score was calculated by using the following formula: $11.2 \times (\ln \text{INR}) + 0.378 \times (\ln \text{total bilirubin}) + 0.957 \times (\ln \text{creatinine}) + 0.643$ [6].

Echocardiographic analysis

Echocardiographic examinations were performed for all patients. The left ventricular ejection fraction (LVEF) was calculated after measuring the end-diastolic and end-systolic left ventricul (LV) volumes in the apical four-chamber and two-chamber views using the modified Simpson's method.

Tricuspid regurjitation (TR) severity was quantified and classified on an ordinal scale as absent, mild, moderate, and severe. To estimate of right atrial (RA) pressure during echocardiography, we used 2-dimensional and Doppler imaging characteristics of the inferior vena cava and hepatic veins and graded as 5, 10, 15, and 20 mmHg. Righ ventricle (RV) systolic pressure was calculated as 4 times the square of the peak trans–tricuspid valve systolic regurgitant velocity (according to the simplified Bernoulli equation) plus the estimated RA pressure [12].

RA and RV enlargement and RV systolic function were semiquantitatively described as normal, mild, moderate, or severe enlargement or dysfunction in accordance with an ordinal qualitative scale based on visual assessment [12].

Treatment

All coronary angiography and PCI procedures were performed via the transfemoral approach by experienced interventional cardiologists. Both the UA and NSTEMI patients underwent coronary angiography with subsequent PCI within the first 48 h. Primary PCI for STEMI was performed according to the current guidelines [13]. The diagnosis of CAD was confirmed by coronary angiography in all patients and consisted of documentation of a significant disease (defined as coronary stenoses ≥50% luminal narrowing in at least one of the major coronary arteries, or an infarct-related artery). Multivessel disease was defined as at least 50% diameter stenosis of two or more epicardial coronary arteries, or left main by visual estimation. Angiographic data of the patients were evaluated from catheter laboratory records. All patients were treated according to good clinical practice and the current guidelines [13, 14]. The type of stent and the use of thrombectomy devices, predilation, poststenting adjunctive balloon inflation, intravascular ultrasound, intra-aortic balloon counterpulsation, or glycoprotein IIb/IIIa inhibitors were all left to the operators' discretion. Both aspirin (100 mg/day) and clopidogrel (75 mg/day) or prasugrel (10 mg/day) or tigacrelor (90 mg twice daily) were maintanied for at least 12 months, followed by indefinite single antiplatelet theraphy in our study. Beta-blockers, angiotensin-converting enzyme inhibitors, and statins were administered according to the European Society of Cardiology guidelines [13, 14].

Definition

According to the criteria of the universal definition of myocardial infarction, diagnosis was established in the presence of an increasing/decreasing pattern in cardiac troponin I values, with at least one measurement above the 99th percentile together with evidence of myocardial ischemia [15]. Additionally, myocardial infarction was classified as STEMI or NSTEMI according to current guidelines [13, 14]. STEMI involves the presence of (1) ST-segment elevation consistent with myocardial infarction of ≥2 mm in adjacent chest leads and/or ST-segment elevation of ≥1 mm in two or more standard leads or new left bundle branch block (LBBB) and (2) positive cardiac necrosis markers. Diagnosis of NSTEMI was established in accordance with current guidelines. Including typical chest pain, serial increased levels of cardiac biomarkers and diagnostic electrocardiographic changes without ST elevation. Furthermore, UA involves (1) the absence of ST-segment elevation consistent with MI or new LBBB, (2) the presence of negative cardiac necrosis markers, and (3) the presence of angina pectoris (or an equivalent type of ischemic discomfort) with any one of the following three features: (a) prolonged (> 20 min) angina occurring at rest, (b) new-onset angina of at least Canadian Cardiovascular Society (CCS) class III severity, or (c) recent acceleration of angina reflected by an increase in severity of at least one CCS class to at least CCS class III [14]. Cardiovascular risk factors (arterial hypertension, diabetes, hypercholesterolemia, and smoking) were defined according to the accepted current criteria.

The primary study end point was defined as occurrence of all-cause total mortality during the median follow-up of 28 months. In addition, cardiac death, myocardial reinfarction, stroke/transient ischemic attack (TIA), target-vessel revascularization (TVR), and heart-failure admission were assessed. Reinfarction was defined according to the third universal definition of myocardial infarction [15]. TVR was defined as any revascularization procedure, including by-pass surgery, involving the initially treated artery. Stroke/ TIA was defined as an acute neurological deficit accompanied by brain imaging compatible with a recent ischemic or hemorrhagic event. Bleeding events were defined using the criteria of the Academic Research Consortium definition [16].

Follow-up

The patients were followed for clinical events such as deaths, MI, stroke, and heart failure during the median follow-up of 28 months. Follow-up data were obtanied from hospital records or by interviewing (in person or by telephone) patients, their families, or their personal physicians.

Statistical analysis

Continuous variables were expressed as mean ± standard deviation, and categorical variables were expressed as number of subjects with percentage of total number. Comparison of parametric values between the two groups was performed using Student's t-test or the Mann-Whitney U-test, as appropriate. A chi-squared test was used to compare categorical variables between the groups. The cumulative survival curves for total mortality were estimated with Kaplan-Meier plots. A log-rank test was used to analyze the significant differences in survival curves. A multivariate Cox regression analysis was performed to identify independent predictors for the primary end point. Factors entered into the multivariate model comprised those with p-values < 0.1 from the univariate analysis and variables with known prognostic value. The predictive values of MELD score and a combination of LVEF and MELD score were estimated by comparing the areas under the receivers operating characteristic (ROC) curve. DeLong's test was used to compare the AUC from each of models [17], which were analysed by use of Analyse-it software programme. Morever, the increased discriminative value after the addition of LVEF to MELD score was also estimated using the Net Reclassification Improvement (NRI) and Integrated Discrimination Improvement (IDI) [18]. Two-sided p-values < 0.05 were considered statistically significant. Statistical tests were performed with SPSS version 16 (SPSS Inc., Chicago, IL, USA).

Results

Baseline characteristics

The mean age was 62.2 ± 12.3 years. Of the 846 patients, 629 (74%) were males and 217 (26%) were females. The median follow-up period was 28 months (inter-quartile range 25th and 75th percentile: 13 to 44 months). The baseline characteristics of the study patients are presented Table 1. Subgroup analysis according to both gender and age was performed. For age, age was categorized as < 65, and ≥ 65 years. Also, this analysis was presented as Additional file 1: Tables S6 to S8 (for gender), and Additional file 2: Tables S9 to S11 (for age).

Non-survivors were older (67 ± 12 vs 62 ± 12 years, $p < 0.001$) and had a higher prevalence of diabetes mellitus (DM) (42 vs 27%, $p < 0.001$). Compared with survivors, history of heart failure, hypertension (HT), previous coronary artery disease (CAD), and higher Killip class were more frequent in non-survivors. On the other hand, use of beta-blockers and angiotensin-converting enzyme inhibitors was lower in non-survivors than survivors (Table 1). Major bleeding rates were higher in non-survivors than survivors (5% vs 2%, $p = 0.039$).

Laboratory findings

The laboratory variables of the groups are shown in Table 2. LVEF was significantly lower in non-survivors than survivors (41.3 ± 11.8% vs 47.5 ± 10.0%, $p < 0.001$). Non-survivors had higher leukocyte counts and higher

Table 1 Baseline characteristics of the study population

Variable	Survivors (*n* = 663)	Non-survivors (*n* = 183)	*P*-value
Age (year)	62 ± 12	67 ± 12	< 0.001
Female n (%)	158 (24)	59 (32)	0.021
History of HF n (%)	11 (2)	15 (8)	< 0.001
Hypertension n (%)	301 (45)	107 (59)	0.002
Diabetes mellitus n (%)	117 (27)	77 (42)	< 0.001
Hyperlipidemia n (%)	94 (14)	31 (17)	0.351
Current smoking n (%)	210 (32)	41 (22)	0.015
Previous CAD n (%)	183 (28)	66 (26)	0.026
Prior stroke/TIA n (%)	21 (3)	19 (10)	< 0.001
Type of ACS n (%)			
STEMI	419 (63)	105 (57)	0.151
NSTEMI	179 (27)	62 (34)	0.102
UA	56 (8)	13 (7)	0.557
Major bleeding n (%)	14 (2)	9 (5)	0.039
Killip class ≥2 n (%)	33 (5)	48 (26)	< 0.001
Medication at discharge			
Beta-blocker n (%)	580 (88)	136 (74)	< 0.001
Statin n (%)	539 (81)	143 (78)	0.339
ACE-I/ARB n (%)	555 (84)	126 (99)	< 0.001
Outcomes			
In-hospital death n (%)	0 (0)	30 (16)	< 0.001
Stroke n (%)	14 (2)	9 (5)	0.039
HF admission n (%)	24 (4)	25 (14)	< 0.001
Myocardial reinfarction n (%)	62 (9)	17 (9)	0.980
TVR n (%)	78 (12)	11 (6)	0.025
Cardiac death n (%)	0 (0)	59 (32)	< 0.001

HF heart failure, *CAD* coronary artery disease, *TIA* transient ischemic attack, *ACE-I* angiotensin-converting enzyme inhibitors, *ARB* angiotensin receptor blocker, *ACS* acute coronary syndrome, *UA* unstable angina, *NSTEMI* non-ST-elevation myocardial infarction, *STEMI* ST-elevation myocardial infarction, *TVR* target vessel revascularization

Table 2 Laboratory results of the study groups

Variable	Survivors (*n* = 663)	Non-survivors (*n* = 183)	*P* value
Peak-troponin-Ia, ng/mL	28 (19–44)	30 (18–51)	0.444[a]
Peak-troponin-I*, ng/mL	1.8 (0.6–4.2)	2.3 (0.5–12.4)	0.853[b]
Total cholesterol	170 ± 40	179 ± 46	0.128
SCr^{*}_{adm} (mg/dl)	0.82 (0.73–1.02)	1.03 (0.79–1.42)	< 0.001
WBC (× 10^3/mm^3)	11 ± 3	12 ± 4	< 0.001
Hemoglobin (g/dl)	12.6 ± 2	11.8 ± 2.2	< 0.001
LVEF (%)	47.5 ± 10.0	41.3 ± 11.8	< 0.001
ALT* (U/L)	32 (21–49)	28 (18–54)	0.420
AST* (U/L)	51 (27–105)	44 (23–129)	0.321
Total bilirubin* (mg/dl)	0.57 (0.40 ± 0.78)	0.60 (0.40–0.90)	0.015
INR	1 ± 0.11	1 ± 0.16	< 0.001
MELD score	7.8 ± 2.4	10.1 ± 4.4	< 0.001

SCr serum creatinine at admission, *WBC* wight blood cell, *LVEF* left ventricular ejection fraction, *ALT* alanine transaminase, *AST* aspartat transaminase, *INR* international normalised ratio, *MELD* model for liver end-stage liver disease
*Comparison was made using Mann-Whitney *U* test at *P* < 0.05, and these values were described by median with inter-quartile range (25th and 75th percentile)
[a]Comparison was made in patients with ST-elevation myocardial infarction
[b]Comparison was made in patients with non-ST-elevation myocardial infarction

levels of sCr than survivors. Moreover, INR and TB level were higher in non-survivors compared with survivors. Serum troponine level was comparable between groups (Table 2).

Compared with survivors, MELD score was higher in non-survivors (10.1 ± 4.4 vs. 7.8 ± 2.4, $p < 0.001$). In the correlation analysis, MELD score was inversely and weakly correlated with LVEF ($r = -0.19$, $p < 0.001$), and hemoglobin ($r = -0.25$, $p < 0.001$), but positively correlated with age ($r = 0.28$, $p < 0.001$).

Angiographic and procedural characteristics

The angiographic and procedural characteristics of the patients are provided in Table 3. Stent use, stent type, and tirofiban use did not differ significantly between the two groups, whereas the rate of multivessel disease was more frequent in non-survivors than survivors (60 vs 45%, $p < 0.001$).

MELD score, LVEF, and clinical outcomes

Table 1 presents the clinical outcomes. Sixteen percent of total deaths was in-hospital death and 32% was due to cardiac causes. Stroke/TIA rate was more prevalent in non-survivors than survivors (5% vs. 2%, $p = 0.039$). Hospitalization for heart failure was also higher in non-survivors than survivors (14% vs. 4%, $p < 0.001$), however TVR rate was lower in non-survivors (12% vs. 6%, $p = 0.025$). Myocardial reinfarction rate was comparable in the groups.

The independent predictors for all-cause death identified using the multivariate Cox regression analysis are presented in Table 4. MELD score and LVEF were independently predictive for all-cause mortality (HR: 1.116, 95%CI: 1.069–1.164, $p < 0.001$; HR: 0.972, 95%CI: 0.958–0.986, $p < 0.001$, respectively, Table 4).

AUC of LEVF for all-cause mortality was 0.659 (0.612–0.715, $p < 0.001$). The analysis of ROC curve showed an area under curve (AUC) of 0.690 for the prediction of all-cause mortality by MELD score of 7.3 (Fig. 1). The patients were divided into two subgroups based on this cut-point of MELD score; low (≤ 7.3) and high-subgroups (> 7.3). In subgroup analyses, in-hospital death (3 vs 0.6%, $p < 0.001$),

Table 3 Angiographic and procedural characteristics of the study population

Variable	Survivors (*n* = 663)	Non-sruvivors (*n* = 183)	*P*-value
Vessel involvement			0.374
LMCA	0(0)	1 (0.6)	
LAD	304 (46)	76 (42)	
CX	99 (15)	23 (13)	
RCA	209 (32)	65 (36)	
Others	51 (8)	19 (10)	
Multi-vessel disease n (%)	296 (45)	110 (60)	< 0.001
Stent use n (%)	634 (96)	173 (95)	0.533
Stent length. mm	21 (18–28)	23 (18–28)	0.722
Stent diameter, mm	3.4 ± 0.6	3.5 ± 0.6	0.887
Stent type			0.141
DES n (%)	67 (10)	10 (6)	
BMS n (%)	583 (90)	168 (94)	
Tirofiban use n (%)	257 (39)	66 (36)	0.506

LMCA left main coronary artery, *LAD* left anterior descending coronary artery, *CX* circumflex coronary artery, *RCA* right coronary artery, *DES* drug-eluting stent, *BMS* bare-metal stent

cardiac death (5 vs 1.5%, $p < 0.001$), and all-cause total mortality (14 vs 18%, $p < 0.001$, Fig. 2) were higher in patients with high MELD score than those with low MELD score. Morever, heart failure admission rate was higher in high-subgroups than low-subgroups (4 vs 2%, $p < 0.001$). There was no significant difference between groups with regard to myocardial reinfarction, stroke/TIA, and TVR rates (5 vs 5%, 7 vs 5%, 2 vs 1%, and 7 vs 4%, respectively, each $p >$ 0.05). Compared with the MELD score alone, the combining LVEF with MELD score was associated significant improvement in the ability to predict mortality (AUC:0.733 vs 0.690, $p < 0.001$, Fig. 1). The addition of LVEF to MELD score significantly improved the reclassification (NRI = 24.6%, Table 5) and the integrated discrimination (IDI: 0.045, $p < 0.001$).

Discussion

This study demonstrated that MELD score and LVEF were associated with increased all-cause mortality in ACS patients treated with PCI who were not on anticoagulant therapy during the median follow-up of 28 months. To the best of our knowledge, this is the first study investigating the combining of LVEF with MELD score for predicting mortality in these patients. Morever, the present study showed that the combined use of LVEF and MELD score was better able to predict all-cause mortality compared with the MELD score alone.

Bilirubin, the end product of heme catabolism, is derived primarily from circulating hemoglobin [19]. Although bilirubin has long been considered a waste product, it is currently recognized as a potent endogenous antioxidant which has the capacity to reduce the reactive oxygen radicals and, prevent the oxidation of low-density lipoprotein cholesterol [20]. A growing number of studies report a negative association between serum bilirubin levels and the prevalence of

Table 4 Independent predictors of all-cause mortality

Variable	Univariate			Multivariate		
	HR	95% CI	*p*-value	HR	95% CI	*p*-value
Age (per 1 year)	1.042	1.029–1.056	< 0.001	1.023	1.008–1.038	0.002
Male	0.663	0.486–0.904	0.009	0.944	0.666–1.354	0.774
Diabetes mellitus	1.780	1.327–2.387	< 0.001	1.384	1.004–1.907	0.047
Hipertension	1.480	1.103–1.986	0.009	0.999	0.719–1.390	0.997
Stroke history	2.602	1.617–4.189	< 0.001	1.954	1.193–3.200	0.008
History of CAD	1.370	1.013–1.852	0.011	1.113	0.804–1.542	0.518
Major bleeding	1.898	0.970–3.713	0.068	0.812	0.395–1.669	0.571
Multi-vessel disease	1.872	1.392–2.518	< 0.001	1.197	0.866–1.654	0.276
Killip class ≥2	5.545	3.981–7.722	< 0.001	4.149	2.907–5.922	< 0.001
LVEF (per 1% change)	0.957	0.945–0.969	< 0.001	0.972	0.958–0.986	< 0.001
Hemoglobin (per 1 mg/dl)	0.805	0.748–0.866	< 0.001	0.887	0.816–0.965	0.005
WBC (per 10^3/L)	1.081	1.043–1.121	< 0.001	1.063	1.024–1.103	0.001
B-blocker use at follow-up	0.489	0.351–0.682	< 0.001	0.638	0.444–0.917	0.015
ACE/ARB use at follow-up	0.452	0.331–0.619	< 0.001	0.989	0.668–1.464	0.956
TVR	0.490	0.266–0.902	0.022	0.765	0.410–1.4128	0.401
MELD[a] score (per 1 point)	1.291	1.222–1.364	< 0.001	1.116	1.069–1.164	< 0.001

HR hazard ratio, *CI* confidence interval, *LVEF* left ventricular ejection fraction, *MELD* model for end-stage liver disease, *WBC* white blood cell, *HDL-C* high-density lipoprotein cholesterol, *ACE-I/ARB* angiotensin-converting enzyme inhibitors/ angiotensin-reseptor blocker, *TVR* target vessel revascularization
[a]Considered as continous variable

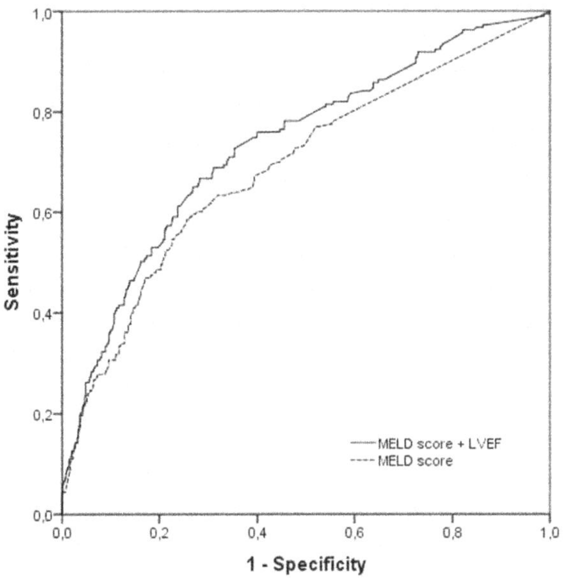

Fig. 1 Receiver operating characteristic (ROC) curves for the MELD score alone and the combining MELD score with LVEF for predicting all-cause total mortality

Table 5 Reclassification of ACS patients who died or who were alive at follow-up based on LVEF status

MELD score without LVEF	MELD score with LVEF			Total
	< 10% risk	10–30% risk	> 30% risk	
Patients who died, no.				
< 10% risk	0	0	0	0
10–30% risk	14	86	31	131
> 30% risk	0	7	45	52
Total no.	14	93	76	183
Patients who were alive, no.				
< 10% risk	0	0	0	0
10–30% risk	149	416	38	603
> 30% risk	0	16	44	60
Total	149	432	82	663

ACS acute coronary syndrome, *MELD* the Model for End-Stage Liver Disease, *LVEF* left ventricular ejection fraction

CAD [21]. Higher serum bilirubin levels were associated with lower Framingham risk scores [21].

The above-mentioned studies were not performed under acute stress condition. On the other hand, heme oxygenase (HO) 1 enzyme activity and its end product bilirubin increase with acute stress [22]. Also, HO-1 levels have a positive correlation with TB levels in patients with acute MI [22]. Celik et al. investigated associations of TB level with the devolopment of post-PCI coronary no-reflow and in-hospital major adverse cardiac events (MACE) [8]. They demonstrated that serum bilirubin levels were independently associated with no-reflow and in-hospital MACE in STEMI patients undergoing PCI. However, in their study, there was no association between TB levels and long-term mortality. In another study by Kaya et al., TB levels were found to be related to severity of coronary artery disease in patients with NSTEMI [23]. They showed that its level was independently associated with high SYNTAX score. In our study, non-survivors had a higher levels of TB compared with survivors. Also, TB was an independent predictor of all-cause mortality at follow-up.

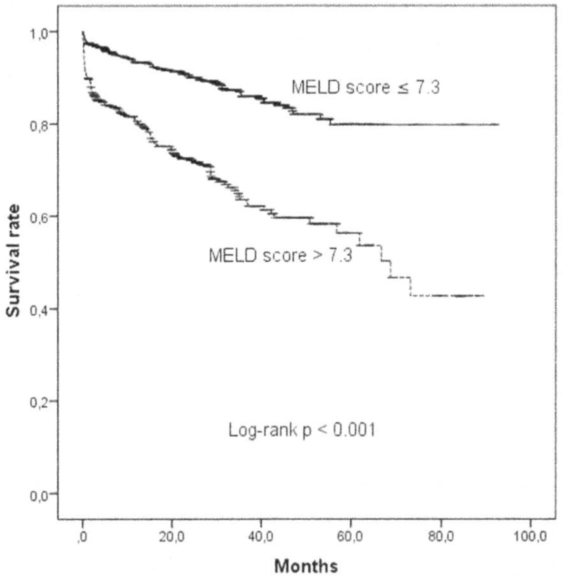

Fig. 2 Kaplan-Meier survival curves of all-cause mortality according to the MELD score

sCr levels has a significant prognostic value in ACS patients. It has been shown that baseline renal dysfunction was associated with a higher mortality in patients with ACS as found in our study [24]. Similarly, renal dysfunction has been shown to be independently associated with mortality STEMI patients treated with primary PCI [25]. Several factors associated with impaired renal function may contribute to the adverse outcome of patients with acute coronary syndrome. These factors include insulin resistance [26], alterations in the extracellular matrix [27], oxidative stress [28], inflammation [29], endothelial dysfunction [30], reninangiotensin-aldosterone system activation [31], and increased plasma levels of fibrinogen and homocysteine [32]. Also, derangements in calcium–phosphate homeostasis and anemia may increase cardiovascular risk by renal dysfunction [33]. All of them are asssociated with accelerated atherosclerosis and endothelial dysfunction. Furthermore, patients with renal dysfunction have a higher prevalence of baseline cardiovascular comorbidities such as diabetes, heart failure, previous MI and stroke and coronary interventions [34]. In addition, diffuse coronary artery disease proven by angiography was more frequent in these patients. All these conditions may related to adverse prognosis in patienst with ACS [35].

A higher INR in the absence of anticogulant use was associated with 6-month mortality in acute PE patients [10, 11]. INR > 1.2 was independent predictor of mortality in those patients. Okada et al. showed an increased INR was independent predictor of all-cause mortality in acute heart failure patients without anticoagulant therapy [10]. In their study, INR > 1.05 was significantly related to mortality. Similarly, an elevated INR was independent predictor of mortality in our population not on anticoagulant therapy. Increased INR may be associated with activated coagulation, inflammation, neurohumoral activation, and hepatic insufficiency [10]. Also, it may represent a serious inflammatory state in ACS.

Prior studies have described an relation EF and advers outcomes after ACS [36]. In a recent study by Wei et al., they demonstrated that LVEF was an independent predictor of in-hospital and 1-year mortality in STEMI patients [37]. It has been shown that LVEF independently predicted major adverse cardiac events in STEMI patients [38]. Similarly, a low LVEF was found to have predictive power for in patients with NSTEMI [39].

As MELD score requires 3 parameters only, it is the simplest score. Morever, serum TB, Cr, and INR can readily obtanied by an easily-accessible and non-invasive blood test and objectively evaluated. Similarly, LVEF can be easily measured with a bedside echocardiogram. Furthermore, these laboratory parameters indicating cardiac, hepatic and renal dysfunction can be associated with mortality in cardiovascular disease as in the aforementioned studies. In our study, non-survivors had a higher MELD score than survivors. Also, stroke/TIA and heart failure admission rates were higher non-survivors compared with survivors, whereas there was no significant difference in rate of myocardial reinfarction between non-survivors and survivors. The patients with a higher MELD score had a higher rate of cardiac death compared with those with low MELD score in our study.

Our study has several limitations. The database analysis is retrospective in nature and therefore has all the associated limitations of a retrospective study. The study can not establish causal relationships and is subject to inherent biases. Also, we did not measure the level of specific coagulation factors such as factor II,VII, and IX in these patients. Contrary to the previous studies, this cut-point used to predict mortality in present study was not consistent with what has been used in the surgical literature [40, 41]. As the current study included patients with ACS, which is a different clinical setting from the reported clinical situation in the previous literature, this may explain the difference in the cut-point used in our study. Thus, further studies are required to validate the prognostic performance and optimal cutoff values of the MELD score in patients with ACS. It has been shown that troponine- I as myocardial injury marker, and Brain Natriuretic Peptide (BNP) as stress biomarker were associated with mortality in both patients with normal LVEF and heart failure [42, 43]. In present study, although troponine-I level was measured, we did not measure the serum level of BNP. Therefore, we did not assess relation of this marker to clinical outcomes. In our study, patients with right ventricle dysfunction or right ventricular dilatation were excluded from this study. Therefore, association hepatic dysfunction with right ventricle was not evaluated. Also, we did not evaluated the association between depressed EF and hepatic dysfunction in this study. Another limitation is that syntax score indicating complexity of coronary artery lesions was not used in the present study. Last, DM was associated with mortality in our study. The DM patients treated with incretin had a significantly lower rate of major cardiovascular events compared to those were not treated by this treatment [44, 45]. As data regarding incretin usage was not present in many patients, its effect on mortality in present study could not be assesed.

Conclusions

The MELD score is a simple score derived from an easily-accessible and non-invasive blood test. Similarly, LVEF may be easily determined by a bedside echocardiogram. They were independently associated with all-cause mortality in ACS patients undergoing PCI who were not receiving previous anticoagulant therapy. Furthermore, adding LVEF to MELD score improved the predictive value for all-cause mortality in these patients.

Abbreviations

ACS: Acute coronary syndrome; BNP: Brain natriuretic peptide; CAD: Coronary artery diseases; CCS: Canadian Cardiovascular Society; DM: Diabetes mellitus; HO 1: Heme oxygenase 1; HT: Hypertension; IDI: Integrated discrimination improvement; INR: International normalized ratio; LBBB: Left bundle branch block;; LVEF: Left ventricular ejection fraction; MACE: Major adverse cardiac events; MELD: Model for End-Stage Liver Disease; NRI: Net reclassification improvement; NSTEMI: Non-ST elevation myokard infarction;
PCI: Percutaneous coronary intervention; PE: Pulmonay embolism; RA: Right atrial; ROC: receivers operating characteristic; RV: Right ventricle; sCr: Serum creatinine; STEMI: ST-elevation myocardial infarction; TB: Total bilirubin;
TIA: transient ischemic attack; TR: Tricuspid regurjitation; TVR: Targetvessel revascularization; UA: Unstable angina

Acknowledgements

Not applicable.

Funding

This research received no grant from any funding agency in the public, commercial or not-for-profit sectors.

Authors' contributions

TK: conception and design of the work; EA: acquisition, analysis, and interpretation of data; AC: drafting the manuscript and revising it critically for important intellectual content: TK and EA: final approval of the version to be published. All authors agreed to beaccountable for all aspects of the work and in ensuring that questions related to the accuracy or integrity of any part of the work are appropriately investigated and resolved. All authors read and approved the final manuscript.

Authors' information

Tuncay Kiris takes responsibility for all aspects of the reliability and freedom from bias of the data presented and their discussed interpretation.

Competing interests

The authors declare that they have no competing interests.

Author details

[1]Department of Cardiology, Izmir Katip Celebi University, Ataturk Training and Research Hospital, 35360 Izmir, Turkey. [2]Department of Cardiology, Balikesir University Faculty of Medicine, 10345 Balikesir, Turkey.

References

1. Braunwald E, Morrow DA. Unstable angina: is it time for a requiem? Circulation. 2013;127(24):2452–7.
2. Braunwald E, Antman EM, Beasley JW, et al. ACC/AHA guidelines for the management of patients with unstable angina and non-STsegment elevation myocardial infarction. A report of the American College of Cardiology/American Heart Association task force on practice guidelines (Committee on the Management of Patients with Unstable Angina). J Am Coll Cardiol. 2000;36(3):970–1062.
3. Pocock S, Bueno H, Licour M, et al. Predictors of one-year mortality at hospital discharge after acute coronary syndromes: a new risk score from the EPICOR (long-teErm follow uP of antithrombotic management patterns in acute CORonary syndrome patients) study. Eur Heart J Acute Cardiovasc Care. 2015;4(6):509–17.
4. Eagle KA, Lim MJ, Dabbous OH, et al.; GRACE investigators. A validated prediction model for all forms of acute coronary syndrome: estimating the risk of 6-month postdischarge death in an international registry. JAMA 2004; 291(22):2727–2733.
5. Kamath PS, Wiesner RH, Malinchoc M, et al. A model to predict survival in patients with end-stage liver disease. Hepatology. 2001;33(2):464–70.
6. Kim MS, Kato TS, Farr M, et al. Hepatic dysfunction in ambulatory patients with heart failure: application of the MELD scoring system for outcome prediction. J Am Coll Cardiol. 2013;61(22):2253–61.
7. Celik T, Kaya MG, Akpek M, et al. Does Serum Bilirubin level on admission predict TIMI flow grade and in-hospital MACE in patients with STEMI undergoing primary PCI. Angiology. 2014;65(3):198–204.
8. Wright RS, Reeder GS, Herzog CA, et al. Acute myocardial infarction and renal dysfunction: a high-risk combination. Ann Intern Med. 2002;137(7):563–70.
9. Okada A, Sugano Y, Nagai T, et al. Prognostic Value of Prothrombin Time International Normalized Ratio in Acute Decompensated Heart Failure- A Combined Marker of Hepatic Insufficiency and Hemostatic Abnormality. Circ J. 2016; Epub ahead of print
10. Wong CC, Ng AC, Lau JK, et al. High mortality in patients presenting with acute pulmonary embolism and elevated INR not on anticoagulant therapy. Thromb Haemost. 2016;115 [Epub ahead of print]
11. van der Vleuten PA, Rasoul S, Huurnink W, van der Horst IC, Slart RH, Reiffers S, Dierckx RA, Tio RA, Ottervanger JP, De Boer MJ, Zijlstra F. The importance of left ventricular function for long-term outcome after primary percutaneous coronary intervention. BMC Cardiovasc Disord. 2008;8:4.
12. Zoghbi WA, Enriquez-Sarano M, Foster E, Grayburn PA, Kraft CD, Levine RA, Nihoyannopoulos P, Otto CM, Quinones MA, Rakowski H, Stewart WJ, Waggoner A, Weismann NJ, American Society of Echocardiography. Recommendations for evaluation of the severity of native valvular regurgitation with two-dimensional and Doppler echocardiography. J Am Soc Echocardiogr. 2003;16:777–802.
13. Steg PG, James SK, Atar D, et al. ESC guidelines for the management of acute myocardial infarction in patients presenting with ST-segment elevation. Task force on the management of ST-segment elevation acute myocardial infarction of the European Society of Cardiology (ESC). Eur Heart J. 2012;33(20):2569–619.
14. Hamm CW, Bassand JP, Agewall S, et al. ESC Committee for practice guidelines. ESC Guidelines for the management of acute coronary syndromes in patients presenting without persistent ST-segment elevation: The Task Force for the management of acute coronary syndromes (ACS) in patients presenting without persistent ST-segment elevation of the European Society of Cardiology (ESC). Eur Heart J. 2011;32(23):2999–3054.
15. Thygesen K, Alpert JS, Jaffe AS, et al. Third universal definition of myocardial infarction. Circulation. 2012;126(16):2020–35.
16. Mehran R, Rao SV, Bhatt DL, et al. Standardized bleeding definitions for cardiovascular clinical trials: a consensus report from the Bleeding Academic Research Consortium. Circulation. 2011;123(23):2736–47.
17. DeLong ER, DeLong DM, Clarke-Pearson DL. Comparing the areas under two or more correlated receiver operating characteristic curves: a nonparametric approach. Biometrics. 1988;44(3):837–45.
18. Pencina MJ, D'Agostino RB Sr, Steyerberg EW. Extensions of net reclassification improvement calculations to measure usefulness of new biomarkers. Stat Med. 2011;30(1):11–21.
19. Vitek L. The role of bilirubin in diabetes, metabolic syndrome, and cardiovascular diseases. Front Pharmacol. 2012;3:55.
20. Shibahara S. The heme oxygenase dilemma in cellular homeostasis: new insights for the feedback regulation of heme catabolism. Tohoku J Exp Med. 2003;200(4):167–86.
21. Kim KM, Kim BT, Park SB, Cho DY, Je SH, Kim KN. Serum total bilirubin concentration is inversely correlated with Framingham risk score in Koreans. Arch Med Res. 2012;43(4):288–93.
22. Okuhara K, Kisaka T, Ozono R, et al. Change in bilirubin level following acute myocardial infarction is an index for heme oxygenase activation. South Med J. 2010;103(9):876–81.
23. Kaya MG, Sahin O, Akpek M, et al. Relation between serum total bilirubin levels and severity of coronary artery disease in patients with non-ST-segment elevation myocardial infarction. Angiology. 2014;65(3): 245–9.
24. Henry RM, Kostense PJ, Bos G, et al. Mild renal insufficiency is associated with increased cardiovascular mortality: the Hoorn study. Kidney Int. 2002; 62(4):1402–7.
25. Ferrer-Hita JJ, Dominguez-Rodriguez A, Garcia-Gonzalez MJ, Abreu-Gonzalez P. Renal dysfunction is an independent predictor of in-hospital mortality in patients with ST-segment elevation myocardial infarction treated with primary angioplasty. Int J Cardiol. 2007;118(2):243–5.
26. Caccamo G, Bonura F, Bonura F, et al. Insulin resistance and acute coronary syndrome. Atherosclerosis. 2010;211(2):672–5.
27. Pai AS, Giachelli CM. Matrix remodeling in vascular calcification associated with chronic kidney disease. J Am Soc Nephrol. 2010;21(10):1637–40.
28. Taki K, Takayama F, Tsuruta Y, Niwa T. Oxidative stress, advanced glycation end product, and coronary artery calcification in hemodialysis patients. Kidney Int. 2006;70(1):218–24.
29. Muntner P, Hamm LL, Kusek JW, et al. The prevalence of nontraditional risk factors for coronary heart disease in patients with chronic kidney disease. Ann Intern Med. 2004;140(1):9–17.
30. Zoccali C. The endothelium as a target in renal diseases. J Nephrol. 2007; 20(12):39–44.
31. Schiele F. Renal dysfunction and coronary disease: a high-risk combination. J Nephrol. 2009;22(1):39–45.
32. Ochodnicky P, Vettoretti S, Henning RH, et al. Endothelial dysfunction in chronic kidney disease: determinant of susceptibility to end-organ damage and therapeutic response. J Nephrol. 2006;19(3):246–58.
33. Luft FC. Renal disease as a risk factor for cardiovascular disease. Basic Res Cardiol. 2000;95(1):I72–6.
34. Hanna EB, Chen AY, Roe MT, Saucedo JF. Characteristics and in-hospital outcomes of patients presenting with non-ST-segment elevation myocardial infarction found to have significant coronary artery disease on coronary angiography and managed medically: stratification according to renal function. Am Heart J. 2012;164(1):52–7.

35. Liu Y, Gao L, Xue Q, et al. Impact of renal dysfunction on long-term outcomes of elderly patients with acute coronary syndrome: a longitudinal, prospective observational study. BMC Nephrol. 2014;15:78.
36. Ng VG, Lansky AJ, Meller S, Witzenbichler B, Guagliumi G, Peruga JZ, Brodie B, Shah R, Mehran R, Stone GW. The prognostic importance of left ventricular function in patients with ST-segment elevation myocardial infarction: the HORIZONS-AMI trial. Eur Heart J Acute Cardiovasc Care. 2014;3(1):67–77.
37. Wei XB, Liu YH, He PC, Jiang L, Zhou YL, Chen JY, Tan N, Yu DQ. Additive prognostic value of left ventricular ejection fraction to the TIMI risk score for in-hospital and long-term mortality in patients with ST segment elevation myocardial infarction. J Thromb Thrombolysis 2016. [Epub ahead of print].
38. Liu KL, Lin SM, Chang CH, Chen YC, Chu PH. Plasma angiopoietin-1 level, left ventricular ejection fraction, and multivessel disease predict development of 1-year major adverse cardiovascular events in patients with acute ST elevation myocardial infarction - a pilot study. Int J Cardiol. 2015; 182:155–60.
39. Bosch X, Théroux P. Left ventricular ejection fraction to predict early mortality in patients with non-ST segment elevation acute coronary syndromes. Am Heart J. 2005 Aug;150(2):215–20.
40. Krafcik BM, Farber A, Eslami MH, et al. The role of Model for End-Stage Liver Disease (MELD) score in predicting outcomes for lower extremity bypass. J Vasc Surg. 2016; https://doi.org/10.1016/j.jvs.2016.01.033. [Epub ahead of print]
41. Morimoto N, Okada K, Okita Y. The model for end-stage liver disease (MELD) predicts early and late outcomes of cardiovascular operations in patients with liver cirrhosis. Ann Thorac Surg. 2013;96(5):1672–8. Am J Cardiol 107(7):965–971
42. Katsanos S, Mavrogenis AF, Kafkas N, Sardu C, Kamperidis V, Katsanou P, Farmakis D, Parissis J. Cardiac Biomarkers Predict 1 Year Mortality in Elderly Patients Undergoing Hip Fracture Surgery. Orthopedics. 2017;40(3):e417–24.
43. Petretta M, Colao A, Sardu C, Scopacasa F, Marzullo P, Pivonello R, Fontanella L, de Caterina M, de Simone A, Bonaduce D. NT-proBNP, IGF I and survival in patients with chronic heart failure. Growth Hormon IGF Res. 2007;17(4):288–96.
44. Marfella R, Sardu C, Balestrieri ML, Siniscalchi M, Minicucci F, Signoriello G, Calabrò P, Mauro C, Pieretti G, Coppola A, Nicoletti G, Rizzo MR, Paolisso G, Barbieri M. Effects of incretin treatment on cardiovascular outcomes in diabetic STEMIpatients with culprit obstructive and multivessel non obstructive-coronary-stenosis. Diabetol Metab Syndr 2018;3. 10:1.
45. Marfella R, Sardu C, Calabrò P, Siniscalchi M, Minicucci F, Signoriello G, Balestrieri ML, Mauro C, Rizzo MR, Paolisso G, Barbieri M. Non-ST-elevation myocardial infarction outcomes in patients with type 2 diabetes with non-obstructive coronary artery stenosis: Effects of incretin treatment. Diabetes Obes Metab. 2017; https://doi.org/10.1111/dom.13122. [Epub ahead of print]

22

Circulating adipocyte fatty acid-binding protein is a predictor of cardiovascular events in patients with stable angina undergoing percutaneous coronary intervention

Wataru Takagi[1], Toru Miyoshi[2*], Masayuki Doi[1], Keisuke Okawa[1], Kazumasa Nosaka[1], Tomoyuki Nishibe[1], Naoaki Matsuo[1], Satoshi Hirohata[3] and Hiroshi Ito[2]

Abstract

Background: Adipocyte fatty acid-binding protein (A-FABP) is expressed in both adipocytes and macrophages. Recent studies have shown that A-FABP is secreted by adipocytes and that the A-FABP concentration is associated with obesity, insulin resistance, and atherosclerosis. We have reported that the coronary atherosclerotic burden is associated with the serum A-FABP concentration. In the present study, we investigated whether the serum A-FABP concentration is associated with prognosis in patients with stable angina pectoris who have undergone percutaneous coronary intervention (PCI).

Methods: This was a prospective single-center trial. In total, 130 patients with stable angina pectoris undergoing their first PCI were enrolled from August 2008 to July 2010 at Kagawa Prefectural Central Hospital. The primary endpoints were cardiovascular death, nonfatal myocardial infarction, nonfatal stroke, revascularization, and hospitalization for heart failure.

Results: During the follow-up (median, 50 months; interquartile range, 23–66 months), 49 cardiovascular events occurred. Kaplan–Meier analysis showed that the cumulative incidence of the primary endpoints in the high A-FABP group (median A-FABP concentration of ≥ 18.6 ng/ml) was greater than that in the low A-FABP group. Cox analysis showed that the A-FABP concentration was an independent predictor of cardiovascular events adjusted for age and the presence of multi-vessel disease (hazard ratio, 1.03; 95% confidence interval, 1.01–1.04; $p = 0.01$).

Conclusion: The serum A-FABP concentration is associated with prognosis in patients with stable angina undergoing PCI, suggesting that the serum A-FABP concentration could be useful for risk assessment of secondary prevention.

Keywords: Adipocyte, Fatty acid, Coronary artery disease, Risk factor

* Correspondence: miyoshit@cc.okayama-u.ac.jp
[2]Department of Cardiovascular Medicine, Okayama University Graduate School of Medicine, Dentistry and Pharmaceutical Sciences, 2-5-1 Shikata-cho, Okayama 700–8558, Japan
Full list of author information is available at the end of the article

Background

Stratification for subsequent cardiovascular events among patients with stable angina pectoris who have undergone percutaneous coronary intervention (PCI) is of considerable interest because of the potential to guide secondary preventive therapies [1, 2].

Adipocyte fatty acid-binding protein (A-FABP), also known as aP2 or FABP-4, is a cytoplasmic protein that is abundantly expressed in mature adipocytes and activated macrophages [3]. Substantial experimental evidence shows that A-FABP plays an important role in metabolic deterioration and the development of atherosclerosis [3–6]. We and other investigators previously reported that a higher circulating A-FABP concentration is an independent risk factor for coronary artery disease [7–9]. Recent studies have shown an association between the circulating A-FABP concentration and future cardiovascular disease in patients with end-stage renal disease [10], prevalent coronary heart disease [11], and acute coronary syndrome [12] as well as in a community-based cohort [13].

The aim of this study was to elucidate the association between the circulating A-FABP concentration and subsequent adverse cardiovascular events in patients with stable angina pectoris who have undergone PCI.

Methods

Patients

This was a prospective, single-center trial including patients with stable angina pectoris undergoing their first PCI. Patents' enrollment was shown in Fig. 1. Four hundred sixty-nine patients underwent PCI from August 2008 to July 2010 at Kagawa Prefectural Central Hospital. Patients were then excluded based on the presence of any of the following criteria: acute coronary syndrome or history of PCI ($n = 148$), New York Heart Association functional classification of ≥ III ($n = 1$), malignant disease with an expected prognosis of <1 year ($n = 2$), chronic inflammatory disease ($n = 1$), and chronic renal failure (serum creatinine concentration of > 2.0 mg/dl) ($n = 9$). As patients who did not provide written informed consent ($n = 3$), 132 patients consented to measurement of blood biomarkers prior to PCI. Of them, patients who had no follow-up data ($n = 2$) were also excluded. Finally, 130 patients were included in the analysis.

This study was approved by the Ethics Committee of Kagawa Prefectural Central Hospital. Written informed consent was provided by all of the patients before the study. The investigation conformed to the principles outlined in the Declaration of Helsinki.

PCI

PCI was performed using conventional techniques by the femoral or radial approach under systemic heparinization and oral administration of aspirin and clopidogrel. The stent type and inflation pressure were chosen at the discretion of the physicians, who were blinded to the study protocol. Procedural success was defined as reduction of stenosis to < 30% of residual narrowing, improvement of ischemic symptoms, and no major in-hospital complications such as death or emergency bypass surgery. After PCI, the patients received aspirin at 100 mg/day indefinitely and clopidogrel at 75 mg. Revascularization of the original stented target lesion was defined as repeated PCI and was performed in the presence of in-

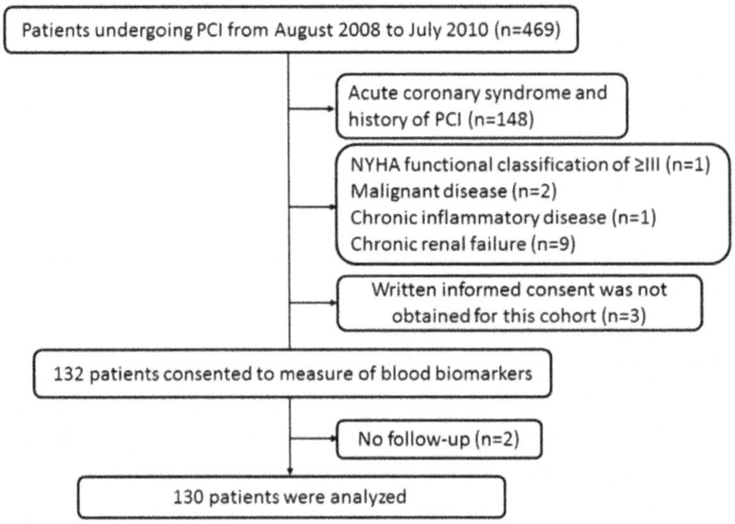

Fig. 1 Patients' enrollment of this study

stent restenosis and any symptoms or objective signs of myocardial ischemia.

Blood sampling

Blood samples were taken after an overnight fast. The serum was separated and stored at −80 °C, and the serum concentration of A-FABP was measured by enzyme-linked immunosorbent assay (BioVendor Laboratory Medicine, Modrice, Czech Republic) [14] during follow-up. With respect to performance, this assay has a < 7% intra-assay and < 5% inter-assay coefficient of variation. Other laboratory parameters were measured using standard laboratory techniques with an automatic analyzer.

Primary endpoints

The primary endpoints were cardiovascular death, nonfatal myocardial infarction and stroke, revascularization, and hospitalization for heart failure. The time to the first primary endpoint was evaluated retrospectively. All endpoints were defined and assessed according to the statement of the American College of Cardiology/American Heart Association Task Force [15]. Myocardial infarction was defined as type 1 or 2 according to the Third Universal Definition of Myocardial Infarction [16]. Elective coronary revascularization was performed only if the invasive fractional flow reserve of a coronary lesion was ≤ 0.80 [17]. Stroke included both ischemic and hemorrhagic types. Data were carefully collected from the clinical charts and by telephone or letter. Diagnoses was confirmed by an investigator who was blinded to the patients' data.

Statistical analysis

Continuous variables are presented as mean ± standard deviation or median (25th, 75th percentiles), and differences between the two groups were evaluated with an unpaired *t*-test or the Mann–Whitney U-test, as appropriate. Categorical variables are presented as number (percentage), and intergroup comparisons were performed using the chi-square test. The Kaplan–Meier analysis of event-free survival during follow-up was based on the median A-FABP concentration. The association between the A-FABP concentration and future events was assessed by Cox proportional hazards analysis. Multivariate Cox proportional hazards analysis was then applied using covariates with p value < 0.1 in the univariate Cox proportional hazards analysis. Based on previous studies [11, 12] that reported estimated event rates of 10% and 30% in patients with low and high A-FABP concentrations, respectively, a population of 144 patients would be needed to detect this difference at α = 0.05 and a power of 0.80. A p value of < 0.05 was considered statistically significant. Statistical analysis was performed using SPSS 24.0 for Windows (IBM Corp., Armonk, NY).

Results

Table 1 shows the patients' baseline characteristics. The patients' age was 72 ± 9 years, and 81% were male. The proportions of patients with hypertension, dyslipidemia, and diabetes mellitus were 76%, 76%, and 50%, respectively. The patients were divided into two groups according to the median A-FABP concentration (18.6 ng/ml). The high A-FABP group had a higher proportion of men ($p = 0.01$) and a higher body mass index ($p < 0.01$) than the low A-FABP group. There were no significant intergroup differences in age; the presence of hypertension, dyslipidemia, diabetes mellitus, or smoking; or the parameters of lipid and glycemic control. Drug therapies, including administration of antihypertensive drugs and statins, were comparable between the low A-FABP and high A-FABP groups. The distribution of the number of diseased vessels was not significantly different between the two groups.

During the median follow-up period of 50 months (interquartile range, 23–66 months), we confirmed 49 cardiovascular events (18 in the low A-FABP group and 31 in the high A-FABP group), including 16 cardiovascular deaths (5 in the low A-FABP group and 11 in the high A-FABP group), 6 strokes (4 in the low A-FABP group and 2 in the high A-FABP group), 18 revascularizations (7 in the low A-FABP group and 11 in the high A-FABP group), and 9 hospitalizations for heart failure (2 in the low A-FABP group and 9 in the high A-FABP group). The follow-up durations in the low and high A-FABP groups did not differ significantly (median [interquartile range]: 50 months [36–75 months] and 48 months [18–66 months], respectively; $p = 0.54$). As shown in Table 2, the estimated total event rate in the high A-FABP group was significantly greater at 1 year than that in the low A-FABP group. Kaplan–Meier survival curves showed that the high A-FABP group had a significantly higher mortality rate than the low A-FABP group (Fig. 2). The Cox proportional hazard regression analysis to predict cardiovascular events included A-FABP concentration, age, men, hypertension, diabetes mellitus, dyslipidemia, smoking, multi-vessel disease, and medications (Table 3). The model demonstrated that the A-FABP concentration was a significant explanatory variable after adjustment for the other parameters, suggesting that a higher A-FABP level is an independent predictor of long-term cardiovascular events (hazard ratio, 1.03; 95% confidence interval, 1.01–1.04; $p = 0.01$).

Discussion

We found that the circulating A-FABP concentration predicts cardiovascular events in patients with stable angina undergoing PCI. Further analysis using a multivariable-adjusted model supported the presence of an independent association between the A-FABP concentration and

Table 1 Patients' characteristics

	All (*n* = 130)	low A-FABP < 18.6 ng/ml (*n* = 65)	high A-FABP ≥ 18.6 ng/ml (*n* = 65)	*p* value (high vs. low)
A-FABP (ng/ml)	18.6 (13.8, 27.3)	14.2 (11.2, 16.8)	25.6 (22.6, 34.7)	
Age (years)	72 ± 9	72 ± 9	71 ± 9	0.77
Men, n (%)	105 (81)	47 (72)	89 (81)	0.01
Body mass index (kg/m^2)	24.5 ± 3.3	23.6 ± 2.8	25.4 ± 3.5	<0.01
Hypertension, n (%)	99 (76)	51 (78)	48 (74)	0.54
Dyslipidemia, n (%)	99 (76)	50 (77)	49 (75)	0.42
Diabetes mellitus, n (%)	65 (50)	33 (51)	32 (49)	0.51
Smoking, n (%)	18 (14)	9 (14)	9 (14)	0.99
LDL cholesterol (mg/dl)	103 ± 28	104 ± 25	102 ± 31	0.64
HDL cholesterol (mg/dl)	43 ± 11	41 ± 10	44 ± 12	0.13
Triglycerides (mg/dl)	141 (102, 181)	132 (97, 187)	148 (118, 178)	0.57
Fasting blood sugar (mg/dl)	99 (92, 119)	99 (92, 119)	100 (92, 120)	0.82
Serum creatinine (mg/l)	0.85 (0.70, 1.00)	0.86 (0.70, 0.96)	0.82 (0.71, 1.01)	0.35
HemoglobinA1c (%)	5.8 (5.3, 6.7)	5.6 (5.2, 6.6)	5.9 (5.3, 6.8)	0.34
hsCRP (mg/l)	0.14 (0.04, 0.36)	0.11 (0.04, 0.34)	0.16 (0.06, 0.41)	0.56
Number of diseased vessels				
One	56 (43)	32 (49)	24 (37)	
Two	42 (32)	21 (33)	21 (32)	0.21
Three	32 (25)	12 (18)	20 (31)	
Medications				
Antiplatelets	130 (100)	65 (100)	65 (100)	1.00
ACEIs/ARBs	70 (54)	35 (54)	35 (54)	0.99
Calcium channel blockers	64 (49)	33 (51)	31 (48)	0.75
β-blockers	39 (30)	16 (25)	23 (35)	0.18
Statins	75 (58)	40 (62)	35 (54)	0.32

Data are expressed as mean ± standard deviation, or number (%), or median (25th, 75th percentiles)
LDL low-density lipoprotein, *HDL* high-density lipoprotein, *A-FABP* adipocyte fatty acid-binding protein, *hsCRP* high-sensitivity C-reactive protein, *ACEI* angiotensin-converting enzyme inhibitor; ARB, angiotensin II receptor blocker

subsequent cardiovascular events. To our knowledge, this is the first long-term prospective study to demonstrate that the circulating A-FABP concentration is linked to clinical cardiovascular outcomes in patients with stable angina undergoing PCI.

Several studies have evaluated the association between the circulating A-FABP concentration and future cardiovascular events. Chow et al. reported that the circulating A-FABP concentration predicted the development of cardiovascular disease in a community-based cohort [13]. Eynatten et al. identified an association between the circulating A-FABP concentration and long-term prognosis in patients with coronary heart disease [11]. In their study, many participants were patients with an old myocardial infarction undergoing coronary artery bypass grafting, PCI, and noninvasive treatment. Other groups reported the usefulness of the circulating A-FABP concentration as a prognostic biomarker in patients with acute coronary syndrome as well as in those with end-stage renal disease [12, 10]. Our study included patients with stable angina pectoris who underwent PCI, which is an advantage in terms of understanding the clinical relevance of the circulating A-FABP concentration in this specific population.

The present study showed that women had higher A-FABP concentrations than men. Sex-related differences in the circulating A-FABP concentration have been reported in several previous studies [8, 14]. The expression of A-FABP in subcutaneous adipose was higher than that in visceral adipose tissue [18]. Men generally have more visceral fat, and women have more subcutaneous fat. Furthermore, the A-FABP concentration has been shown to be negatively correlated with the free testosterone concentration in women [19], suggesting that testosterone suppresses the expression of A-FAPB. The differences in the regional fat distribution and sex hormones may explain the sex-related difference.

The underlying mechanisms involved in the association between the circulating A-FABP concentration and

Table 2 Primary endpoints at 1 and 3 years

	low A-FABP	high A-FABP	*p* value[a] (high vs. low)
At 1 year			
Total events	4 (6%)	15 (23%)	0.006
Cardiovascular death	0 (0%)	4 (7%)	0.035
Nonfatal myocardial infarction	0 (0%)	0 (0%)	N/A
Nonfatal stroke	0 (0%)	1 (1%)	0.317
Revascularization	2 (3%)	7 (12%)	0.063
Hospitalization for heart failure	2 (3%)	3 (5%)	0.596
At 3 years			
Total events	15 (23%)	23 (35%)	0.084
Cardiovascular death	4 (7%)	7 (13%)	0.249
Nonfatal myocardial infarction			
Nonfatal stroke	3 (5%)	2 (4%)	0.765
Revascularization	6 (10%)	9 (15%)	0.288
Hospitalization for heart failure	2 (3%)	5 (9%)	0.204

Data are expressed as number and Kaplan–Meier estimated event rates at 1 year and 3 years
[a]Log-rank test was performed for comparison between two groups
A-FABP adipocyte fatty acid-binding protein

future cardiovascular events remain unclear. However, there are several potential explanations. First, A-FABP derived from adipose tissue or activated macrophages may directly influence the vasculature. Previous experimental studies have shown that A-FABP induces smooth muscle cell proliferation and inhibits the expression/activation of endothelial nitric oxide synthase in vascular endothelial cells [20, 21]. Another study showed that A-FABP locally produced by perivascular fat and macrophages in vascular plaques contributes to the development

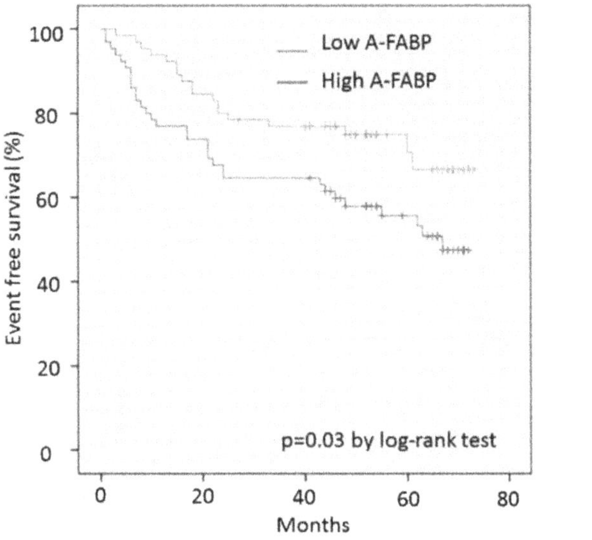

		0	20	40	60	(Months)
No. at risk	Low A-FABP	65	55	49	18	
	High A-FABP	65	48	42	23	

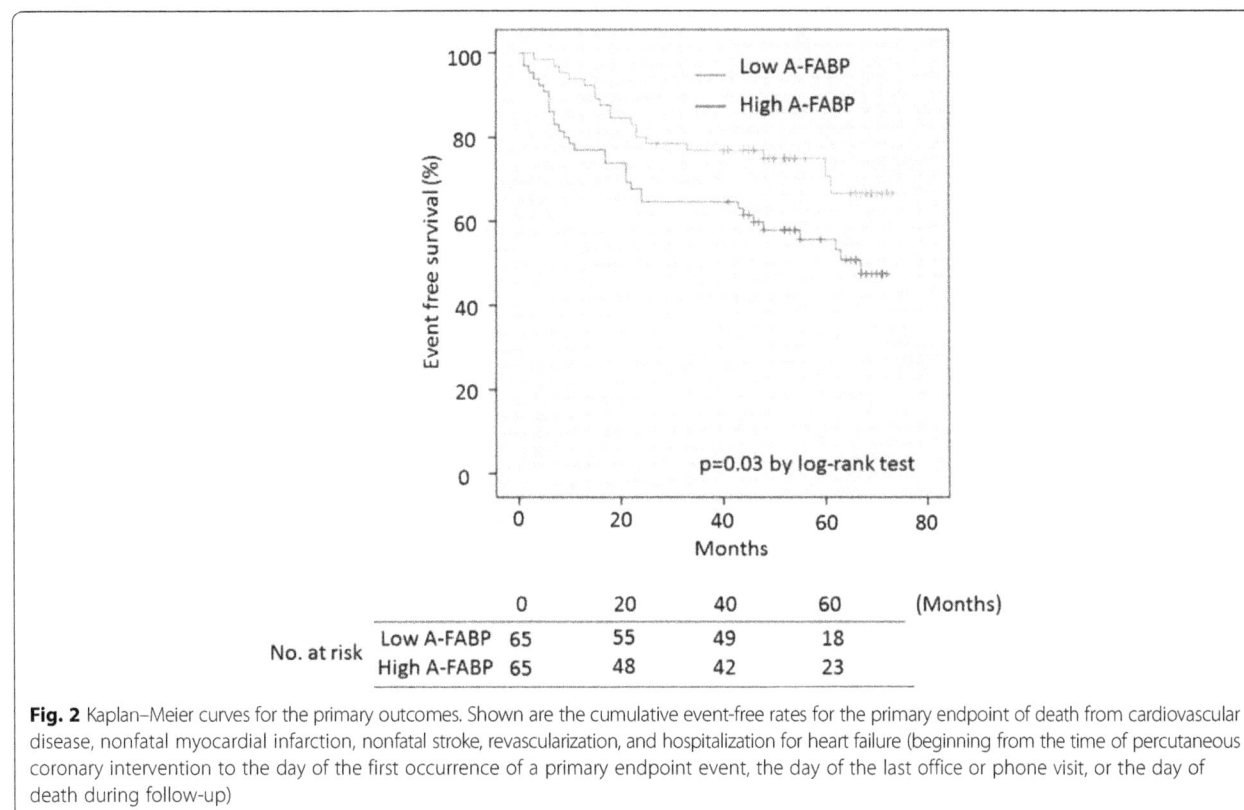

Fig. 2 Kaplan–Meier curves for the primary outcomes. Shown are the cumulative event-free rates for the primary endpoint of death from cardiovascular disease, nonfatal myocardial infarction, nonfatal stroke, revascularization, and hospitalization for heart failure (beginning from the time of percutaneous coronary intervention to the day of the first occurrence of a primary endpoint event, the day of the last office or phone visit, or the day of death during follow-up)

Table 3 Multivariate analysis

	Univariate		Multivariate	
	Hazard ratio (95%CI)	*p* value	Hazard ratio (95%CI)	*p* value
A-FABP, per 1 ng/ml	1.02 (1.01–1.03)	< 0.01	1.03 (1.01–1.04)	0.01
Age, per 1 year	1.04 (1.01–1.07)	< 0.01	1.04 (1.01–1.08)	0.01
Men	1.41 (0.56–2.36)	0.72	–	
Hypertension	1.47 (0.71–3.04)	0.29	–	
Diabetes mellitus	1.01 (0.58–1.77)	0.97	–	
Dyslipidemia	0.86 (0.46–1.62)	0.64	–	
Smoking	0.99 (0.44–2.20)	0.98	–	
Multivessel disease	1.71 (0.95–3.08)	0.08	1.71 (0.95–3.10)	0.08
CCBs	1.09 (0.63–1.92)	0.75	–	
ACEIs/ARBs	1.54 (0.87–2.72)	0.14	–	
Statins	1.25 (0.62–2.52)	0.53	–	
Hypoglycemic agents	0.63 (0.32–1.23)	0.18	–	

CI confidence interval, *A-FABP* adipocyte fatty acid-binding protein, *CCBs* calcium channel blockers, *ACEI* angiotensin-converting enzyme inhibitor, *ARB* angiotensin II receptor blocker. Multivariate Cox proportional hazards analysis was then applied using covariates with p value < 0.1 in the univariate Cox proportional hazards analysis

of coronary atherosclerosis [22]. Second, the presence of a high circulating A-FABP concentration is a consequence of accumulation of cardiometabolic risks. Our clinical studies showed that the A-FABP concentration is associated with the body mass index; concentrations of triglycerides, high-density lipoprotein cholesterol, adiponectin, and C-reactive protein; and the homeostasis model assessment–insulin resistance value [8, 14, 23–25]. Thus, the circulating A-FABP concentration is closely associated with obesity, insulin resistance, and type 2 diabetes. However, in the present study, the multivariate analysis revealed that the circulating A-FABP concentration was an independent factor associated with future cardiovascular events. In addition, a genotype–phenotype study showed that carriers of the T-87C polymorphism at the A-FABP locus have a reduced risk for coronary heart disease [26]. Basically, A-FABP works as a chaperon of fatty acids in cells. Thus, interaction of A-FABP and its modulation of cardiovascular risk factors may be another explanation.

We demonstrated the usefulness of the baseline circulating A-FABP concentration as a predictor of future cardiovascular events. Meanwhile, the circulating A-FABP concentration can be modified. We previously reported that an angiotensin II receptor blocker reduced the serum A-FABP concentration in hypertensive patients [23]. Other groups showed that the A-FABP concentration decreased by an omega-3 fatty acid [27], a statin [28], and a dipeptidyl peptidase 4 inhibitor [29] and possibly increased by a sodium-glucose cotransporter 2 inhibitor [30]. Experimental studies have identified several compounds that directly block A-FABP [31–33], but no clinical applications are available. The impact of changes in the circulating A-FABP concentration on cardiovascular events remains unknown. Further studies are required to evaluate the direct impact of changes in the circulating A-FABP concentration on clinical outcomes.

Limitations

This study has several limitations. First, a small number of patients were enrolled. Second, we included only Japanese patients with stable angina undergoing PCI; therefore, our findings cannot be extrapolated to other ethnic groups or patients without cardiovascular disease. In addition, we excluded patients with acute coronary syndrome, history of PCI, a New York Heart Association functional classification of ≥ III, malignant disease with an expected prognosis of < 1 year, chronic inflammatory disease, and chronic renal failure (serum creatinine concentration of > 2.0 mg/dl). Our findings cannot be applied to all patients with stable angina pectoris undergoing PCI. The results must therefore be interpreted with caution. Third, most of the differences between the two groups occurred in the "soft" endpoints of revascularization and hospitalization for heart failure. Thus, it is possible that A-FABP is more closely associated with symptoms or other laboratory results that would result in more intense treatment approaches rather than disease progression itself. Fourth, our study design precluded the investigation of a direct causal relationship. To determine this causal relationship, long-term interventional studies involving therapeutic agents that reduce A-FABP expression or action such as A-FABP inhibitors are warranted.

Conclusions

The circulating A-FABP concentration is a predictor of subsequent cardiovascular events in patients with stable angina who have undergone PCI. This finding suggests that the circulating A-FABP concentration has the potential to guide secondary preventive therapies.

Abbreviations

A-FABP: Adipocyte fatty acid-binding protein; PCI: Percutaneous coronary intervention

Acknowledgements

We are grateful to Michiyo Ishikawa for her scientific input, discussion, and contributions.

Funding

This work was supported by JSPS KAKENHI Grant Number 15 K09157.

Authors' contributions

WT, TM, MD, KO, KN, TN, NM, SH, HI each made substantial contributions to conception and design, or acquisition of data, or analysis and interpretation of data; was involved in drafting the manuscript or revising it critically for important intellectual content. All authors had read and approved the final manuscript.

Competing interests

The authors declare that they have no competing interests.

Author details

[1]Department of Cardiology, Kagawa Prefectural Central Hospital, Takamatsu, Japan. [2]Department of Cardiovascular Medicine, Okayama University Graduate School of Medicine, Dentistry and Pharmaceutical Sciences, 2-5-1 Shikata-cho, Okayama 700–8558, Japan. [3]Department of Medical Technology, Okayama University Graduate School of Health, Okayama, Japan.

References

1. Fihn SD, Gardin JM, Abrams J, Berra K, Blankenship JC, Dallas AP, et al. ACCF/AHA/ACP/AATS/PCNA/SCAI/STS Guideline for the diagnosis and management of patients with stable ischemic heart disease: a report of the American College of Cardiology Foundation/American Heart Association Task Force on Practice Guidelines, and the American College of Physicians, American Association for Thoracic Surgery, Preventive Cardiovascular Nurses Association, Society for Cardiovascular Angiography and Interventions, and Society of Thoracic Surgeons. J AM Coll Cardiol. 2012;60(24):e44–e164.
2. Yusuf S, Rangarajan S, Teo K, Islam S, Li W, Liu L, et al. Cardiovascular risk and events in 17 low-, middle-, and high-income countries. N Engl J Med. 2014;371(9):818–27.
3. Hotamisligil GS, Johnson RS, Distel RJ, Ellis R, Papaioannou VE, Spiegelman BM. Uncoupling of obesity from insulin resistance through a targeted mutation in aP2, the adipocyte fatty acid binding protein. Science. 1996;274(5291):1377–9.
4. Gold C. A primary mesothelioma involving the rectovaginal septum and associated with beryllium. J Pathol Bacteriol. 1967;93(2):435–42.
5. Boord JB, Maeda K, Makowski L, Babaev VR, Fazio S, Linton MF, et al. Adipocyte fatty acid-binding protein, aP2, alters late atherosclerotic lesion formation in severe hypercholesterolemia. Arterioscler Thromb Vasc Biol. 2002;22(10):1686–91.
6. Makowski L, Boord JB, Maeda K, Babaev VR, Uysal KT, Morgan MA, et al. Lack of macrophage fatty-acid-binding protein aP2 protects mice deficient in apolipoprotein E against atherosclerosis. Nat Med. 2001;7(6):699–705.
7. Bao Y, Lu Z, Zhou M, Li H, Wang Y, Gao M, et al. Serum levels of adipocyte fatty acid-binding protein are associated with the severity of coronary artery disease in Chinese women. PLoS One. 2011;6(4):e19115.
8. Doi M, Miyoshi T, Hirohata S, Nakamura K, Usui S, Takeda K, et al. Association of increased plasma adipocyte fatty acid-binding protein with coronary artery disease in non-elderly men. Cardiovasc Diabetol. 2011;10:44.
9. Rhee EJ, Lee WY, Park CY, KW O, Kim BJ, Sung KC, et al. The association of serum adipocyte fatty acid-binding protein with coronary artery disease in Korean adults. Eur J Endocrinol. 2009;160(2):165–72.
10. Furuhashi M, Ishimura S, Ota H, Hayashi M, Nishitani T, Tanaka M, et al. Serum fatty acid-binding protein 4 is a predictor of cardiovascular events in end-stage renal disease. PLoS One. 2011;6(11):e27356.
11. von Eynatten M, Breitling LP, Roos M, Baumann M, Rothenbacher D, Brenner H. Circulating adipocyte fatty acid-binding protein levels and cardiovascular morbidity and mortality in patients with coronary heart disease: a 10-year prospective study. Arterioscler Thromb Vasc Biol. 2012;32(9):2327–35.
12. Reiser H, Klingenberg R, Hof D, Cooksley-Decasper S, Fuchs N, Akhmedov A, et al. Circulating FABP4 is a prognostic biomarker in patients with acute coronary syndrome but not in asymptomatic individuals. Arterioscler Thromb Vasc Biol. 2015;35(8):1872–9.
13. Chow WS, Tso AW, Xu A, Yuen MM, Fong CH, Lam TH, et al. Elevated circulating adipocyte-fatty acid binding protein levels predict incident cardiovascular events in a community-based cohort: a 12-year prospective study. J Am Heart Assoc. 2013;2(1):e004176.
14. Miyoshi T, Onoue G, Hirohata A, Hirohata S, Usui S, Hina K, et al. Serum adipocyte fatty acid-binding protein is independently associated with coronary atherosclerotic burden measured by intravascular ultrasound. Atherosclerosis. 2010;211(1):164–9.
15. Hicks KA, Tcheng JE, Bozkurt B, Chaitman BR, Cutlip DE, Farb A *et al.*: 2014 ACC/AHA Key Data Elements and Definitions for Cardiovascular Endpoint Events in Clinical Trials: A Report of the American College of Cardiology/American Heart Association Task Force on Clinical Data Standards (Writing Committee to Develop Cardiovascular Endpoints Data Standards). Circulation 2015, 132(4):302–361.
16. Thygesen K, Alpert JS, Jaffe AS, Simoons ML, Chaitman BR, White HD, et al. Third universal definition of myocardial infarction. Circulation. 2012;126(16):2020–35.
17. Tonino PA, De Bruyne B, Pijls NH, Siebert U, Ikeno F, Van't Veer M, et al. Fractional flow reserve versus angiography for guiding percutaneous coronary intervention. N Engl J Med. 2009;360(3):213–24.
18. Fisher RM, Eriksson P, Hoffstedt J, Hotamisligil GS, Thorne A, Ryden M, et al. Fatty acid binding protein expression in different adipose tissue depots from lean and obese individuals. Diabetologia. 2001;44(10):1268–73.
19. Doganay M, Ozyer SS, Var T, Tonguc E, Gun Eryilmaz O, Ozer I, et al. Associations between adipocyte fatty acid-binding protein and clinical parameters in polycystic ovary syndrome. Arch Gynecol Obstet. 2015;291(2):447–50.
20. Aragones G, Saavedra P, Heras M, Cabre A, Girona J, Masana L. Fatty acid-binding protein 4 impairs the insulin-dependent nitric oxide pathway in vascular endothelial cells. Cardiovasc Diabetol. 2012;11:72.
21. Girona J, Rosales R, Plana N, Saavedra P, Masana L, Vallve JC. FABP4 induces vascular smooth muscle cell proliferation and migration through a MAPK-dependent pathway. PLoS One. 2013;8(11):e81914.
22. Furuhashi M, Fuseya T, Murata M, Hoshina K, Ishimura S, Mita T, et al. Local Production of Fatty Acid-Binding Protein 4 in Epicardial/Perivascular Fat and Macrophages Is Linked to Coronary Atherosclerosis. Arterioscler Thromb Vasc Biol. 2016;36(5):825–34.
23. Miyoshi T, Doi M, Hirohata S, Kamikawa S, Usui S, Ogawa H, et al. Olmesartan reduces arterial stiffness and serum adipocyte fatty acid-binding protein in hypertensive patients. Heart Vessel. 2011;26(4):408–13.
24. Kajiya M, Miyoshi T, Doi M, Usui S, Iwamoto M, Takeda K, et al. Serum adipocyte fatty acid-binding protein is independently associated with complex coronary lesions in patients with stable coronary artery disease. Heart Vessel. 2013;28(6):696–703.
25. Iwamoto M, Miyoshi T, Doi M, Takeda K, Kajiya M, Nosaka K, et al. Elevated serum adipocyte fatty acid-binding protein concentrations are independently associated with renal dysfunction in patients with stable angina pectoris. Cardiovasc Diabetol. 2012;11:26.
26. Tuncman G, Erbay E, Hom X, De Vivo I, Campos H, Rimm EB, et al. A genetic variant at the fatty acid-binding protein aP2 locus reduces the risk for hypertriglyceridemia, type 2 diabetes, and cardiovascular disease. Proc Natl Acad Sci U S A. 2006;103(18):6970–5.
27. Furuhashi M, Hiramitsu S, Mita T, Omori A, Fuseya T, Ishimura S, et al. Reduction of circulating FABP4 level by treatment with omega-3 fatty acid ethyl esters. Lipids Health Dis. 2016;15:5.
28. Karpisek M, Stejskal D, Kotolova H, Kollar P, Janoutova G, Ochmanova R, et al. Treatment with atorvastatin reduces serum adipocyte-fatty acid binding protein value in patients with hyperlipidaemia. Eur J Clin Investig. 2007;37(8): 637–42.

23

In-hospital major arrhythmias, arrhythmic death and resuscitation after successful primary percutaneous intervention for acute transmural infarction

Marco Albanese[1,3,4*], Korhan Alpaslan[1], Taoufik Ouarrak[2], Peter Merguet[1], Steffen Schneider[2] and Wolfgang Schöls[1]

Abstract

Background: Transmural acute myocardial infarction (AMI) is associated with a high risk for ventricular arrhythmia before, during and after treatment. Consequently, it is recommended that patients diagnosed with transmural AMI be monitored in a cardiac care unit (CCU) so life-threatening arrhythmias can be treated promptly. We examined the incidence and timing of in-hospital malignant ventricular arrhythmias, sudden cardiac or arrhythmic death (SCD/AD) and resuscitation requirements in patients with transmural AMI recovering from percutaneous coronary intervention (PCI) undertaken within 12 h of symptom onset and without antecedent thrombolysis.

Methods: This was a retrospective cohort study using the Duisburg Heart Center (Germany) cardiac patient registry. In total, 975 patients met the inclusion criteria. The composite endpoint was post-PCI ventricular fibrillation or tachycardia, SCD/AD or requirement for resuscitation. We compared the demographic and clinical characteristics of patients who met the composite endpoint with those who did not, recorded the timing of endpoint episodes, and used multivariable logistic regression analysis to identify factors associated with the endpoint criteria.

Results: There was no significant difference in the length of CCU or hospital stay between the groups. In-hospital mortality was 6.5%, and the composite endpoint was met in 7.4% of cases. Malignant ventricular tachyarrhythmia occurred in 2.8% of the patients, and SCD/AD occurred in 0.3% of the cases. There was a biphasic temporal distribution of endpoint events; specifically, 76.7% occurred < 96 h after symptom onset, and 12.6% occurred 240–360 h after symptom onset. Multivariable regression analysis identified positive associations between an endpoint episode and the following: age (odds ratio [OR] 1.03, 95% confidence interval [CI] 1.01–1.05] per year); left ventricular ejection fraction (LVEF) < 30% (OR 3.66, 95% CI 1.91–6.99); peak serum creatine phosphokinase concentration (OR 1.01, 95% CI 1.00–1.02 per 100 U/dl); leucocytosis (OR 1.86, 95% CI 1.04–3.32), and coronary thrombus (OR 1.85, 95% CI 1.04–3.27).

Conclusions: Most post-PCI malignant ventricular arrhythmias, SCD/AD and resuscitation episodes occurred within 96 h of transmural AMI (76.7%). A substantial minority (12.6%) of these events arose 240–360 h after symptom onset. Further study is needed to establish the influence of age, LVEF < 30%, peak serum creatine phosphokinase concentration, leucocytosis and coronary thrombus on post-PCI outcomes after transmural AMI.

Keywords: Myocardial infarction, Arrhythmias, cardiac, Ventricular fibrillation, Tachycardia, ventricular, Resuscitation, Death, sudden, cardiac

* Correspondence: m.albanese@hin.ch
[1]Herzzentrum Duisburg, Gerrickstr. 21, D-47137 Duisburg, Germany
[3]Klinik für Kardiologie und Angiologie, Herzzentrum Duisburg, Gerrickstr. 21, 47137 Duisburg, Germany
Full list of author information is available at the end of the article

Background

Transmural acute myocardial infarction (AMI) is associated with a high risk for life-threatening arrhythmias in the early phase of an ischaemic event [1]. Current guidelines suggest that patients with transmural AMI be admitted to the intensive cardiac care unit (CCU) for 24–48 h after symptom onset [2]. Admission to the CCU allows prompt resuscitation in the event of cardiac arrest but has a substantial impact on treatment costs [3]. Although several models exist for predicting early complications in AMI, major arrhythmias have not been addressed in these models [4].

Mechanical reperfusion has become the treatment of choice for transmural AMI. Compared with thrombolysis, reperfusion has been shown to achieve higher rates of the best grade of coronary flow (Thrombolysis in Myocardial Infarction [TIMI] grade 3) and to reduce the incidence of recurrent ischaemia and reinfarction as well as infarct size, thus preserving left ventricular ejection fraction (LVEF) [5–7]. Nonetheless, there are limited data on the potential therapeutic benefit of primary percutaneous coronary intervention (PCI) in terms of the incidence of in-hospital malignant arrhythmias in patients with acute ST-elevation MI (STEMI). The incidence of in-hospital ventricular arrhythmias was not reported in large clinical trials, such as PRAGUE-2 or DANAMI-2 [7, 8]. A meta-analysis of large clinical trials indicates that the incidence of ventricular fibrillation (VF) appears to be lower in patients treated with PCI compared with that in patients treated with thrombolysis [1]. Several single-centre reports have yielded conflicting results on the incidence of in-hospital arrhythmias after primary PCI for acute STEMI. According to Giglioli and colleagues, no in-hospital life-threatening arrhythmias occurred after PCI; most life-threatening arrhythmias arose in the catheterization laboratory [9, 10]. Similarly, in a Swiss study, most arrhythmias occurred in the catheterization laboratory, nearly all within 24 h; a report from Germany revealed that 90% of fatal events occurred within the first 48 h [11, 12].

In our clinical practice, we were struck by the sudden cardiac death (SCD) of a 40-year-old patient 96 h after symptom onset in an otherwise apparently uncomplicated anterior STEMI. This patient satisfied none of the predictive factors, such as LVEF < 40%, commonly used for risk stratification. To better understand the timing of and risk factors for major arrhythmias in a current patient population treated by PCI, we retrospectively analysed the data of 975 patients treated at our tertiary care centre. Our analysis differed from that in the Swiss and German single-centre studies referred to above. As the analysis was limited to patients treated by primary PCI within 12 h of symptom onset and *without* antecedent thrombolysis, our cohort was a homogenous patient population that had only been exposed to the therapeutic consequences of PCI. In addition, we defined transmural AMI using angiographic evidence of an occluded vessel to ensure identification of transmural infarctions without ST-elevation on the surface electrocardiogram (ECG). A STEMI and this well-defined non-ST-elevation myocardial infarction (NSTEMI) subgroup were thus included in our cohort, as they represent a common pathoanatomical substrate associated with an increased risk of fatal events. We sought to establish whether 48 h of monitoring was sufficient to prevent fatal events and to determine whether clinical predictors of the occurrence of fatal events in our patient population differed from those described in previous publications.

Our primary objective was to determine the timing and total burden of in-hospital major arrhythmias after successful primary PCI for transmural AMI undertaken within 12 h of symptom onset without antecedent thrombolysis. The secondary objective was to identify clinical predictors associated with the occurrence of the combined endpoint of ventricular tachycardia (VT), SCD or arrhythmic death (SCD/AD) and resuscitation in the early phase of acute transmural infarction.

Methods

Study patients and data collection

This was a retrospective cohort study using our institution's cardiac patient registry, into which data are input on discharge from hospital or after in-hospital death. Data collection began on January 1, 2005, and ended on May 17, 2011. We selected patients with symptom onset < 12 h before performance of PCI and evidence of transmural AMI as reflected by ST-segment elevation in at least two contiguous leads or the presence of left bundle branch block (LBBB) on the surface ECG or by angiographic evidence of AMI as determined by the presence of an occluded vessel. This definition of transmural AMI was chosen to ensure that transmural infarctions without ST-elevation were not missed; for example, left circumflex or right coronary artery occlusion without ST-elevation in the appropriate leads. Patients were excluded if they had undergone antecedent thrombolysis, if they were not treated by primary PCI, if primary PCI was not successful or if coronary artery bypass surgery was performed. Cardiogenic shock was not an exclusion criterion. The selection of patients in the cohort is shown in Fig. 1.

All patients were treated by a single group of cardiologists at the Duisburg Heart Centre, Duisburg, Germany, a tertiary care centre. Approximately 70% of the patients were admitted directly, with the remainder transferred from primary or secondary care centres where PCI was not available.

Catheterization and percutaneous coronary intervention

Patients were treated with an oral loading of 300 mg clopidogrel. Further medical therapy was given, and the choice of bare metal or drug-eluting stents was made according

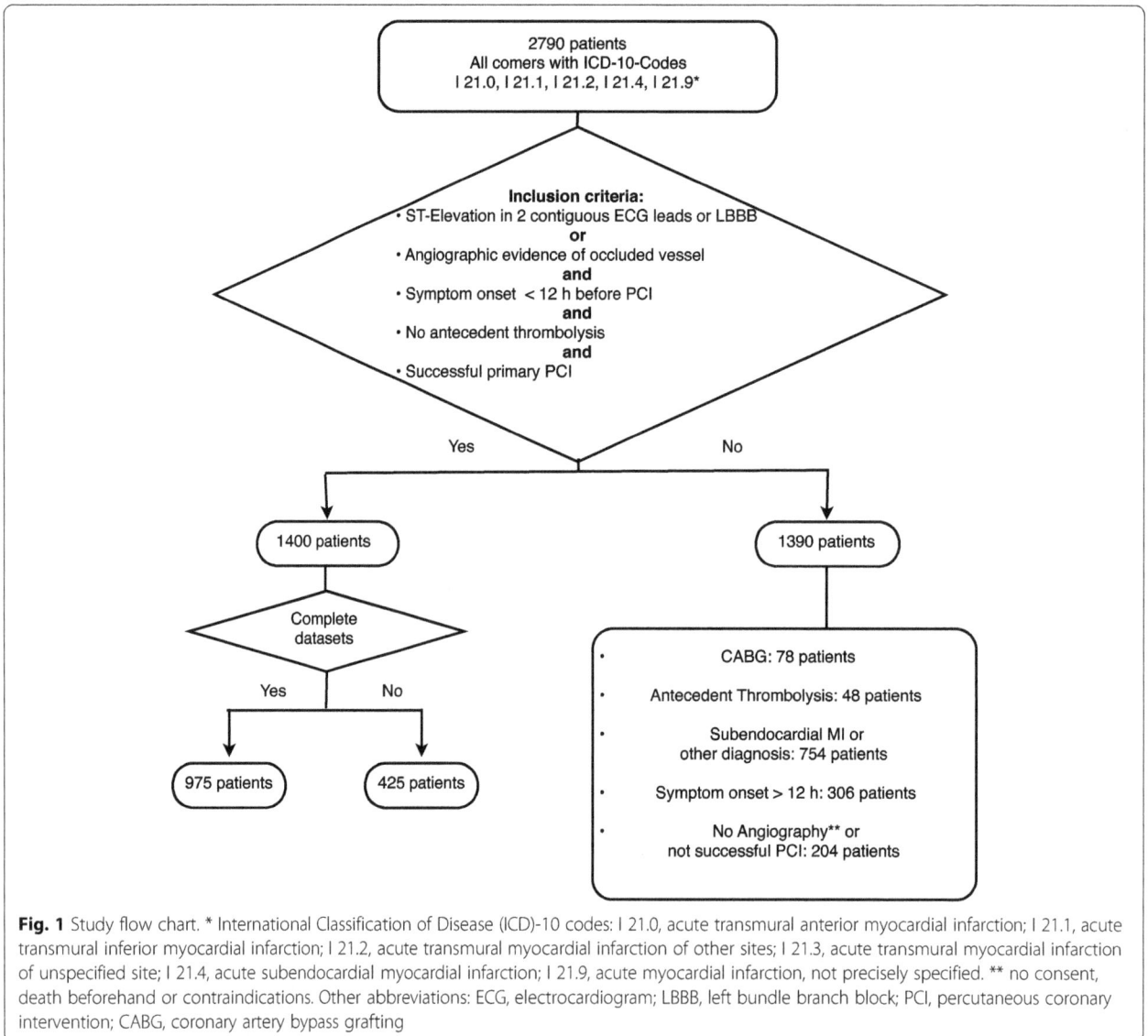

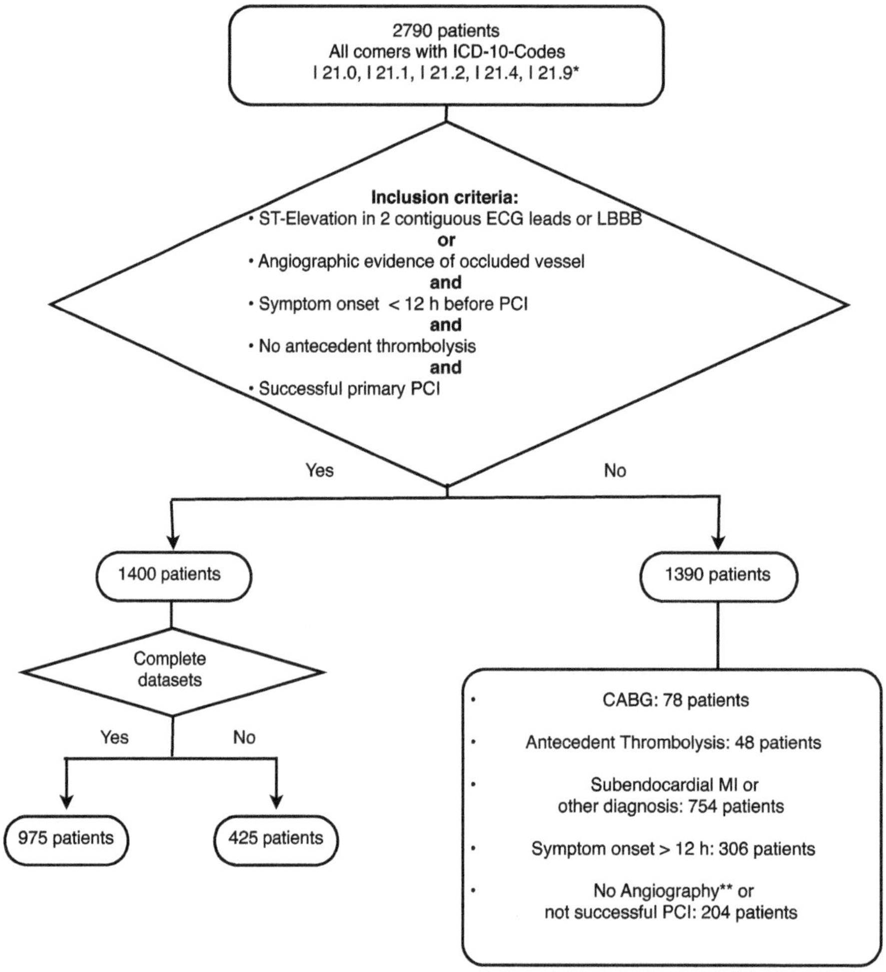

Fig. 1 Study flow chart. * International Classification of Disease (ICD)-10 codes: I 21.0, acute transmural anterior myocardial infarction; I 21.1, acute transmural inferior myocardial infarction; I 21.2, acute transmural myocardial infarction of other sites; I 21.3, acute transmural myocardial infarction of unspecified site; I 21.4, acute subendocardial myocardial infarction; I 21.9, acute myocardial infarction, not precisely specified. ** no consent, death beforehand or contraindications. Other abbreviations: ECG, electrocardiogram; LBBB, left bundle branch block; PCI, percutaneous coronary intervention; CABG, coronary artery bypass grafting

to current national guidelines. Treatment with glycoprotein IIb/IIIa inhibitors or bivalirudin was performed at the cardiologist's discretion. In most cases, only culprit lesions were treated by primary PCI, i.e., only the lesion of the infarct-related artery (IRA) was treated directly by angioplasty and stent delivery. Patients with cardiogenic shock instead underwent the most complete revascularization possible; specifically, all stenosed segments, including those vessels that were not the IRA, were treated by multiple PCIs during the acute intervention. Angioplasty success was defined as < 50% stenosis and a TIMI flow of grade 2 or 3; coronary thrombus was identified on angiography and by TIMI flow.

Endpoints and definitions

The primary combined endpoints were the occurrence and timing of in-hospital ventricular arrhythmia, SCD/AD or resuscitation after primary PCI. All endpoints were either monitored or witnessed by experienced personnel or were ascertained by autopsy. Malignant ventricular arrhythmia or malignant tachyarrhythmia included VF or VT with haemodynamic compromise, and SCD was an unexpected death resulting from heart disease occurring within 1 h of symptom onset or unwitnessed overnight. Arrhythmic death was an unexpected death resulting from arrhythmia other than SCD or VT, i.e., complete heart block (CHB), pulseless electrical activity (PEA) or asystole. Resuscitation was defined as cardiocirculatory arrest followed by basic/advanced life support according to International Liaison Committee on Resuscitation (ILCOR) or American Heart Association (AHA) guidelines. Cardiac arrest was assessed by experienced medical and paramedic personnel based on telemetry detection of heart rhythm, blood pressure monitoring and pulse oxymetry or, in late events, on clinical evaluation. Any episodes before or during catheterization were not taken into account. Telephone follow-up was undertaken for the 7% of patients who had been transferred to other hospitals after primary PCI. No other follow-up was performed in this study, which focused on in-hospital events and the possible prevention of such events.

According to hospital policy, all patients were transferred to the CCU after PCI and were then continuously monitored for complex arrhythmia for a minimum of 48 h. Telemetry was used to monitor high-risk patients after transfer to the ward. Endpoints occurring throughout the entire hospital stay were analysed, and an autopsy was performed in unclear cases.

Normal left ventricular function was defined as an LVEF > 50%, slightly impaired function was defined as 40–50%, moderately impaired function was defined as 30–40% and severely impaired function was defined as < 30%. Contrast ventriculography or echocardiography was used to estimate LVEF immediately after admission.

Statistical analysis

Absolute numbers and proportions (expressed as percentages) are used to describe the patient population. Medians (with quartiles) or means (with standard deviations) were calculated as appropriate. Categorical values were compared using the chi-square test, and continuous variables were compared using the two-tailed Wilcoxon rank sum test.

Multivariable logistic regression analysis was performed to identify independent predictors of the combined endpoint. The regression analysis took into account all events recorded. All baseline parameters previously reported to be associated with a higher risk for acute coronary syndrome were used as independent parameters in the model (Table 2) [4, 5]. *P* values< 0.05 were considered statistically significant. All *p* values were results of two-tailed tests. All analyses were performed using the SAS statistics programme (version 9.2; SAS Institute Inc., Cary, NC).

Results

Patient and treatment characteristics

The demographic and clinical characteristics of the patient population are shown in Table 1; the majority underwent PCI < 4 h after symptom onset (89.3%), and one or more stents were deployed in 98.7% of the cases (drug-eluting stents were deployed in 12.6% of the cases). Left ventricular function was severely impaired in 9.3% of the patient population. The mean duration of hospitalization was 10 d (range 7–35 d). Length of hospital stay was not associated with the occurrence of the combined endpoint. There was no statistically significant difference in the duration of CCU stay or of telemetric monitoring between patients who did or did not meet the composite endpoint.

The combined endpoint was observed in 7.4% of patients. PEA and VT were the most common malignant arrhythmias. Resuscitation was undertaken in 7.1% of the patients. By analysing the patient population according to the presence or absence of the combined endpoint, we observed the following. Patients who met the endpoint criteria were older, more frequently had a history of previous MI and peripheral arterial disease, more often took aspirin, and were more frequently diagnosed with anterior STEMI, atrial fibrillation or LBBB on admission. Serum troponin and creatine phosphokinase (CK) concentrations were almost doubled, and a higher proportion had an elevated white blood cell count (WBC) compared with those who did not meet the composite endpoint.

During coronary intervention, patients who subsequently met the composite endpoints were found to have a more extensive coronary thrombus, and there was a tendency towards more frequent use of glycoprotein IIb/IIIa inhibitors. More patients with severely impaired LVEF (< 30%) or who required vasopressor support subsequently met the combined endpoint. There was no difference in coronary status or time to reperfusion between the two groups. Although the difference in stent deployment rate was statistically significant ($P < 0.05$), it was not considered relevant because of the small difference in absolute numbers (97.2 vs 99.5%).

Descriptive analysis of the data showed that 27.5% of the patients who met the endpoint underwent early perfusion (< 90 min), 64.9% underwent intermediate perfusion (1.5–4 h), and 7.6% underwent late reperfusion (> 4 h). There was no significant difference in the proportions who developed VT (21.6, 18.6 and 18.6%, respectively) or AD (32.5, 32.2 and 41.9%, respectively) or who required resuscitation (45.9, 49.2 and 41.9%, respectively).

Predictors of the composite endpoint

Of the 12 original candidate variables, five remained statistically significant in the multivariate analysis and formed a final set of predictor variables (Table 2). These variables were age, WBC > 10,000/l, coronary thrombus, LVEF < 30% and peak serum CK concentration. The presence of atrial fibrillation was not a significant predictor ($P = 0.051$).

Temporal distribution of endpoints and correlation with endpoint predictors

We observed a biphasic distribution of events: a total of 62.7% of the combined endpoints occurred within the first 48 h of symptom onset, and a total of 76.7% were recorded within 96 h of symptom onset. Between 240 and 360 h following symptom onset, the incidence of the combined endpoint was 12.0%. A smaller number of endpoint events occurred later in the clinical course (Fig. 2).

Table 1 Baseline demographic and clinical characteristics of patients included in the study

	Total	Patients with composite endpoint	Patients without composite endpoint	*P*-value
Demographics				
Total, %	975	72 (7.4%)	903 (92.6%)	
Female, %	29.2% (285/975)	33.3% (24/72)	28.9% (261/903)	0.45
Age, (years)	62 (52–73)	68 (53–78)	62 (52–72)	< 0.05
Clinical presentation				
BMI, kg/m^2	27 (25–30)	26 (25–29)	28 (25–30)	< 0.03
Adiposity (BMI > 30), %	24.0% (220/916)	12.7% (8/63)	24.9% (212/853)	< 0.05
Medical history				
Previous MI, %	14.0% (135/961)	24.3% (17/70)	13.2% (118/891)	< 0.05
Previous PCI, %	12.5% (120/960)	14.3% (10/70)	12.4% (110/890)	0.64
Previous CABG, %	3.3% (32/962)	7.1% (5/70)	3.0% (27/892)	0.06
Previous stroke, %	3.0% (29/963)	4.3% (3/70)	2.9% (26/893)	0.52
Hypertension, %	71.4% (688/964)	70.4% (50/71)	71.4% (638/893)	0.85
Hypercholesterolemia, %	74.9% (719/960)	59.7% (43/72)	76.1% (676/888)	< 0.01
Diabetes mellitus, %	24.0% (234/975)	29.1% (21/72)	23.5% (213/903)	0.27
Current smoker, %	46.9% (449/958)	31.9% (22/69)	48.0% (427/889)	< 0.01
PAD, %	5.7% (54/946)	13.0% (9/69)	5.1% (45/877)	< 0.01
Aspirin on admission, %	23.7% (221/957)	37.1% (26/70)	22.0% (195/887)	< 0.01
Laboratory on admission				
Potassium, mmol/L	4.0 (3.7–4.3)	4.2 (3.8–4.7)	4.0 (3.7–4.3)	< 0.05
Creatinine, mg/dl	0.9 (0.8–1.1)	1.1 (0.9–1.4)	0.9 (0.8–1.1)	< 0.0001
Elevated CRP (≥5×), %	10.3% (76/741)	14.3% (8/56)	9.9% (68/685)	0.30
WBC > 10.000 μl, %	57.0% (547/960)	72.0% (52/72)	55.7% (495/885)	< 0.01
HbA1c, %	8.4 ± 7.5	10.4 ± 13.8	8.1 ± 6.4	0.9
ECG on admission				
anterior STEMI, %	39.5% (383/970)	55.6% (40/72)	38.5% (343/891)	< 0.05
AF, %	4.4% (42/968)	10.3% (7/71)	3.9% (35/890)	< 0.01
LBBB, %	1.8% (17/965)	5.5% (4/72)	1.5% (13/888)	< 0.05
AV block, %	3.9% (38/968)	4.1% (3/72)	3.9% (35/820)	0.97
Coronary angiogram and intervention				
Three-vessel disease, %	27.3% (266/975)	31.9% (23/72)	26.9% (243/903)	0.36
Time to reperfusion < 4 h, %	89.3% (868/972)	92.4% (67/72)	89.6% (795/893)	0.35
Coronary thrombus, %	19.2% (187/973)	33.3% (24/72)	18.2% (163/894)	< 0.01
Stent implantation, %	98.7% (956/969)	97.2% (70/72)	99.5% (886/890)	< 0.05
GPIIa-IIIb antagonist, %	2.9% (28/965)	6.9% (5/72)	2.6% (23/887)	0.05
Bivalirudin, %	15.0% (145/968)	20.3% (15/72)	14.5% (130/889)	0.17
Clinical course				
CCU stay, h	46 (32–54)	49 (20–169)	46 (33–52)	0.17
Routine hospital ward stay, h	150 (120–193)	170 (105–200)	150 (120–193)	0.60
Telemetric monitoring, h	47 (33–66)	50 (13–192)	47 (33–58)	0.26
Use of vasopressors, %	12.5% (122/975)	83.5% (60/72)	6.9% (62/896)	< 0.0001
Maximum troponin value, U/L	3.4 (1.5–6.4)	5.9 (1.7–14.1)	3.3 (1.5–6.1)	< 0.01
Maximum CK value, mg/dl	1413 (549–2822)	2178 (609–4513)	1351 (545–2706)	< 0.01
Clinical outcome				

Table 1 Baseline demographic and clinical characteristics of patients included in the study *(Continued)*

	Total	Patients with composite endpoint	Patients without composite endpoint	*P*-value
EF < 30%, %	9.3% (80/857)	43.4% (23/53)	7.1% (57/804)	< 0.0001
Death	6.5% (63/974)	72.2% (52/72)	1.2% (11/896)	< 0.0001
Cardiac death, % of total	88.9% (56/63)	96.2% (50/52)	54.5% (6/11)	< 0.001

Troponin was assayed as troponin T (normal < 0.01 U/L)
Abbreviations: *BMI* body mass index, *MI* myocardial infarction, *PCI* percutaneous coronary intervention, *CABG* coronary artery bypass grafting, *PAD* peripheral artery disease, *CRP* C-reactive protein, *WBC* white blood cell count, *Hba1c* glycated hemoglobin, *STEMI* ST-elevation MI, *AF* atrial fibrillation, *LBBB* left bundle branch block, *AV* atrioventricular, *GP* glycoprotein, *CCU* coronary care unit, *CK* creatine phosphokinase (normal < 250 mg/dl), *EF* ejection fraction

Specifically, 12.7% of malignant ventricular arrhythmias and 21.6% of resuscitations occurred within the first 48 h of symptom onset. In addition, 13.4% of VT/VF and 31.7% of resuscitations were recorded within 96 h of symptom onset. Between 240 and 360 h following symptom onset, the incidence of ventricular arrhythmia was 1.4% and that of resuscitation was 4.2%. In the first 48 h after AMI, 25.4% of the SCD/AD episodes were observed, and a total of 31.7% occurred within 96 h of symptom onset. The incidence of SCD/AD between 240 and 360 h following symptom onset was 7%. The exact timing of events is shown in Table 3 (*supplemental data).*

Due to the low number of events, it was not possible to calculate a risk score. Therefore, we analysed the data for the presence of predictor variables in patients with endpoints that occurred > 48 h after admission. In 90.0% of the patients with endpoints > 48 h after admission, a minimum of two or more predictors was present (data not shown).

Secondary outcomes

Total in-hospital mortality was 6.5%. Most of the deaths were from a cardiac cause (88.9%) and 77.0% were due to arrhythmia. A minority of cardiac deaths (8.7%) occurred unobserved late in the clinical course (> 96 h after admission). Patients experiencing sustained VT or VF had in-hospital mortality rates of 15.4 and 93.3%, respectively. Only 0.8% developed CHB after successful PCI. Among the patients who developed PEA, VF, CHB or asystole, cardiogenic shock was present in 86.7% of patients with PEA and 53.3% of patients with VF (Table 4).

Discussion

Key findings

The primary objective of this study was to determine the total burden and timing of in-hospital major arrhythmias and of the combined endpoint of ventricular arrhythmia, SCD/AD or resuscitation after successful primary PCI for transmural AMI within 12 h of symptom onset. Malignant ventricular tachyarrhythmia occurred in 2.8% of the patients, bradyarrhythmia occurred in 1.1%, PEA occurred in 2.6%, asystole occurred in 0.8% and SCD occurred in 0.3%. The combined endpoint was met in 7.4% of patients. We observed a biphasic distribution of events, with 76.7% of endpoints occurring within 96 h of symptom onset and 12.6% occurring 240–360 d after AMI. Occasional events were, however, observed throughout the hospital stay.

Table 2 Predictors of the composite endpoint in patients with acute myocardial infarction (multivariate analysis)

	ß Coefficient	*P* value	Odds ratio (95% CI)
Female	0.3059	0.6699	0.878 (0.48–1.59)
Age, years	0.0118	0.008	1.032 (1.008–1.05)
PAD	0.4613	0.4581	1.408 (0.57–3.47)
anterior STEMI, %	0.2774	0.4000	1.263 (0.73–2.17)
AF, %	0.4641	0.0514	2.470 (0.99–6.13)
LBBB, %	0.7615	0.3608	2.006 (0.45–8.92)
Coronary thrombus, %	0.2909	0.0339	1.853 (1.04–3.27)
EF < 30%	0.3307	< 0.0001	3.656 (1.91–6.99)
Creatinine, mg/dl	0.0037	0.9077	1.000 (0.99–1.00)
WBC > 10.000 µl	0.0118	0.0354	1.863 (1.04–3.32)
Maximum troponin value, U/L	0.0009	0.7892	1.000 (0.99–1.00)
Maximum CK value, 100 U/dl	0.0032	< 0.0001	1.014 (1.00–1.02)

Abbreviations: *CI* confidence intervals, *PAD* peripheral artery disease, *STEMI* ST-elevation myocardial infarction, *AF* atrial fibrillation, *LBBB* left bundle brunch block, *EF* ejection fraction, *WBC* white blood cell count, *CK* creatine phosphokinase

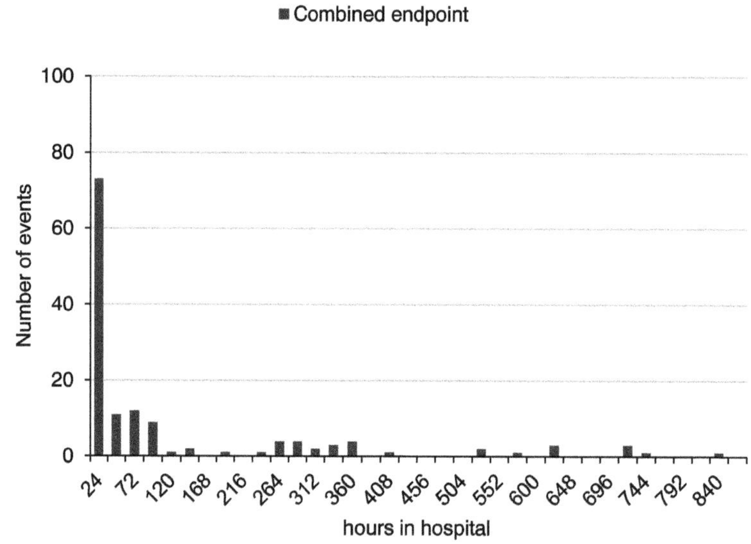

Fig. 2 Distribution of time of events of the combined endpoint in transmural AMI after reperfusion by primary PCI without antecedent thrombolysis. The combined endpoint comprises VT, resuscitation and SCD/arrhythmic death. Multiple events per patient were possible: 24 h: 73; 48 h: 16; 72 h: 11; 96 h: 9; 120 h: 1; 144 h: 2; 168 h: 0; 192 h: 1; 216 h: 0; 240 h: 1; 264 h: 4; 288 h: 4; 312 h: 2; 336 h: 3; 360 h: 4; 384 h: 0; 408 h: 1; 432 h: 0; 456 h: 0; 480 h: 0; 504 h: 0; 528 h: 1; 552 h: 0; 576 h: 1; 600 h: 0; 624 h: 3; 648 h: 0; 672 h: 0; 696 h: 0; 720 h: 3; 744 h: 1; 768 h: 0; 792 h: 0; 816 h: 0; 840 h: 1

The secondary objective was to identify clinical predictors associated with the occurrence of the combined endpoint, ventricular arrhythmia, SCD/AD or resuscitation in the early phase of acute transmural infarction. Due to the low number of events, we were unable to reliably identify clinical predictors but observed positive associations between the combined endpoint and age, severely impaired LVEF, peak serum CK concentration, leucocytosis and coronary thrombus in the multivariable regression analysis.

Comparison with other studies

It is difficult to compare our findings with other studies on PCI, which were designed differently and had different endpoints. In some studies, more time elapsed between symptom onset and PCI than in our cohort. In other studies, the occurrence of endpoints before and during cardiac catheterization were taken into account, and the length of observation time and the differentiation of arrhythmias were not the same in all studies.

Table 3 Occurrence of the specific components of the combined endpoint in time

Adverse event	24 h	48h	72 h	96 h	120 h	144 h	168 h	192 h	216 h	240 h
VT/VF	18		1							
SCD/AD	25	11	5	4	1	1				1
Resuscitation	30	5	5	5		1		1		
Adverse event	264 h	288 h	312 h	336 h	360h	384 h	408h	432h	456h	480h
VT/VF		1		1			1			
SCD/AD	3	1	2		3					
Resuscitation	1	2		2	1					
Adverse event	504 h	528 h	552 h	576 h	600h	624h	648h	672h	696h	720h
VT/VF						1				1
SCD/AD		1		1		1				
Resuscitation						1				2
Adverse event	744h	768h	792h	816 h	840h					
VT/VF										
SCD/AD	1				1					
Resuscitation										

Depicted are absolute numbers and multiple events per patient were possible. A total of 142 events divided into specfic events as follows: a) Ventricular tachycardia (VT) 24 events b) SCD/arrhythmic death 62 events c) Resuscitation 56 events

Table 4 In-hospital arrhythmias: relationship to cardiogenic shock and relative mortality

Malignant arrhythmia	% of total[a]	Cardiogenic shock[b]	Mortality[b]
Tachyarrhythmia			
sustained VT, %	1.3%	15.4%	15.4%
VF, %	1.5%	53.3%	93.3%
Bradyarrhythmia			
CHB, %	0.8%	37.5%	62.5%
Bradyarrhythmia absoluta, %	0.2%	0%	0%
Sinus arrest,	0.1%	0%	0%
SCD, %	0.3%	0%	100%
PEA, %	2.6%	86.7%	100%
Asystole, %	0.8%	53.8%	84.6%

VT ventricular tachycardia, *VF* ventricular fibrillation, *CHB* complete heart block, *SCD* sudden cardiac death, *PEA* pulseless electrical activity
[a] with respect to entire study population
[b] with respect to cases of VT, VF, CHB, Bradyarrhythmia absoluta, sinus arrest, SCD, PEA, Asystole

The studies were, however, broadly comparable regarding study populations, concomitant medications, techniques and stents used.

The incidences of sustained VT or VF and SCD in our registry were 2.8 and 0.3%, respectively. The total burden of in-hospital malignant ventricular arrhythmias in our registry was therefore similar to or lower than that described in other reports of transmural AMI treated by primary PCI. In a similarly designed study by Giglioli et al., only episodes of VF were recorded, which occurred in 0.6% of patients after cardiac catheterization; however, the absence of reports on other endpoints makes a direct comparison with their findings difficult. In our study, the time to reperfusion was less than 4 h after symptom onset in 89.3% of the patients, and the results are probably best compared with the following two studies, which both included patients with STEMI treated with primary PCI within 6 h of symptom onset. Mehta et al. reported in the APEX-AMI trial that 2.0% of patients developed VT or VF after cardiac catheterization [13]. Furthermore, Mehta et al. undertook an analysis of outcomes from the HORIZONS-AMI trial and reported that 5.2% of patients developed VT/VF after PCI [14]. Only a limited comparison is possible with the following studies because the time to primary PCI after symptom onset was longer in those studies. An analysis by Ohlow of an observational registry of patients with STEMI treated with primary PCI within 24 h of symptom onset revealed that the incidence of malignant arrhythmia was 4.7%; however, the investigators did not state where the arrhythmias occurred, and they observed endpoints only during the CCU stay [12]. A single-centre retrospective cohort study of patients with STEMI treated with primary PCI within 24 h of symptom onset undertaken by Cricri and colleagues reported a comparable number of patients (2.6%) who developed VT or VF after cardiac catheterization [11].

There are limited data on the potential therapeutic benefit of primary PCI compared to thrombolysis in terms of the incidence of in-hospital malignant arrhythmias in patients with acute STEMI. The incidence of malignant ventricular arrhythmia in our cohort was less than the VF or sustained VT incidence of 10.2% reported in the GUSTO-I study, a large randomized clinical trial investigating thrombolysis with streptokinase in patients with STEMI within 6 h of symptom onset [15]. This observation corroborates the hypothesis of PCI being superior to thrombolysis.

We observed a predominantly biphasic distribution of composite endpoint events, with 76.7% occurring within 96 h of symptom onset and 12.6% occurring between 240 and 360 h. This biphasic pattern differs from the more monophasic distribution observed in the thrombolysis era as well as in studies of major arrhythmias after successful primary angioplasty for acute STEMI. In the GUSTO-1 thrombolysis trial, 39 and 55% of in-hospital deaths occurred within 24 and 48 h of randomization, respectively, while 84% of malignant arrhythmias occurred within 48 h of randomization [16]. In study settings similar to ours with patients treated within 6 h of symptom onset, Mehta and colleagues found, in retrospective analyses of the APEX-AMI study population and in the prospective HORIZONS-AMI trial, that 70 and 85%, respectively, of VT-associated fatal events occurred within the first 48 h of leaving the catheterization laboratory [13, 14]. In the two studies that included patients with STEMI treated with primary PCI within 24 h of symptom onset, a different temporal distribution was observed. In the study of Cricri and colleagues, most of the malignant arrhythmias (sustained VT, VF or bradycardia necessitating cardiac pacing) developed in the catheterization laboratory, and nearly all of these arrhythmias occurred within 24 h [11].

Ohlow and colleagues reported 90% of VTs occurring within the first 48 h [12].

Our secondary objective was to identify clinical predictors associated with the occurrence of the combined endpoint of VT, SCD or arrhythmic death, and resuscitation in the early phase of acute transmural infarction. These predictors would a) identify patients at high risk for the combined endpoint at the time of hospitalization and b) identify patients at risk despite the apparent lack of established risk factors, e.g., cardiogenic shock.

The variables used for our logistic regression modelling were based on observations from prior studies of risk stratification and include patient demographic and clinical characteristics, measures of the acuity and angiographic presentation of the MI, and indicators of the type and extent of myocardial ischaemia and necrosis [4, 5]. Our results indicate that age, severely impaired LVEF, peak serum CK concentration, leucocytosis and the presence of coronary thrombus were positively associated with the combined endpoint. In patients treated by primary PCI in the APEX-AMI trial as well as those in the study of Ohlow and colleagues, a post-procedural TIMI flow of less than grade 3 was associated with VT or VF [12, 13]. In the APEX-AMI trial, leucocytosis was also a predictor of ventricular arrhythmia [13]. A similar observation was also made by Rahimi et al. in patients with NSTEMI [17].

In several studies from the thrombolysis era, age, severely impaired LVEF and peak serum CK concentration have also been consistently associated with a higher incidence of VF or VT during or immediately after AMI. An analysis of the Holter Registry data from the Cardiac Arrhythmia Suppression Trials showed that age and reduced LVEF were independent predictors of the incidence and frequency of VT [18]. The analysis by Ruiz-Bailén and colleagues of the ARIAM Database also showed that age and peak CK concentration were associated with VF [19]. In the study by Mont and colleagues of patients with AMI who were referred to a CCU after thrombolysis, serum CK-MB fraction concentration, Killip class and bifascicular block were independent predictors of the development of sustained monomorphic tachycardia [20].

We also reported on secondary outcomes and found that in our 'real-world' single-centre registry of patients with acute transmural infarction treated with primary PCI, total in-hospital mortality was 6.5%, which is consistent with other reports. In similarly designed retrospective single-centre studies by Giglioli et al. and Kozieradzka et al., in-hospital mortality was 5.9% and 30-d mortality was 6.3% [4, 10]. A more recent small single-centre study in China showed that mortality was 8.6% in patients aged > 60 years compared with 1.5% in the non-elderly group [21]. In our cohort, 15% of patients with sustained VT and 93% of patients with VF died, resulting in a mortality rate among those who developed a ventricular arrhythmia twice that in a retrospective cohort study of 2317 patients with AMI reported by Henkel et al. (mortality rate 38%) and the APEX-AMI study (mortality rate 33%) [1, 13]. The incidence of bradyarrhythmia in our cohort was also lower than that in other reports; specifically, only 1.3% of the patients developed bradyarrhythmia (with 0.8% of the cases being CHB), while Giglioli et al. reported an incidence of 6.3% [10].

Possible mechanisms and explanations

Our observation of a biphasic temporal distribution of the combined endpoint can be explained by the nature of our chosen endpoint, which comprised episodes of all major ventricular arrhythmias, SCD/AD and resuscitation not only during the initial phase when patients were continuously monitored in the CCU but also during the entire hospital stay. In addition, we did not consider any events that occurred before or during cardiac catheterization [9, 11]. Other potential explanations are that the time to PCI was longer (up to 24 h) in other studies [11, 12], and thus, myocardial necrosis may have been more pronounced in these studies. Furthermore, our population was unselected, unlike trials of study drugs/drug-eluting stents, such as the APEX-AMI and HORIZONS-AMI trials, in which some potential participants were excluded [13, 14].

The multivariate analysis identified variables associated with the composite endpoint that differed from those of other studies, potentially because our endpoint included all ventricular arrhythmias, SCD/AD and resuscitation episodes, while other studies used only ventricular arrhythmias and CHB as the endpoint. Furthermore, leucocytosis, elevated CK concentration and severely impaired LVEF would not have been a consequence of staged or advanced infarctions in our cohort, as we only included patients with < 12 h of symptoms in whom necrosis and reactive inflammation would not have become established. In addition, 92.4% of our patients underwent primary PCI within 4 h of symptom onset.

It is challenging to explain the relatively high mortality rate of those who developed arrhythmia in our cohort. We cannot conclude that adverse outcomes were due to cardiogenic shock and VF alone, as > 40% of the patients in our cohort who died after an episode of VF did not exhibit symptoms or signs of low cardiac output.

Barron et al. concluded in the retrospective analyses of a TIMI 10 thrombolysis study that an elevated WBC was associated with reduced epicardial blood flow and myocardial perfusion, thromboresistance (arteries open later and have a greater thrombus burden), and a higher incidence of new congestive heart failure and death [22]. Our data therefore seem to suggest that inflammation and the WBC itself may also be directly correlated with coronary thrombosis, impaired perfusion, and reperfusion injury in the PCI era.

Study strengths and limitations

Our cohort comprised 975 multi-ethnic patients with a clearly defined pathophysiological substrate (transmural AMI) and therapy (only primary PCI for reperfusion of the occluded vessel). In this cohort, we found a lower incidence of in-hospital major arrhythmia, SCD/AD and resuscitation but a higher mortality rate and biphasic temporal distribution of those who met the composite endpoint. Multivariable regression analysis showed positive associations between several factors and the combined endpoint. Due to the low number of events, we were unable to develop and calculate a risk score for the occurrence of the combined endpoint. The low number of events may be a consequence of the retrospective nature of this study.

A major concern may relate to the period in which data were collected (2005–2011) and the procedural aspects, i.e., the P2Y12 inhibition provided (Clopidogrel) and the very low percentage of implanted DES during primary PCI (12.6%) in our study. In the EUROMAX trial, the choice of prasugrel or ticagrelor over clopidogrel was not associated with differences in acute stent thrombosis or 30-day ischaemic outcomes after PCI [23]. Furthermore, in the PRAGUE-18 study, prasugrel and ticagrelor were found to be similarly effective during the first year after MI, and economically motivated early post-discharge switches to clopidogrel were not associated with an increased risk of ischaemic events [24]. The low percentage of implanted DES (all first generation) in our study should not be of concern because a meta-analysis [25], cost analysis data [26], cohort registries [27] as well as single-centre studies [28] have shown that the only benefit of DES is the reduction of target vessel revascularization. Total mortality and MACE or stent thrombosis are not superior in patients with STEMI receiving bare metal stents (BMS), although a trend toward lower mortality may be seen with everolimus-eluting stents (EES) [29]. Furthermore, in the Norwegian Coronary Stent (NORSTENT) trial, patients (26% with STEMI) were randomized to the DES or BMS group. There were no differences in the incidence of the primary endpoint (a composite of death from any cause or non-fatal spontaneous MI) after a median follow-up of 5 years [30].

Another limitation is the potential lack of generalizability of this single-centre study, which may not reflect outcomes achieved by other teams in different settings. Furthermore, observational studies may generate only a hypothesis that remains to be proven in a randomized controlled trial [31].

Conclusions

In this population of patients with acute transmural myocardial infarction treated with early PCI, we found that the total burden of malignant ventricular arrhythmias was reduced but that the mortality rate of those who developed these arrhythmias was substantially higher. Reperfusion by PCI resulted in a biphasic distribution of all major ventricular arrhythmias, SCD/AD or resuscitation. This result differed from the single peak pattern described in previous studies with thrombolysis as well as with primary PCI.

Nearly one-third of malignant arrhythmias and/or deaths occur late in the clinical course, and predictors are necessary to prevent such events. Due to the low numbers of events and the retrospective nature of this study, more evidence of the predictive value of the identified variables is needed before firm conclusions can be drawn. At this point, we would not recommend any change in clinical practice, as there is no basis for an algorithm to identify patients at risk. Our findings should, however, prompt a multi-centre study to examine the predictors that we have identified in greater detail, to establish a risk scoring system, and to investigate the influence of preventive measures, such as longer periods of monitoring and the use of wearable defibrillator vests.

Abbreviations

AD: Arrhythmic death; AMI: Acute myocardial infarction; BMS: Bare metal stent; CCU: Coronary care unit; CHB: Complete heart block; CK: Creatine phosphokinase; DES: Drug-eluting stent; ECG: Electrocardiogram; EES: Everolimus-eluting stent; EF: Ejection fraction; ICU: Intensive care unit; IRA: Infarct-related artery; LAD: Left anterior descending; LBBB: Left bundle branch block; LV: Left ventricular; LVEF: Left ventricular ejection fraction; M: Myocardial infarction; NSTEMI: Non-ST-elevation myocardial infarction; PAD: Peripheral artery disease; PCI: Percutaneous coronary interventions; PEA: Pulseless electric activity; SCD: Sudden cardiac death; STEMI: ST-elevation myocardial infarction; TIMI: Thrombolysis in myocardial infarction; VF: Ventricular fibrillation; VT: Ventricular tachycardia; WBC: White blood cell count

Acknowledgements

The authors thank Dunja Schulenburg and Dirk Böhm for their help with the collection of data, technical assistance and management of the databases.

Funding

This work was supported by a grant from the German Cardiac Society financed by GlaxoSmithKline.

Authors' contributions

MA was responsible for the study conception and design, interpretation of the data, and drafting of the manuscript. PM and KA collected, analysed and interpreted the data. TO and SS were responsible for the statistical analysis and data interpretation. WS examined and revised the manuscript for intellectual content and gave final approval of the manuscript submitted. All authors read and approved the final version of the manuscript.
committee declared that no ethics approval or consent was necessary (Ärztekammer Nordrhein, Germany; reference number 19–2013).

Competing interests

The authors declare that they have no financial or non-financial competing interests regarding the research conducted.

Author details

[1]Herzzentrum Duisburg, Gerrickstr. 21, D-47137 Duisburg, Germany. [2]Stiftung Institut für Herzinfarktforschung, Bremserstraße 79 - Haus, MD-67063 Ludwigshafen a. Rh, Germany. [3]Klinik für Kardiologie und Angiologie, Herzzentrum Duisburg, Gerrickstr. 21, 47137 Duisburg, Germany. [4]Present address: Herzzentrum Hirslanden Zentralschweiz, Klinik St. Anna, St. Anna Str. 32, CH-6006 Luzern, Switzerland.

References

1. Henkel DM, Witt BJ, Gersh BJ, Jacobsen SJ, Weston SA, Meverden RA, et al. Ventricular arrhythmias after acute myocardial infarction: a 20-year community study. Am Heart J. 2006;151:806–12.
2. Hasin Y, Danchin N, Filippatos GS, Heras M, Janssens U, Leor J, et al. Recommendations for the structure, organization, and operation of intensive cardiac care units. Eur Heart J. 2005;26:1676–82.
3. Kaul P, Newby LK, Fu Y, Mark DB, Califf RM, Topol EJ, et al. International differences in evolution of early discharge after acute myocardial infarction. Lancet. 2004;363:511–7.
4. Kozieradzka A, Kaminski KA, Maciorkowska D, Olszewska M, Dobrzycki S, Nowak K, et al. GRACE, TIMI, Zwolle and CADILLAC risk scores–do they predict 5-year outcomes after ST-elevation myocardial infarction treated invasively? Int J Cardiol. 2011;148:70–5.
5. TIMI Study Group. The thrombolysis in myocardial infarction (TIMI) trial. Phase I findings. N Engl J Med. 1985;312:932–6.
6. Keeley EC, Boura JA, Grines CL. Primary angioplasty versus intravenous thrombolytic therapy for acute myocardial infarction: a quantitative review of 23 randomised trials. Lancet. 2003;361:13–20.
7. Widimsky P, Budesinsky T, Vorac D, Groch L, Zelizko M, Aschermann M, et al. Long distance transport for primary angioplasty vs immediate thrombolysis in acute myocardial infarction. Final results of the randomized national multicentre trial–PRAGUE-2. Eur Heart J. 2003;24:94–104.
8. Busk M, Maeng M, Rasmussen K, Kelbaek H, Thayssen P, Abildgaard U, et al. The Danish multicentre randomized study of fibrinolytic therapy vs. primary angioplasty in acute myocardial infarction (the DANAMI-2 trial): outcome after 3 years follow-up. Eur Heart J. 2008;29:1259–66.
9. Giglioli C, Margheri M, Valente S, Comeglio M, Lazzeri C, Romano SM, et al. The incidence and timing of major arrhythmias following successful primary angioplasty for acute myocardial infarction. Ital Heart J. 2005;6:28–34.
10. Giglioli C, Margheri M, Valente S, Comeglio M, Lazzeri C, Chechi T, et al. Timing, setting and incidence of cardiovascular complications in patients with acute myocardial infarction submitted to primary percutaneous coronary intervention. Can J Cardiol. 2006;22:1047–52.
11. Cricri P, Trachsel L, Muller P, Wackerlin A, Reinhart W, Bonetti P. Incidence and time frame of life-threatening arrhythmias in patients with ST-segment elevation myocardial infarction undergoing primary percutaneous coronary intervention. Swiss Med Wkly. 2012;8:13604.
12. Ohlow M, Geller J, Richter S, Farah A, Muller S, Fuhrmann J, et al. Incidence and predictors of ventricular arrhythmias after ST-segment elevation myocardial infarction. Am J Emerg Med. 2012;30:580–6.
13. Mehta R, Starr A, Lopes R, Hochman J, Widimsky P, Pieper K, et al. Incidence of and outcomes associated with ventricular tachycardia or fibrillation in patients undergoing primary percutaneous coronary intervention. JAMA. 2009;301:1779–89.
14. Mehta R, Yu J, Piccini J, Tcheng J, Farkouh M, Reiffel J, et al. Prognostic significance of postprocedural sustained ventricular tachycardia or fibrillation in patients undergoing primary percutaneous coronary intervention (from the HORIZONS-AMI trial). Am J Cardiol. 2012;109:805–12.
15. Newby K, Thompson T, Stebbins A, Topol E, Califf R, Natale A. Sustained ventricular arrhythmias in patients receiving thrombolytic therapy: incidence and outcomes. The GUSTO Investigators. Circ. 1998;98:2567–73.
16. Lee KL, Woodlief LH, Topol EJ, Weaver WD, Betriu A, Col J, et al. Predictors of 30-day mortality in the era of reperfusion for acute myocardial infarction. Results from an international trial of 41,021 patients. GUSTO-I investigators. Circ. 1995;91:1659–68.
17. Rahimi K, Watzlawek S, Thiele H, Secknus MA, Hayerizadeh BF, Niebauer J, et al. Incidence, time course, and predictors of early malignant ventricular arrhythmias after non-ST segment elevation myocardial infarction in patients with early invasive treatment. Eur Heart J. 2006;27:1706–11.
18. Josephson R, Papa L, Brooks M, Morris M, Akiyama T, Greene H. Effect of age on postmyocardial infarction ventricular arrhythmias (Holter registry data from CAST I and CAST II). Cardiovascular arrhythmia suppression trials. Am J Cardiol. 1995;76:710–3.
19. Ruiz-Bailen M, Aguayo de Hoyos E, Ruiz-Navarro S, Issa-Khozouz Z, Reina-Toral A, Diaz-Castellanos MA, et al. Ventricular fibrillation in acute myocardial infarction in Spanish patients: results of the ARIAM database. Crit Care Med. 2003;31:2144–51.
20. Mont L, Cinca J, Blanch P, Blanco J, Figueras J, Brotons C, et al. Predisposing factors and prognostic value of sustained monomorphic ventricular tachycardia in the early phase of acute myocardial infarction. J Am Coll Cardiol. 1996;28:1670–6.
21. Su Y, Cai X, Geng H, Sheng H, Fan M, Pan M. In-hospital clinical outcomes of elderly patients (>/=60 years) undergoing primary percutaneous coronary intervention. Int J Clin Exp Med. 2015;8:11244–51.
22. Barron H, Cannon C, Murphy S, Braunwald E, Gibson C. Association between white blood cell count, epicardial blood flow, myocardial perfusion, and clinical outcomes in the setting of acute myocardial infarction: a thrombolysis in myocardial infarction 10 substudy. Circ. 2000;102:2329–34.
23. Huber K, Ducrocq G, Hamm CW, Van 't Hof A, Lapostolle F, Coste P, et al. Early clinical outcomes as a function of use of newer oral P2Y12 inhibitors versus clopidogrel in the EUROMAX trial. Open Heart. 2017;4:e000677.
24. Motovska Z, Hlinomaz O, Kala P, Hromadka M, Knot J, Varvarovsky I, et al. 1-year outcomes of patients undergoing primary angioplasty for myocardial infarction treated with prasugrel versus ticagrelor. J Am Coll Cardiol. 2018; 71:371–81.
25. Wang L, Wang H, Dong P, Li Z, Wang Y, Duan N, et al. Long-term outcomes of drug-eluting versus bare-metal stent for ST-elevation myocardial infarction. Arq Bras Cardiol. 2014;102:529–38.
26. Stella SF, Gehling Bertoldi E, Polanczyk CA. Contemporary context of drug-eluting stents in Brazil: a cost utility study. Med Decis Mak. 2016;36:1034–42.
27. Natsuaki M, Morimoto T, Furukawa Y, Nakagawa Y, Kadota K, Yamaji K, et al. Late adverse events after implantation of sirolimus-eluting stent and bare-metal stent: long-term (5-7 years) follow-up of the coronary revascularization demonstrating outcome study-Kyoto registry Cohort-2. Circ Cardiovasc Interv. 2014;7:168–79.
28. Lee VW, Cheng FW, Choi AY, Fong ST, Yu CM, Yan BP. Clinical, humanistic, and economic outcomes between drug-eluting stent (DES) and bare metal stent (BMS): 18-month follow-up study. J Med Econ. 2017;20:239–45.
29. Iqbal MB, Nadra IJ, Ding L, Fung A, Aymong E, Chan AW, et al. Long-term outcomes following drug-eluting stents versus bare metal stents for primary percutaneous coronary intervention: a real-world analysis of 11,181 patients from the British Columbia cardiac registry. Catheter Cardiovasc Interv. 2016; 88:24–35.
30. Bonaa KH, Mannsverk J, Wiseth R, Aaberge L, Myreng Y, Nygard O, et al. Drug-eluting or bare-metal stents for coronary artery disease. N Engl J Med. 2016;375:1242–52.
31. Ziff OJ, Lane DA, Samra M, Griffith M, Kirchhof P, Lip GY, et al. Safety and efficacy of digoxin: systematic review and meta-analysis of observational and controlled trial data. BMJ. 2015;351:h4451.

24

Effect of intracoronary agents on the no-reflow phenomenon during primary percutaneous coronary intervention in patients with ST-elevation myocardial infarction

Xiaowei Niu[1], Jingjing Zhang[2], Ming Bai[3], Yu Peng[3], Shaobo Sun[4] and Zheng Zhang[3*]

Abstract

Background: Despite the restoration of epicardial flow after primary percutaneous coronary intervention (PPCI), myocardial reperfusion remains impaired in a significant proportion of patients. We performed a network meta-analysis to assess the effect of 7 intracoronary agents (adenosine, anisodamine, diltiazem, nicorandil, nitroprusside, urapidil, and verapamil) on the no-reflow phenomenon in patients with ST-elevation myocardial infarction (STEMI) undergoing PPCI.

Methods: Database searches were conducted to identify randomized controlled trials (RCTs) comparing the 7 agents with each other or with standard PPCI. Outcome measures included thrombolysis in myocardial infarction flow grade (TFG), ST-segment resolution (STR), left ventricular ejection fraction (LVEF), major adverse cardiovascular events (MACEs), and adverse events.

Results: Forty-one RCTs involving 4069 patients were analyzed. The addition of anisodamine to standard PPCI for STEMI was associated with improved post-procedural TFG, more occurrences of STR, and improvement of LVEF. The cardioprotective effect of anisodamine conferred a MACE-free survival benefit. Additionally, nitroprusside was regarded as efficient in improving coronary flow and clinical outcomes. Compared with standard care, adenosine, nicorandil, and verapamil improved coronary flow but had no corresponding benefits regarding cardiac function and clinical outcomes. The ranking probability for the 7 treatment drugs showed that anisodamine consistently ranked the highest in efficacy outcomes (TFG < 3, STR, LVEF, and MACEs). No severe adverse events, such as hypotension and malignant arrhythmia, were observed in patients treated with anisodamine. Network meta-regression analysis showed that age, the time to reperfusion, and study follow-up did not affect the treatment effects.

Conclusions: The intracoronary administration of anisodamine appears to improve myocardial reperfusion, cardiac function, and clinical outcomes in patients with STEMI undergoing PPCI. Given the limited quality and quantity of the included studies, more rigorous RCTs are needed to verify the role of this inexpensive and well-tolerated regimen.

Keywords: Percutaneous coronary intervention, No reflow phenomenon, Intracoronary; pharmacology, Meta-analysis

* Correspondence: zhangccu@163.com
[3]Department of Cardiology, the First Hospital of Lanzhou University, Donggang West Road, No. 1, Lanzhou, Gansu 730000, China
Full list of author information is available at the end of the article

Background

Primary percutaneous coronary intervention (PPCI) is the preferred reperfusion therapy for ST-elevation myocardial infarction (STEMI) [1]. Despite the restoration of epicardial flow after PPCI, impaired myocardial perfusion, known as the no-reflow phenomenon (NR), remains observed in a significant proportion of patients [2]. The NR after PPCI for the treatment of STEMI contributes to infarct size expansion, reduced ventricular function, and increased mortality [3–5]. Several potential mechanisms have been hypothesized to cause NR, including embolization of atherothrombotic material, vasoconstriction, activation of the inflammatory cascade, neutrophil plugging, platelet aggregation, toxic free-radical generation, and myocardial edema [2, 6]. A basic understanding of the process has contributed to several pharmacological drugs proposed to improve myocardial reperfusion after PPCI, such as adenosine, diltiazem, nicorandil, nitroprusside, urapidil, and verapamil [2, 6]. A number of meta-analyses have been conducted to assess whether intracoronary adenosine, diltiazem, nitroprusside, nicorandil, and verapamil can reduce NR and improve clinical outcomes after PPCI. However, these meta-analyses were limited in size and yielded inconclusive results [7]. After the most recent meta-analyses were published [8–12], new randomized controlled trials (RCTs) on this subject have been published, and these additional data may help reduce the amount of uncertainty surrounding the treatment effects. Anisodamine, unlike the aforementioned vasodilators, is a muscarinic cholinergic antagonist [13]. Basic and clinical studies have shown that anisodamine can increase blood pressure and coronary perfusion pressure and improve microcirculation, making it a potentially useful drug for preventing NR [14–16]. However, the value of anisodamine in improving myocardial reperfusion after PPCI has not been studied in any previous meta-analysis.

Traditional pairwise meta-analyses are limited for simultaneously synthesizing all evidence because head-to-head comparisons between treatments are often unavailable [17]. Bayesian network meta-analysis combines direct and indirect comparisons and forms hierarchies for the efficacy of various treatments [18]. Thus, this technique better informs clinicians regarding the optimal use of candidate agents in clinical practice. In this study, we performed standard pairwise and Bayesian network meta-analyses to comprehensively evaluate available intracoronary agents as adjuncts to PPCI, to estimate the relative efficacy and safety of the various agents, and to provide a hierarchy of treatments for the outcomes of interest.

Methods

Study search strategy

PubMed, Embase, Web of Science, and CENTRAL databases were searched systematically, as well as the references of eligible studies and recent reviews from inception to December 31, 2016. The keywords and corresponding Medical Subject Headings (Mesh) were as follows: "adenosine", "anisodamine", "calcium channel blockers", "diltiazem", "verapamil", "nicorandil", "nitroprusside", "urapidil", "vasodilator agents", "intracoronary", "myocardial infarction", and "percutaneous coronary intervention". No limits regarding language and publication type were applied.

Selection criteria

The inclusion criteria were as follows: (i) RCTs involving patients with STEMI undergoing PPCI; (ii) studies that evaluated intracoronary administration of any of the drugs (adenosine, anisodamine, diltiazem, verapamil, nicorandil, nitroprusside, and urapidil) and compared the active drugs to each other or a control (standard PPCI without the use of the aforementioned active drugs); and (iii) trials that reported data on any of the outcomes of interest: thrombolysis in myocardial infarction flow grade (TFG) < 3 [19], ST-segment resolution (STR) defined as at least a 50–70% resolution of ST-segment elevation on an electrocardiogram after PPCI compared with the baseline measurement [20], left ventricular ejection fraction (LVEF), major adverse cardiovascular events (MACEs), and adverse events (AEs). Indicators of reperfusion (TFG and STR) were measured after PPCI. For LVEF outcome, we pooled the data assessed in-hospital to 1 month after PPCI because the data were available in most studies. MACEs was evaluated at the longest available follow-up. The exclusion criteria were as follows: (i) trials containing only one of the aforementioned treatments, (ii) duplicate reporting, and (iii) sub-studies of the RCTs.

Data collection and quality assessment

On the basis of the title, abstract, or full-texts, two independent investigators assessed the studies for eligibility in three screening stages and then extracted data based on the pre-specified forms. The following information was included: (i) the designs of trials and inclusion criteria, (ii) patient characteristics at baseline, (iii) features of the interventions, and (iv) outcomes as aforementioned. Different reviewers independently assessed the methodological quality of eligible trials using the criteria of the Cochrane Handbook [21]. For missing or unclear information, we attempted to contact the original trial authors by e-mail. All divergences were resolved by consensus or adjudication by a third reviewer.

Statistical analysis

Two investigators cross-checked the data from all the identified studies. Standard pairwise and network meta-analyses were performed to obtain estimates for outcomes, and these estimates were presented as odds ratios (ORs) or mean differences (MDs) with 95% CIs for dichotomous or continuous data, respectively. First, we conducted the standard pairwise meta-analysis using STATA 11.0 software (Stata Corp., College Station, Texas, USA). A random-effect model was preferred because of the anticipated variety in study populations. Statistical heterogeneity was evaluated using the Cochrane Q test and I^2 statistic (I^2 values >75% represented significant heterogeneity). Funnel plots were used to evaluate the publication bias of each endpoint. A 0.5 zero-cell correction was used so that studies with no events would still be included for analyses [21]. Second, we performed Bayesian network meta-analysis and meta-regression using WinBUGS 1.4.3 software (MRC Biostatistics Unit, Cambridge, UK) [22]. A random-effect model was used to compare treatments using Markov chain Monte Carlo methods with Gibbs sampling from 150,000 iterations obtained after a 90,000 iteration burn-in phase. Model convergence was assessed graphically according to Gelman and Rubin. Model fit was evaluated by comparing a posterior mean residual deviance to the number of independent data points. The inconsistency of the network was assessed by contrasting estimates from the network analysis with the direct comparison meta-analysis of each node (node splitting). A Bayesian P value >0.05 from the method represented the presence of consistency between direct and indirect comparisons. In addition, we used the surface under the cumulative ranking curve (SUCRA) to rank the treatments for each outcome. SUCRA expressed as percentages would be 100% when a treatment has a high likelihood of being best and 0% when a treatment has a high likelihood of being worst [18]. Network meta-regression analysis was performed to explore the effects of potential treatment modifying covariates, including mean age, the time to reperfusion, and duration of follow-up. In this analysis, an identical interaction effect across all treatments with respect to the control was assumed [23]. The 95% CIs for the interaction coefficient excluded zero, suggesting an interaction effect between the covariates and the treatment effects [23]. The deviance information criterion (DIC) was used to compare fit between the covariate adjusted and unadjusted models for the same data. Differences in the DIC ≥ 3 were considered meaningful [23]. Results were stratified by the type of control group (placebo or conventional PPCI alone) and median duration of follow-up. Given that MACE definition was not identical in all trials, we performed a sensitivity analysis to evaluate treatments by restricting to studies with a relatively uniform definition of MACEs. Data plotting was performed using R 3.3.1 software (R Core Team, Vienna, Austria) [24]. The results were statistically significant with a two-sided $P < 0.05$. We performed this meta-analysis according to the Preferred Reporting Items for Systematic Reviews and Meta-Analyses (PRISMA) statement and Cochrane Handbook guidelines [21, 25].

Results

Study selection and characteristics of the included trials

Of 905 potentially eligible trials, 41 RCTs involving 4069 patients were included in this network meta-analysis (Fig. 1) [26–66]. Seven drug classes were administered intracoronarily during PPCI, including adenosine (n = 1006), anisodamine (n = 208), diltiazem (n = 88), verapamil (n = 181), nicorandil (n = 217), nitroprusside (n = 551), and urapidil (n = 49). The network of available treatment comparisons is shown in Fig. 2. Nineteen studies used placebo (saline solution) as a comparator, whereas 20 studies used conventional PPCI alone as the comparator. Participants were enrolled at a mean age of 61 years, and male participants accounted for 78% of the total population. The time to reperfusion from the onset of symptoms ranged from 116 min to 546 min across studies and the median time to reperfusion across all studies was 273 min. The proportion of patients with multivessel disease ranged from 15 to 65% across 14 studies and the median proportion of patients with multivessel disease across 14 studies was 52% [30, 36–38, 43–45, 50, 51, 54, 55, 59, 61, 65]. Twenty-seven studies reported the incidence of MACEs within a 6-month follow-up, one trial reported within an 8-month follow-up, and four trials reported within a 12-month follow-up. Studies that evaluated adenosine, anisodamine, diltiazem, verapamil, nicorandil, nitroprusside, and urapidil treatments had median follow-up periods of 6 months, 4.5 months, 3.5 months, 1 month, 2 months, 6 months, and 1 month, respectively. Eight RCTs used the relatively uniform definition of MACEs including death, reinfarction, and revascularization. The main characteristics of the identified trials are detailed in Table 1. A summary of outcomes for each agent is listed in Table 2.

Overall, the methodological quality of the included trials was not high (Table 1). The risk of bias was low for random sequence generation in 13 trials (32%), allocation concealment in 8 trials (20%), blinding of participants and personnel in 5 trials (12%), blinding of outcome assessment in 24 trials (59%), incomplete outcome data in 25 trials (61%), selective reporting in 38 trials (93%), and other sources of bias in 38 trials (93%).

TFG < 3

In the network meta-analysis, 37 studies with 3909 patients contributed to the analysis of TFG < 3 after PPCI. The incidence of TFG < 3 was higher in the control group than in the anisodamine (OR 4.19, 95%CI 1.90–9.02), verapamil (OR 3.82, 95%CI 2.01–7.65), nicorandil (OR 3.27, 95%CI 1.63–6.93), nitroprusside (OR 1.85, 95%CI 1.23–2.86), and

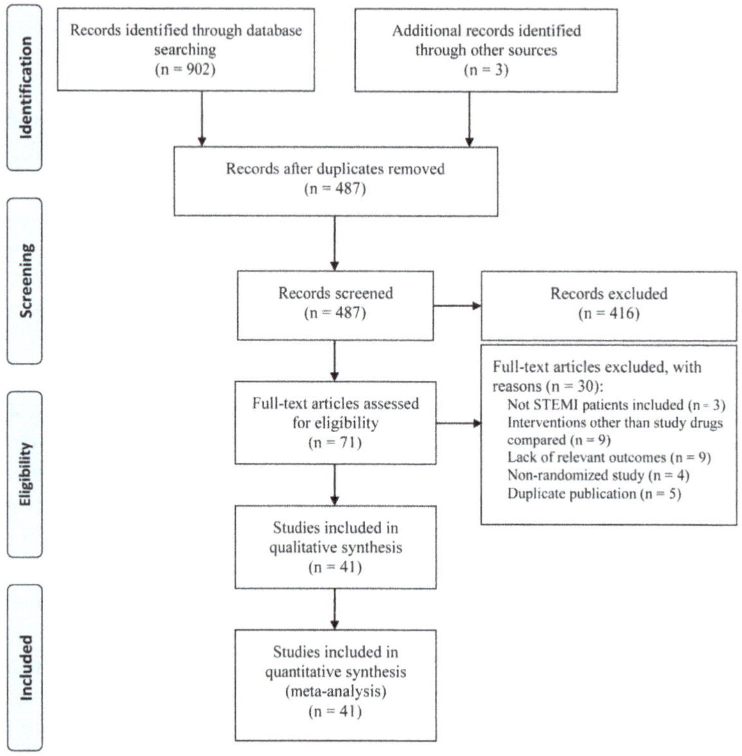

Fig. 1 Flow chart of study selection

adenosine (OR 1.46, 95%CI 1.03–2.06) groups. Adenosine was associated with a significantly increased risk of TFG < 3 compared with anisodamine (OR 2.46, 95%CI 1.00–5.71) and verapamil (OR 2.24, 95%CI 1.09–4.83). In the SUCRA analysis, the hierarchy for treatment efficacy for TFG < 3 (highest to lowest rank) was anisodamine, followed by verapamil, nicorandil, diltiazem, nitroprusside, adenosine,

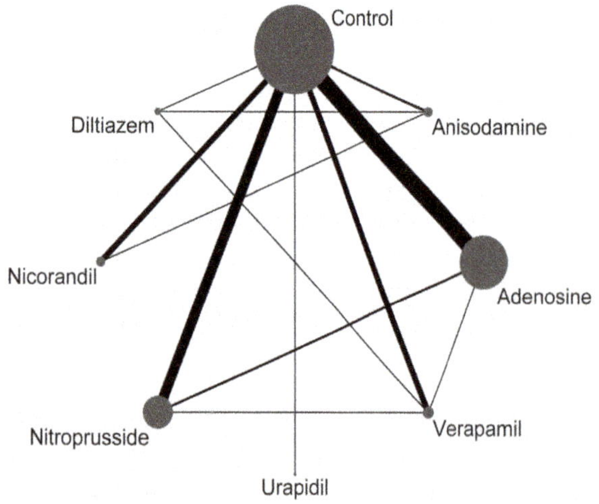

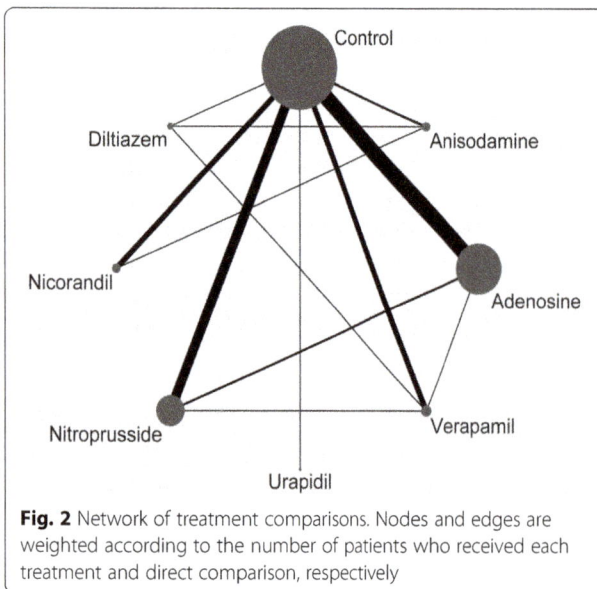

Fig. 2 Network of treatment comparisons. Nodes and edges are weighted according to the number of patients who received each treatment and direct comparison, respectively

urapidil, and the control. In the traditional pairwise meta-analysis, there was no significant heterogeneity for any treatment effect across strata (all $I^2 < 75\%$; $P_{het} > 0.10$). Similar results were observed between the control group and the adenosine (OR 1.46, 95%CI 1.03–2.06), anisodamine (OR 2.80, 95%CI 1.25–6.24), nicorandil (OR 2.95, 95%CI 1.43–6.06), nitroprusside (OR 1.93, 95%CI 1.15–3.26), and verapamil (OR 3.15, 95%CI 1.50–6.59) groups. All comparisons analyzed in the network and pairwise meta-analyses are shown in Fig. 3.

STR

Twenty-one studies with 2902 patients contributed to the evidence network for STR analysis. The control group was associated with a lower rate of STR compared with the anisodamine (OR 0.29, 95%CI 0.14–0.57), nicorandil (OR 0.29, 95%CI 0.11–0.72), and adenosine (OR 0.61, 95%CI 0.44–0.79) groups. Nitroprusside was associated with a significantly reduced rate of STR compared with anisodamine (OR 0.36, 95%CI 0.17–0.82) and nicorandil (OR 0.37, 95%CI 0.14–1.00). As indicated by the SUCRA value, anisodamine ranked the highest, and the control ranked the lowest, indicating that anisodamine was most likely to be the best treatments for this outcome. For pairwise meta-analysis, results of the comparison between the control group and the adenosine (OR 0.65, 95%CI 0.49–0.86), anisodamine (OR 0.38, 95%CI 0.19–0.74), and

Table 1 Description of included studies

Study	Year	Sample size (n)	Type of intervention	Dose of active drugs	Control definition	Outcomes	MACE definition	Age (years)	Men (%)	Time to reperfusion (min)	Follow-up (mo)	Quality of study A	B	C	D	E	F	G
Abdelaziz[26]	2017	30/30	Verapamil/ Nitroprusside	180 μg/ 750 μg	-	TFG, STR, LVEF, MACEs, AEs	Cardiac death, MI, TVR, or HF	53	73	311	1	⊕	⊕	⊕	⊕	⊕	⊕	⊕
Akagi[27]	2006	10/10	Nicorandil/ Control	2 mg	Conventional PPCI alone	LVEF	-	65	75	223	1	?	?	?	?	?	⊕	⊕
Akturk[28]	2014	15/16/ 15	Verapamil/ Adenosine/ Control	1.5 mg/ 240 μg	Saline solution	TFG, STR, LVEF, MACEs	Death	58	83	225	6	⊕	?	?	⊕	?	⊕	⊕
Amit[29]	2006	48/50	Nitroprusside/ Control	60 μg	Saline solution	TFG, STR, MACEs, AEs	Death, MI or TVR	62	87	221	6	⊕	?	?	⊕	?	⊕	⊕
Bai[30]	2016	104/36	Anisodamine/ Control	1-4 mg	Saline solution	TFG, STR, LVEF, MACEs	Cardiac death, MI, TVR, or malignant arrhythmia	61	76	355	3	?	?	?	?	?	⊕	⊕
Chen[31]	2015	26/26/ 26	Anisodamine/ Nicorandil/ Control	2 mg/ 2 mg	Conventional PPCI alone	TFG, STR, LVEF, MACEs	Death, MI or TVR	59	69	430	1	?	?	?	⊕	⊕	⊕	⊕
Chen[32]	2008	22/21	Urapidil/ Control	5 mg	Saline solution	LVEF	-	63	67	-	In-hospital	?	?	?	?	?	⊕	⊕
Darahim[33]	2014	20/40	Adenosine/ Control	6 mg	Saline solution	TFG, STR, LVEF, MACEs, AEs	Death or MI	52	73	254	In-hospital	?	?	?	⊕	⊕	⊕	⊕
Desmet[34]	2011	56/54	Adenosine/ Control	4 mg	Saline solution	TFG, STR, LVEF, MACEs, AE	Death, HF, or malignant arrhythmia	61	82	204	12	⊕	⊕	⊕	⊕	?	⊕	⊕
Fan[35]	2007	24/23	Anisodamine/ Control	1 mg	Conventional PPCI alone	LVEF, MACEs	Cardiac death, MI, TVR, or malignant arrhythmia	63	77	-	6	?	?	?	?	?	⊕	⊕
Fokkema[36]	2009	226/222	Adenosine/ Control	120 μg twice	Saline solution	TFG, STR, MACEs, AEs	Death, MI or TVR	62	75	173	1	?	?	?	⊕	⊕	⊕	⊕
Garcia[37]	2014	100/97	Adenosine/ Control	4.5 mg	Saline solution	TFG, STR, LVEF, MACEs, AEs	Death, MI, TVR, or HF	59	86	211	6	⊕	?	?	⊕	⊕	⊕	⊕
Grygier[38]	2011	35/35	Adenosine/ Control	1 mg + 2 mg twice	Saline solution	TFG, STR, LVEF, MACEs, AEs	Death, MI, TVR, or HF	65	63	249	1	?	?	?	⊕	⊕	⊕	⊕
Hamza[39]	2014	25/25	Verapamil/ Control	100 μg	Conventional PPCI alone	TFG, LVEF, MACEs	Death, MI or TVR	53	88	355	In-hospital	?	?	?	?	⊕	⊕	⊕
Hendler[40]	2006	10/10/ 10/10	Nitroprusside/ Adenosine/ Verapamil/ Control	100-500 μg/ 60-120 μg/ 100-500 μg/	Conventional PPCI alone	TFG, LVEF	-	62	80	120	1	?	?	?	⊕	⊕	⊕	⊕
Huang[41]	2012	34/34/ 34	Diltiazem/ Verapamil/ Control	400 μg/ 200 μg	Conventional PPCI alone	TFG, STR, LVEF, MACEs	Death, MI or TVR	65	77	324	1	⊕	⊕	?	⊕	⊕	⊕	⊕
Ji[42]	2007	23/27	Adenosine/ Control	300 μg	Saline solution	TFG, LVEF, AEs	-	60	82	268	1	?	?	?	⊕	⊕	⊕	⊕
Lee[43]	2008	37/36	Nicorandil/ Control	2 mg twice	Conventional PPCI alone	TFG, MACEs	Death, MI or TLR	58	84	350	1	?	?	?	?	⊕	⊕	⊕
Li[44]	2016	130/128	Adenosine/ Control	2 mg twice	Saline solution	TFG, STR, LVEF, MACEs	Cardiac death, MI, TVR, or HF	61	76	220	1	⊕	⊕	?	⊕	⊕	⊕	⊕
Marzilli[45]	2000	27/27	Adenosine/ Control	4 mg	Saline solution	TFG, MACEs	Cardiac death, MI, HF, recurrent angina	60	80	116	In-hospital	?	?	?	⊕	⊕	⊕	⊕
Miyazawa[46]	2006	35/35	Nicorandil/ Control	2 mg	Conventional PPCI alone	TFG, LVEF, MACEs	Death, MI, TLR, or HF	62	81	422	8	?	?	?	⊕	?	⊕	⊕
Nameki[47]	2004	13/14	Nicorandil/ Control	4 mg	Conventional PPCI alone	TFG, LVEF, MACEs	Death	63	81	381	3	?	?	?	⊕	⊕	⊕	⊕
Nayel[48]	2013	20/20	Nitroprusside/ Control	100-300 μg	Conventional PPCI alone	TFG	-	-	-	-	In-hospital	?	?	?	?	?	?	?
Nazir[49]	2016	82/79/ 86	Adenosine/ Nitroprusside/ Control	1 mg + 2 mg twice/ 250 μg twice	Conventional PPCI alone	TFG, STR, LVEF, MACEs, AEs	Death, MI, TLR, or HF	59	80	151	6	⊕	⊕	?	⊕	⊕	⊕	⊕
Niccoli[50]	2013	80/80 /80	Adenosine/ Nitroprusside/ Control	120 μg + 2 mg/60 μg +100 μg	Saline solution	TFG, STR, MACEs, AEs	Death, MI, TLR, or HF	64	75	278	1	⊕	⊕	?	⊕	⊕	⊕	⊕
Ota[51]	2006	31/27	Nicorandil/ Control	1-2 mg	Conventional PPCI alone	TFG, STR	-	63	78	241	In-hospital	?	?	?	?	⊕	⊕	⊕
Pan[52]	2009	46/46	Nitroprusside/ Control	100 μg	Conventional PPCI alone	TFG, MACEs	Death, MI, or revascularization	53	83	492	6	?	?	?	⊕	?	⊕	⊕
Peng[53]	2014	54/54	Anisodamine/ Diltiazem	1 mg 2 mg	-	TFG, STR, LVEF, MACES, AEs	Death, MI, or TVR	63	79	522	6	⊕	⊕	?	⊕	?	⊕	⊕
Petronio[54]	2005	30/30	Adenosine/ Control	4 mg	Conventional PPCI alone	TFG, STR, LVEF, MACEs, AEs	Death	59	85	179	6	⊖	?	?	⊕	?	⊕	⊕
Sai[55]	2011	44/43	Nitroprusside/ Control	200 μg	Conventional PPCI alone	TFG	-	-	-	-	In-hospital	?	?	?	?	?	?	?
Shinozaki[56]	2010	34/35	Nitroprusside/ Control	120 μg	Conventional PPCI alone	TFG	-	-	-	-	In-hospital	?	?	?	?	?	?	?
Stoel[57]	2008	27/22	Adenosine/ Control	60 mg	Saline solution	STR, MACEs	Death, MI, HF, or revascularization	67	65	223	12	?	?	⊕	?	⊕	⊕	⊕
Sung[58]	2008	37/36	Nicorandil/ Control	2 mg twice	Conventional PPCI alone	TFG, MACEs	Death, MI, or TLR	58	84	-	1	?	?	?	?	⊕	⊕	⊕
Taniyama[59]	1997	20/20	Verapamil/ Control	0.5 mg	Conventional PPCI alone	TFG, LVEF	-	64	78	441	1	?	?	?	⊕	⊕	⊕	⊕
Tong[60]	2013	130/128	Adenosine/ Control	2 mg twice	Saline solution	TFG, STR, MACEs, AEs	Death, MI, TVR, or HF	61	76	320	12	⊕	?	?	⊕	⊕	⊕	⊕
Yamada[61]	2016	28/24	Nicorandil/ Control	0.2 mg/kg	Conventional PPCI alone	TFG, LVEF	-	66	87	396	In-hospital	?	?	?	?	⊕	⊕	⊕
Yang[62]	2016	80/40	Nitroprusside/ Control	100 μg	Conventional PPCI alone	TFG	-	63	68	546	In-hospital	⊕	⊕	?	⊕	⊕	⊕	⊕
Yao[63]	2009	27/27	Urapidil/ Control	12.5 mg	Saline solution	TFG, STR, LVEF, MACEs, AEs	Cardiac death, MI, HF, malignant arrhythmia, or recurrent angina	61	61	240	1	⊖	?	⊕	?	⊕	⊕	⊕
Zhao[64]	2013	80/82	Nitroprusside/ Control	100 μg	Saline solution	TFG, STR, LVEF, MACEs, AEs	Cardiac death, MI, or TVR	64	79	345	6	?	?	?	?	?	⊕	⊕
Qiao[65]	2009	47/44	Verapamil/ Control	200 μg	Saline solution	TFG, LVEF, MACEs	Cardiac death, MI, HF, recurrent angina	62	84	306	3	⊕	?	⊕	?	?	⊕	⊕
Wang[66]	2008	14/14	Adenosine/ Control	500 μg	Saline solution	TFG, AEs	-	47	82	-	In-hospital	?	?	?	?	⊕	⊕	⊕

TFG, TIMI flow grade; STR, ST-segment resolution; LVEF, left ventricular ejection fraction; MACEs, major adverse cardiovascular events; AEs, adverse events; PPCI, primary percutaneous coronary intervention; MI, myocardial infarction; HF, heart failure; TVR, target vessel revascularization; TLR, target lesion revascularization. A, Random sequence generation; B, Allocation concealment; C, Blinding of participants and personnel; D, Blinding of outcome assessment; E, Incomplete outcome data; F, Selective

Table 2 Summary of outcomes for each agent

Type of intervention	Outcomes										
	TFG < 3		STR		LVEF			MACEs		AEs	
	Events	Total	Events	Total	Mean	SD	Total	Events	Total	Events	Total
Adenosine	82	978	538	931	48.80	11.72	502	115	959	258	796
Anisodamine	18	184	140	184	58.78	10.31	208	11	208	29	158
Diltiazem	20	88	43	88	54.21	12.33	88	12	88	19	54
Nicorandil	7	207	33	57	55.18	11.75	112	20	148	–	–
Nitroprusside	57	551	191	317	51.46	12.44	199	26	363	50	317
Urapidil	1	27	25	27	54.32	6.65	49	0	27	4	27
Verapamil	26	181	34	79	52.56	12.48	181	18	151	3	30
Control	263	1693	608	1219	50.57	10.88	943	228	1478	87	1008

TFG, TIMI flow grade; STR, ST-segment resolution; LVEF, left ventricular ejection fraction; MACEs, major adverse cardiovascular events; AEs, adverse events

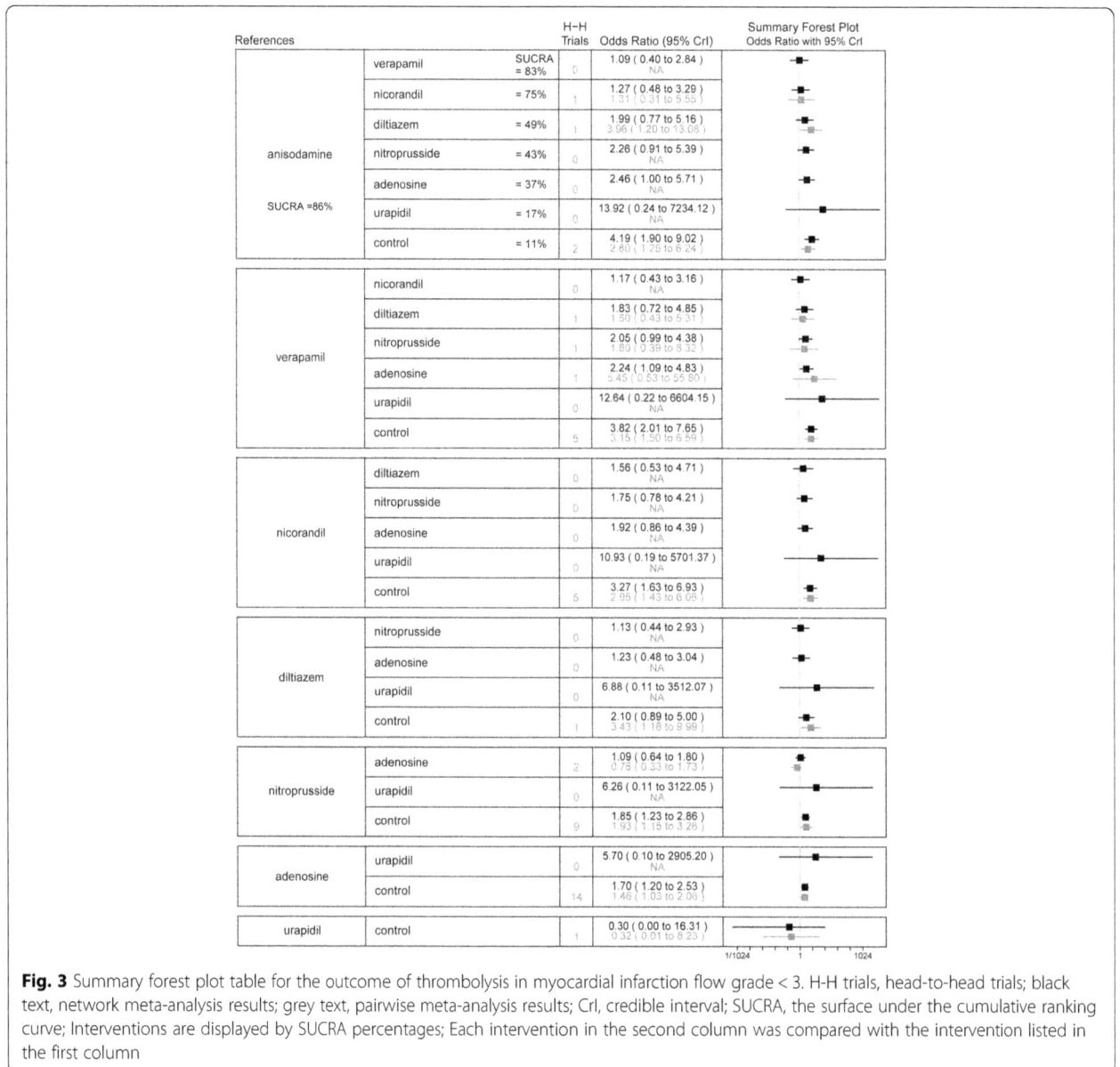

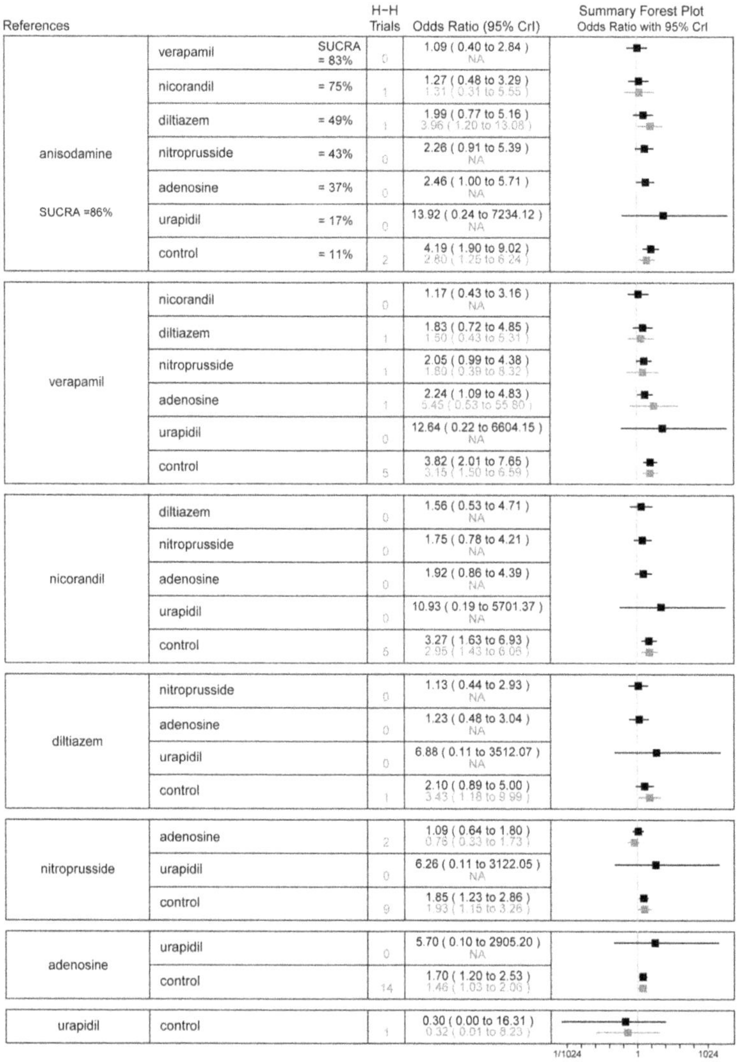

Fig. 3 Summary forest plot table for the outcome of thrombolysis in myocardial infarction flow grade < 3. H-H trials, head-to-head trials; black text, network meta-analysis results; grey text, pairwise meta-analysis results; CrI, credible interval; SUCRA, the surface under the cumulative ranking curve; Interventions are displayed by SUCRA percentages; Each intervention in the second column was compared with the intervention listed in the first column

nicorandil (OR 0.31, 95%CI 0.12–0.80) groups were similar to those of the network meta-analysis. There was no significant heterogeneity for any treatment effect across strata (all $I^2 < 75\%$; $P_{het} > 0.05$). The network and pairwise treatment comparisons are shown in Fig. 4.

LVEF

Twenty-seven studies with 2282 patients were involved in the network meta-analysis for LVEF. Standard care had a significantly lower LVEF after PPCI compared to anisodamine (MD -6.05, 95%CI -9.01 to -3.12) and nitroprusside (MD -3.06, 95%CI -6.18 to -0.27) therapy. Compared to the anisodamine group, the verapamil (MD -4.22, 95%CI -8.07 to -0.39), adenosine (MD -5.54, 95%CI -9.06 to -2.04), diltiazem (MD -5.71, 95%CI -10.29 to-1.12), and nicorandil (MD -6.23, 95%CI -9.90 to -2.48) groups had a significantly lower LVEF. Results of the SUCRA analysis showed that anisodamine was most possibly the best treatment, whereas the control was rated as the least effective treatment. Similarly, results of the pairwise meta-analysis showed that standard care had a lower LVEF than anisodamine (MD -5.05, 95%CI -6.69 to -3.41). However, there was a statistically significant difference in LVEF between the control and urapidil groups (MD -3.83, 95%CI -5.97 to -1.70). Results of the comparison between the control and nitroprusside were no longer significant, but the trend favored nitroprusside. Low heterogeneity was observed for the aforementioned analyses, except for analysis of the control versus nitroprusside ($I^2 = 95\%$; $P_{het} < 0.05$). The network and pairwise treatment comparisons are shown in Fig. 5.

References			H-H Trials	Odds Ratio (95% CrI)
anisodamine SUCRA =86%	nicorandil	SUCRA = 83%	1	1.00 (0.36 to 2.73) 1.00 (0.25 to 3.97)
	urapidil	= 65%	0	0.74 (0.14 to 4.42) NA
	verapamil	= 50%	0	0.51 (0.21 to 1.25) NA
	adenosine	= 47%	0	0.47 (0.23 to 1.02) NA
	diltiazem	= 40%	1	0.45 (0.20 to 1.03) 0.30 (0.13 to 0.68)
	nitroprusside	= 24%	0	0.36 (0.17 to 0.82) NA
	control	= 6%	2	0.29 (0.14 to 0.57) 0.38 (0.19 to 0.74)
nicorandil	urapidil		0	0.74 (0.12 to 4.82) NA
	verapamil		0	0.51 (0.17 to 1.54) NA
	adenosine		0	0.48 (0.19 to 1.26) NA
	diltiazem		0	0.45 (0.15 to 1.43) NA
	nitroprusside		0	0.37 (0.14 to 1.00) NA
	control		2	0.29 (0.11 to 0.72) 0.31 (0.12 to 0.80)
urapidil	verapamil		0	0.69 (0.12 to 3.71) NA
	adenosine		0	0.65 (0.12 to 3.15) NA
	diltiazem		0	0.61 (0.10 to 3.40) NA
	nitroprusside		0	0.49 (0.09 to 2.44) NA
	control		1	0.39 (0.07 to 1.79) 0.41 (0.11 to 1.59)
verapamil	adenosine		1	0.94 (0.48 to 1.86) 0.64 (0.15 to 2.78)
	diltiazem		1	0.89 (0.39 to 2.06) 0.89 (0.34 to 2.31)
	nitroprusside		1	0.72 (0.35 to 1.47) 3.33 (0.99 to 11.14)
	control		2	0.57 (0.29 to 1.08) 0.30 (0.13 to 0.70)
adenosine	diltiazem		0	0.95 (0.42 to 2.13) NA
	nitroprusside		2	0.77 (0.49 to 1.18) 0.68 (0.47 to 1.02)
	control		12	0.61 (0.44 to 0.79) 0.65 (0.49 to 0.86)
diltiazem	nitroprusside		0	0.80 (0.35 to 1.88) NA
	control		1	0.64 (0.29 to 1.35) 0.37 (0.14 to 1.01)
nitroprusside	control		4	0.80 (0.51 to 1.16) 0.83 (0.56 to 1.23)

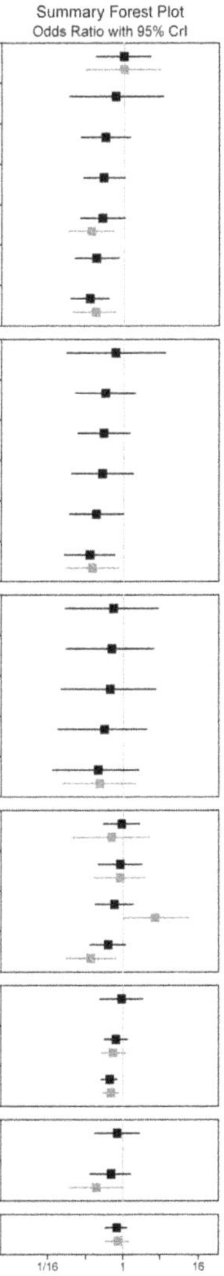

Fig. 4 Summary forest plot table for the outcome of ST-segment resolution. H-H trials, head-to-head trials; black text, network meta-analysis results; grey text, pairwise meta-analysis results; CrI, credible interval; SUCRA, the surface under the cumulative ranking curve; Interventions are displayed by SUCRA percentages; Each intervention in the second column was compared with the intervention listed in the first column

MACEs

Twenty-nine studies with 3422 patients were included in the network meta-analysis for MACEs. Compared with anisodamine, nitroprusside (OR 3.62, 95%CI 1.27–10.74), nicorandil (OR 4.59, 95%CI 1.42–15.12), adenosine (OR 4.94, 95%CI 1.93–14.00), verapamil (OR 5.00, 95%CI 1.58–16.28), and the control (OR 6.56, 95%CI 2.69–17.16) were associated with a significant increase in the risk of MACEs. The incidence of MACEs was higher in the control group than in the nitroprusside group (OR 1.82, 95%CI 1.06–3.15). Results of the SUCRA analysis showed that anisodamine was superior to all other candidate interventions for decreasing the risk of MACEs. In the standard pairwise meta-analysis, we observed similar results between the control and anisodamine (OR 6.02, 95%CI 2.29–15.84), nitroprusside (OR 1.94, 95%CI 1.03–3.66) groups. There was no significant heterogeneity for any treatment effect across strata (all $I^2 < 75\%$; $P_{het} > 0.05$). The network and pairwise treatment comparisons are shown in Fig. 6.

AEs

AEs were reported in 17 RCTs, including flushing, thirst, hypotension, bradycardia, tachycardia, bronchospasm, atrioventricular block, dyspnea, and chest pain. Fortunately, these AEs were almost always transient, and none of the studies reported any long-lasting sequelae. As there were clear differences regarding the definition of AEs for each individual agent, the network meta-analysis was not conducted. Results of the pairwise meta-analysis showed that adenosine therapy was associated with a higher rate of AEs than control therapy (OR 4.69, 95%CI

References			H-H Trials	Mean Difference (95% CrI)
anisodamine SUCRA =96%	urapidil	SUCRA = 76%	0	−2.18 (−7.50 to 3.06) NA
	nitroprusside	= 71%	0	−3.00 (−6.98 to 1.30) NA
	verapamil	= 54%	0	−4.22 (−8.07 to −0.39) NA
	adenosine	= 31%	0	−5.54 (−9.06 to −2.04) NA
	diltiazem	= 31%	1	−5.71 (−10.29 to −1.12) −8.00 (−12.85 to −3.15)
	nicorandil	= 21%	1	−6.23 (−9.90 to −2.48) −7.50 (−9.82 to −5.18)
	control	= 20%	3	−6.05 (−9.01 to −3.12) −5.05 (−6.69 to −3.41)
urapidil	nitroprusside		0	−0.80 (−5.96 to 4.64) NA
	verapamil		0	−2.03 (−7.15 to 3.02) NA
	adenosine		0	−3.36 (−8.16 to 1.50) NA
	diltiazem		0	−3.50 (−9.59 to 2.56) NA
	nicorandil		0	−4.07 (−9.30 to 1.41) NA
	control		2	−3.85 (−8.25 to 0.52) −3.83 (−5.97 to −1.70)
nitroprusside	verapamil		2	−1.23 (−4.78 to 1.97) −0.73 (−9.13 to 7.67)
	adenosine		2	−2.55 (−5.91 to 0.48) −2.23 (−8.05 to 3.59)
	diltiazem		0	−2.73 (−7.86 to 2.14) NA
	nicorandil		0	−3.26 (−7.49 to 0.90) NA
	control		3	−3.06 (−6.18 to −0.27) −5.11 (−10.80 to 0.36)
verapamil	adenosine		2	−1.32 (−4.32 to 1.72) −0.85 (−7.20 to 5.50)
	diltiazem		1	−1.48 (−5.93 to 3.03) 0.80 (−3.79 to 5.39)
	nicorandil		0	−2.02 (−5.93 to 2.12) NA
	control		6	−1.83 (−4.42 to 0.77) −1.40 (−3.57 to 0.77)
adenosine	diltiazem		0	−0.16 (−4.79 to 4.48) NA
	nicorandil		0	−0.71 (−4.26 to 3.06) NA
	control		10	−0.50 (−2.52 to 1.46) −0.34 (−2.27 to 1.57)
diltiazem	nicorandil		0	−0.53 (−5.54 to 4.65) NA
	control		1	−0.33 (−4.59 to 3.85) −0.30 (−4.14 to 3.54)
nicorandil	control		5	0.20 (−3.02 to 3.18) −0.17 (−3.27 to 2.93)

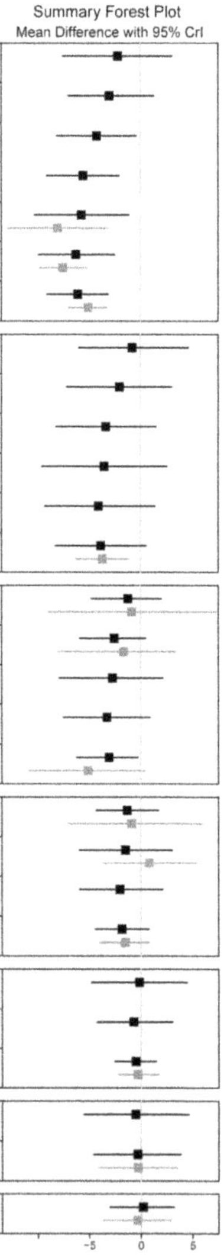

Fig. 5 Summary forest plot table for the outcome of left ventricular ejection fraction. H-H trials, head-to-head trials; black text, network meta-analysis results; grey text, pairwise meta-analysis results; CrI, credible interval; SUCRA, the surface under the cumulative ranking curve; Interventions are displayed by SUCRA percentages; Each intervention in the second column was compared with the intervention listed in the first column

References		SUCRA	H-H Trials	Odds Ratio (95% CrI)	Pairwise (grey)
anisodamine SUCRA =97%	diltiazem	= 65%	1	3.00 (0.96 to 9.76)	2.84 (0.83 to 9.70)
	nitroprusside	= 62%	0	3.62 (1.27 to 10.74)	NA
	nicorandil	= 45%	1	4.59 (1.42 to 15.12)	2.08 (0.18 to 24.51)
	adenosine	= 40%	0	4.94 (1.93 to 14.00)	NA
	verapamil	= 39%	0	5.00 (1.58 to 16.28)	NA
	urapidil	= 37%	0	6.69 (0.14 to 324.70)	NA
	control	= 15%	3	6.56 (2.69 to 17.16)	6.02 (2.29 to 15.84)
diltiazem	nitroprusside		0	1.20 (0.34 to 4.28)	NA
	nicorandil		0	1.52 (0.38 to 6.09)	NA
	adenosine		0	1.64 (0.51 to 5.54)	NA
	verapamil		1	1.66 (0.48 to 5.93)	1.55 (0.24 to 9.91)
	urapidil		0	2.23 (0.04 to 112.30)	NA
	control		1	2.18 (0.71 to 6.98)	2.13 (0.36 to 12.51)
nitroprusside	nicorandil		0	1.26 (0.46 to 3.30)	NA
	adenosine		2	1.37 (0.77 to 2.48)	1.36 (0.34 to 5.52)
	verapamil		1	1.39 (0.56 to 3.36)	0.48 (0.04 to 5.63)
	urapidil		0	1.82 (0.04 to 82.34)	NA
	control		5	1.82 (1.06 to 3.15)	1.94 (1.03 to 3.66)
nicorandil	adenosine		0	1.08 (0.46 to 2.74)	NA
	verapamil		0	1.09 (0.37 to 3.45)	NA
	urapidil		0	1.47 (0.03 to 69.45)	NA
	control		5	1.44 (0.65 to 3.31)	1.21 (0.61 to 2.44)
adenosine	verapamil		1	1.01 (0.44 to 2.23)	0.75 (0.14 to 4.09)
	urapidil		0	1.34 (0.03 to 59.72)	NA
	control		13	1.33 (0.92 to 1.90)	1.38 (0.94 to 1.98)
verapamil	urapidil		0	1.32 (0.03 to 61.81)	NA
	control		3	1.32 (0.62 to 2.84)	1.05 (0.49 to 2.23)
urapidil	control		1	1.00 (0.02 to 43.09)	1.00 (0.02 to 52.29)

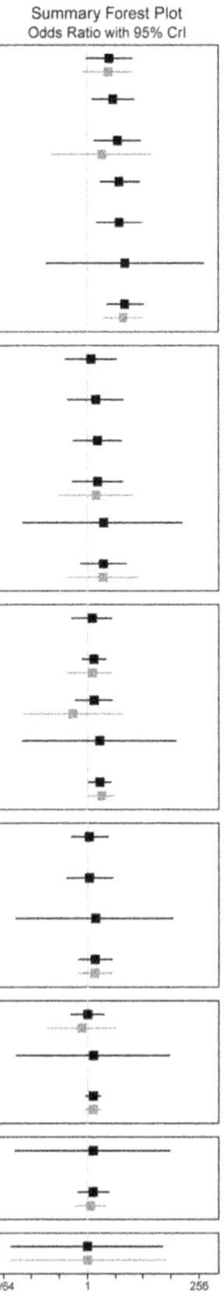

Fig. 6 Summary forest plot table for the outcome of major adverse cardiovascular events. H-H trials, head-to-head trials; black text, network meta-analysis results; grey text, pairwise meta-analysis results; CrI, credible interval; SUCRA, the surface under the cumulative ranking curve; Interventions are displayed by SUCRA percentages; Each intervention in the second column was compared with the intervention listed in the first column

1.82–12.08). There was no statistically significant difference in AEs with anisodamine (OR 0.30, 95%CI 0.00–21.04) and nitroprusside (OR 1.23, 95%CI 0.69–2.19) compared with control therapy. There was also no significant between-study heterogeneity for these analyses (all $I^2 < 75\%$; $P_{het} > 0.05$).

Meta-regression analysis

In network meta-regression analyses (Table 3), we explored the effects of mean age and the time to reperfusion on outcomes: TFG < 3, STR, LVEF, and MACEs, respectively. Since studies reported MACEs at a wide range of follow-up, we also used network meta-regression to adjust for the difference in follow-up periods. The 95% CIs of the interaction coefficients included zero in each adjusted model. None of the covariate adjusted models showed significant improvement in the DIC compared with the unadjusted models.

Subgroup analysis

For TFG < 3, STR, LVEF, and MACE outcomes, subgroup analysis did not reveal any significant effect modification by the type of control group (all P values for interaction > 0.05). For MACE outcome, the analysis stratified by the median duration of follow-up did not yield significantly different results in the two periods (≤ 4.5 months and > 4.5 months). The results of subgroup analysis are presented in Additional file 1: Table S1, Figures S1 and S2.

Sensitivity analysis

Sensitivity analysis was restricted to studies with the relatively uniform definition of MACEs. The pooled risk

Table 3 Model fit statistics for the covariate adjustment analyses

Covariate adjusted RE Binomial logit model	Statistic	
	Interaction coefficient, median (95% CrI)	DIC difference between adjusted and unadjusted models of the same data
Outcome: TFG < 3		
Age	0.37 (−0.30, 1.05)	0.4
Time of reperfusion	−0.14 (−0.86, 0.71)	1.1
Outcome: STR		
Age	0.24 (−0.49, 0.95)	1.0
Time of reperfusion	0.61 (−0.12, 1.27)	0.1
Outcome: LVEF		
Age	1.88 (−1.59, 5.10)	0.6
Time of reperfusion	3.34 (−1.89, 8.11)	1.0
Follow-up	−0.75 (−3.78, 2.24)	0.5
Outcome: MACEs		
Age	0.15 (−0.71, 1.04)	1.1
Time of reperfusion	−0.49 (−1.41, 0.38)	0.1
Follow-up	0.25 (−0.35, 0.91)	0.5

TFG, TIMI flow grade; STR, ST-segment resolution; LVEF, left ventricular ejection fraction; MACEs, major adverse cardiovascular events; CrI, credible interval; DIC, deviance information criterion; RE, random effect

estimates in the sensitivity analysis did not change substantially in comparison with the estimates from the main analysis that included all trials reporting MACE outcome (Additional file 1: Figure S3).

Additional analyses

Visual inspection of the funnel plots did not show asymmetry for any of the analyzed outcomes. The Gelman-Rubin plot confirmed an adequate convergence of the model for each network analysis. Model evaluation indicated adequate fit, as the posterior mean residual deviance was similar to the number of data points in each analysis. There was no evidence of statistical inconsistency between direct and indirect estimates based on the node-splitting method ($P > 0.05$).

Discussion

Through the present meta-analysis comprising 41 RCTs involving 4069 patients, we found that the addition of anisodamine to standard PPCI for STEMI was associated with improved post-procedural coronary flow, more occurrences of STR, and improvement of LVEF. The cardioprotective effect of anisodamine conferred a MACE-free survival benefit. Among the 7 treatment strategies, anisodamine was superior to the other treatments in efficacy outcomes (TFG < 3, STR, LVEF, and MACEs). Severe or life-threatening AEs were not observed in patients treated with anisodamine. Nitroprusside was also regarded as effective for improving coronary flow and clinical outcomes. Additionally, the intracoronary administration of adenosine, nicorandil, and verapamil exerted some cardioprotection in patients with STEMI undergoing PPCI.

The present network meta-analysis included all available RCTs involving intracoronary agents (adenosine, anisodamine, diltiazem, nicorandil, nitroprusside, urapidil, and verapamil) as adjuncts to PPCI. This study took into account the most recent studies and had the largest sample size to date among meta-analyses assessing the effect of intracoronary agents on NR in patients with STEMI undergoing PPCI. Demonstration of the improvement in indicators of myocardial reperfusion is a key step to the investigation of improved clinical outcomes for intracoronary agents as adjuncts to PPCI [7]. Our network meta-analysis, by evaluating surrogate outcomes (TFG, STR, and LVEF) and the composite clinical endpoint (MACEs), provided a comprehensive insight into the use of 7 intracoronary agents during PPCI. However, most included RCTs were designed to assess angiographic or electrocardiographic outcomes, thus partly leading to a limited number of participants. Although angiographic and electrocardiographic indicators of myocardial reperfusion are well-known prognostic factors [4, 5], the improvement in surrogate markers does not always correspond to improved clinical outcomes. For example, aspiration thrombectomy was considered a simple way to remove the thrombus before stent deployment, thereby improving coronary reperfusion. However, recent trials have demonstrated a lack of benefit of thrombus aspiration on clinical outcomes and suggested possible harm from an increased risk of stroke [67, 68]. Therefore, our finding should be viewed as hypothesis generating, given the limitations of the current available evidence.

Anisodamine, a muscarinic cholinergic antagonist, has been reported with multiple pharmacological effects in basic and clinical studies [13–16, 69, 70]. First, anisodamine inhibits the acetylcholine receptor and modulates the balance between sympathetic and vagus nerve activity during myocardial ischemia/reperfusion [13]. Numerous studies have shown that anisodamine can increase blood pressure and heart rate, and further increase the coronary perfusion pressure [16, 69]. The action of anisodamine is especially appealing, because it can help improve coronary microcirculation and has practical importance. Clinicians often have concerns about hypotension and bradycardia, although they are short-lived after the intracoronary administration of vasodilators. Anisodamine may be a promising drug to address these safety concerns. Second, anisodamine has a similar role to a calcium channel blocker. Anisodamine can prevent intracellular calcium overload, reduce lipid superoxidation, inhibit oxygen free radical formation, and relieve microvascular spasms [70]. Finally, anisodamine decreases post-ischemia/reperfusion myocardial swelling, which can reduce capillary compression from surrounding edematous myocytes [14, 15]. This is the first meta-analysis of RCTs of anisodamine to demonstrate a significant benefit of adjuvant anisodamine over standard care in patients with STEMI undergoing PPCI. Our results showed that anisodamine could significantly improve myocardial reperfusion (reflected by TFG and STR) and cardiac function (reflected by LVEF). Importantly, these effects were translated into improvement of composite clinical outcome (MACEs). Moreover, the analyses of rank probabilities revealed that of 7 treatment strategies, anisodamine consistently ranked the highest in improving TFG, promoting post-procedure STR, ameliorating LVEF, and decreasing the risk of MACEs, which made it the most efficacious drugs according to our results. Therefore, anisodamine may be regarded as an effective, well-tolerated, and possibly cost-effective regimen (currently about a dollar per 10 mg) for prevention of NR. However, it should be noted that this evidence was based on relatively small head-to-head RCTs. Large, high-quality RCTs are needed to fully evaluate the role of anisodamine as an adjunct to reperfusion in patients with STEMI.

Nitroprusside is a direct donor of nitric oxide, which is a potent vasodilator of the resistance arteriolar circulation and has anti-platelet and anti-inflammatory effects [71]. Zhao et al. analyzed 7 studies involving 781 patients who were treated with nitroprusside [12]. They assessed TFG < 3, STR, and MACEs, and their results were consistent with our findings. However, this previous meta-analysis included a retrospective study, which may have introduced bias. Our results included all RCTs to date with 4 additional summarized trials [49, 56, 57, 64]. Moreover, our meta-analysis expands previous evidence by demonstrating that the intracoronary administration of nitroprusside significantly increased LVEF after PPCI compared to standard care. We also found that nitroprusside was inferior to anisodamine for improving STR.

Adenosine is an endogenous nucleoside that modulates numerous physiological processes, such as antagonizing platelets and neutrophils, reducing calcium overload and oxygen free radicals, and inducing vasodilation [7]. Two recent meta-analyses have evaluated the role of adenosine in patients with STEMI undergoing PPCI [8, 9]. Our findings are consistent with the results of these 2 previous meta-analyses, which showed that adenosine use was associated with fewer occurrences of TFG < 3 and more occurrences of STR. However, we failed to observe the significant improvement of LVEF and benefit of the MACE endpoint for adenosine. The reason for these conflicting results may be that we included new trials [44, 49]. In the well-conducted REFLO-STEMI trial, Nazir et al. concluded that adenosine did not reduce the infarct size or NR [49]. Furthermore, they found that there were significantly worse outcomes for the adenosine group than for the control, mainly due to an excess of heart failure events. Although the findings were hypothesis generating and difficult to explain, the new data challenge the role of adenosine in PPCI and should be re-evaluated in a meta-analysis. Our updated meta-analysis showed that adenosine had no benefits in terms of LVEF and MACE endpoints, but adenosine use increased the reperfusion indices without having a harmful effect on cardiovascular outcomes other than AEs. On the basis of our results, it is still necessary to perform larger well-powered studies to definitively assess the role of adenosine in this clinical scenario.

Diltiazem and verapamil, two non-dihydropyridine calcium channel blockers, have been shown to produce endothelium-independent vasodilation and reduce calcium overload within intracellular compartments [72]. Wang et al. pooled 8 RCTs with 494 participants and found that verapamil or diltiazem was associated with a significantly improved TFG and reduced incidence of MACEs [10]. In this meta-analysis, however, verapamil and diltiazem were classified as the same group and the three included trials evaluated the effect of oral diltiazem, which might affect the results. In the current study, we separately analyzed the role of intracoronary verapamil or diltiazem. Our results based on RCTs suggest that diltiazem adjunctive therapy did not improve any outcomes studied in patients with STEMI. Although verapamil had a beneficial effect on coronary flow after PPCI, it was not associated with consistent advantages on other outcomes (STR, LVEF, and MACEs).

Nicorandil is a hybrid of nitrates and an adenosine triphosphate-sensitive potassium channel opener [73]. The mechanisms for the beneficial actions of nicorandil have been postulated, including dilation of resistance arteries, reduction of reactive oxygen species production in mitochondria, and attenuation of polymorphonuclear leukocytes activation during ischemia/reperfusion [73]. Recent meta-analysis has indicated that nicorandil was associated with improvement of coronary flow and LVEF in patients with STEMI undergoing PPCI [11]. However, the results could have been confounded by the intracoronary and intravenous administrations of nicorandil. Results of our meta-analysis showed that intracoronary nicorandil therapy leads to improvement in TFG and STR after PPCI. Unfortunately, this did not translate into significant improvement in cardiac function and clinical outcomes.

As a selective adrenoceptor blocker, urapidil may help attenuate the vasoconstrictive tendency of the coronary circulation observed after PPCI [74]. Only 2 RCTs compared urapidil with a control, and urapidil improved ventricular function in both studies. In our network meta-analysis, urapidil did not show any benefits in TFG, STR, and MACEs. For LVEF, the result of our pairwise meta-analysis showed significant improvement, whereas the result of the network meta-analysis indicated a favorable trend when intracoronary urapidil was used during PPCI. However, the relatively small sample size (49 patients) can make it difficult to interpret the data. The results for urapidil should be interpreted with caution.

It is clinically relevant to further investigate the effect of confounding factors such as age, the time to reperfusion, and duration of follow-up on the intervention effect. Ageing has been shown to be associated with reduced efficacy of cardioprotective therapies [75]. The total ischemic time was the major determinant of myocardial damage in patients with STEMI [6]. The present study evaluated MACEs at follow-up ranged from in-hospital to 12 months. Compared to studies with a longer follow-up period, those with shorter follow-up period may be inadequate for determining the differences in MACEs. Network meta-regression can be used to estimate interactions of treatment with study-level characteristics when treatment effects are heterogeneous [23]. Our meta-regression analyses suggested that the results of network meta-analysis were not confounded by age, the time to reperfusion, and duration of follow-up. However, more studies are needed to confirm these results of meta-regression analyses. Additionally, large, well-designed RCTs have shown that complete revascularization was associated with a reduction of MACEs compared with treatment of the culprit lesion only in patients with STEMI and multivessel disease [76]. This reduction was mainly driven by fewer repeat revascularizations, because all-cause mortality and non-fatal reinfarction did not differ between groups. In the present meta-analysis, the median proportion of patients with multivessel disease across 14 included studies was 52%. However, few of included studies provided data about the proportion of patients undergoing complete revascularization. Therefore, we did not perform meta-regression analysis to adjust the results of network meta-analysis for complete revascularization. We suggest that future research should investigate the impact of complete revascularization on the intervention effect. Epinephrine has beta-2 receptor agonist properties leading to the potent coronary vasodilator effect and beta-1 agonist properties mediating chronotropic and inotropic effects on the heart. Pilot studies have shown that the intracoronary administration of epinephrine reversed refractory NR in patients with STEMI [77]. We did not evaluate the safety and efficacy of epinephrine in the present study due to a lack of relevant RCTs. Additional data from RCTs are warranted to assess the effect of epinephrine on NR during PPCI.

A main strength of the present meta-analysis is that it provides the most comprehensive analysis to date of the likelihood of a range of adjunctive pharmacotherapies to prevent or reduce NR. Our results are based on mixed comparisons of multiple treatments and report treatment rankings for 7 types of intracoronary drugs. The findings from our meta-analysis can offer positive evidence regarding the use of anisodamine as an adjunct to PPCI, and pave the way for further RCTs to confirm this beneficial role of anisodamine in patients with STEMI.

Our study has several limitations. First, the present meta-analysis is based on the data of existing publications, and we could not fully assess the potential influences of comorbidities and cardiovascular medications. Second, we did not include other measures of myocardial perfusion, such as the corrected TIMI frame count, myocardial blush grade, and TIMI myocardial perfusion grade. These indices are not commonly used in clinical practice and were unavailable in most of the included studies. TFG and STR, classical indicators of reperfusion, are closely related to short-term and long-term clinical outcomes of patients with STEMI [4, 5]. Third, drug protocols varied across the eligible studies. It was difficult for us to ascertain the optimal drug protocols. Fourth, the sample size in each study was relatively small, and the CI for certain outcomes was wide because of low event rates or the absence of events. Finally, the quality of trials included in our analysis was not high.

Conclusions

The present network meta-analysis, combining both direct and indirect evidences, showed that the intracoronary administration of anisodamine could improve myocardial reperfusion, cardiac function, and clinical outcomes in patients with STEMI undergoing PPCI. However, due to the limited quality and quantity of the included studies, the finding that anisodamine was a useful adjunct to reperfusion therapy should be viewed as hypothesis generating rather than conclusive. More rigorous RCTs are needed to verify the role of this inexpensive and well-tolerated regimen.

Abbreviations

AEs: Adverse events; LVEF: left ventricular ejection fraction; MACEs: Major adverse cardiovascular events; NR: No-reflow phenomenon; PPCI: Primary percutaneous coronary intervention; RCTs: Randomized controlled trials; STEMI: ST-elevation myocardial infarction; STR: ST-segment resolution; TFG: Thrombolysis in myocardial infarction flow grade

Acknowledgements

We would like to thank Dr. Ge Long, the Evidence-based Medicine Center of Lanzhou University, for his help in statistical analysis.

Funding
We have no support or funding to report.

Authors' contributions
XN and ZZ conceived of the study and its design. JZ and MB performed the database search, collected the study and assessed the study quality. JZ and YP corrected and organized the collected data. XN, SS, and ZZ performed the statistical analysis and drafted the manuscript. XN, JZ, MB, YP, SS, and ZZ revised the manuscript. All authors read and approved the final manuscript.

Competing interests
The authors declare that the research was conducted in the absence of any commercial or financial relationships that could be construed as a potential conflict of interests.

Author details
[1]The First School of Clinical Medicine, Lanzhou University, Tianshui South Road, No. 222, Lanzhou, Gansu 730000, China. [2]Baiyin Second People's Hospital, Gongyuan Road, No. 509, Baiyin, Gansu 730900, China. [3]Department of Cardiology, the First Hospital of Lanzhou University, Donggang West Road, No. 1, Lanzhou, Gansu 730000, China. [4]Key Lab of Prevention and Treatment for Chronic Disease, Gansu University of Chinese Medicine, Dingxi East Road, No. 35, Lanzhou, Gansu 730000, China.

References

1. O'Gara PT, Kushner FG, Ascheim DD, Casey DE Jr, Chung MK, de Lemos JA, et al. 2013 ACCF/AHA guideline for the management of ST-elevation myocardial infarction: a report of the American College of Cardiology Foundation/American Heart Association task force on practice guidelines. Circulation. 2013;127(4):e362–425.
2. Feher A, Chen SY, Bagi Z, Arora V. Prevention and treatment of no-reflow phenomenon by targeting the coronary microcirculation. Rev Cardiovasc Med. 2014;15(1):38–51.
3. Hamirani YS, Wong A, Kramer CM, Salerno M. Effect of microvascular obstruction and intramyocardial hemorrhage by CMR on LV remodeling and outcomes after myocardial infarction: a systematic review and meta-analysis. JACC Cardiovasc Imaging. 2014;7(9):940–52.
4. Sattur S, Sarwar B, Sacchi TJ, Brener SJ. Correlation between markers of reperfusion and mortality in ST-elevation myocardial infarction: a systematic review. J Invasive Cardiol. 2014;26(11):587–U50.
5. Niccoli G, Cosentino N, Spaziani C, Loria V, Fracassi F, Roberto M, et al. Concordance of angiographic and electrocardiographic indexes of microvascular obstruction: myocardial haemorrhage role. J Cardiovasc Med (Hagerstown). 2016;17(5):382–91.
6. Jaffe R, Charron T, Puley G, Dick A, Strauss BH. Microvascular obstruction and the no-reflow phenomenon after percutaneous coronary intervention. Circulation. 2008;117(24):3152–6.
7. Kumbhani DJ, de Lemos JA. Finding an effective treatment for microvascular obstruction in STEMI: a road to perdition? Eur Heart J. 2016; 37(24):1920–2.
8. Polimeni A, De Rosa S, Sabatino J, Sorrentino S, Indolfi C. Impact of intracoronary adenosine administration during primary PCI: a meta-analysis. Int J Cardiol. 2016;203:1032–41.
9. Gao Q, Yang B, Guo Y, Zheng F. Efficacy of adenosine in patients with acute myocardial infarction undergoing primary percutaneous coronary intervention: a PRISMA-compliant meta-analysis. Medicine (Baltimore). 2015; 94(32):e1279.
10. Wang L, Cheng Z, Gu Y, Peng D. Short-term effects of verapamil and diltiazem in the treatment of no reflow phenomenon: a meta-analysis of randomized controlled trials. Biomed Res Int. 2015;2015:382086.
11. Wu M, Huang Z, Xie H, Zhou Z. Nicorandil in patients with acute myocardial infarction undergoing primary percutaneous coronary intervention: a systematic review and meta-analysis. PLoS One. 2013;8(10):e78231.
12. Zhao S, Qi G, Tian W, Chen L, Sun Y. Effect of intracoronary nitroprusside in preventing no reflow phenomenon during primary percutaneous coronary intervention: a meta-analysis. J Interv Cardiol. 2014;27(4):356–64.
13. Poupko JM, Baskin SI, Moore E. The pharmacological properties of anisodamine. J Appl Toxicol. 2007;27(2):116–21.
14. Xing K, Fu X, Jiang L, Wang Y, Li W, Gu X, et al. Cardioprotective effect of anisodamine against myocardial ischemia injury and its influence on cardiomyocytes apoptosis. Cell Biochem Biophys. 2015;73(3):707–16.
15. Yin XL, Shen H, Zhang W, Yang Y. Inhibition of endoplasm reticulum stress by anisodamine protects against myocardial injury after cardiac arrest and resuscitation in rats. Am J Chin Med. 2011;39(5):853–66.
16. Fu XH, Fan WZ, Gu XS, Wei YY, Jiang YF, Wu WL, et al. Effect of intracoronary administration of anisodamine on slow reflow phenomenon following primary percutaneous coronary intervention in patients with acute myocardial infarction. Chin Med J. 2007;120(14):1226–31.
17. Song F, Altman DG, Glenny A-M, Deeks JJ. Validity of indirect comparison for estimating efficacy of competing interventions: empirical evidence from published meta-analyses. BMJ. 2003;326(7387):472.
18. Salanti G, Ades AE, Ioannidis JP. Graphical methods and numerical summaries for presenting results from multiple-treatment meta-analysis: an overview and tutorial. J Clin Epidemiol. 2011;64(2):163–71.
19. TIMI Study Group. The thrombolysis in myocardial infarction (TIMI) trial. Phase I findings. N Engl J Med. 1985;312(14):932–6.
20. Schroder R. Prognostic impact of early ST-segment resolution in acute ST-elevation myocardial infarction. Circulation. 2004;110(21):e506–10.
21. Higgins JPT, Green S. Cochrane handbook for systematic reviews of interventions version 5.1.0. The Cochrane Collaboration, 2011. Available from www. cochrane-handbook.org.
22. Dias S, Sutton AJ, Ades AE, Welton NJ. Evidence synthesis for decision making 2: a generalized linear modeling framework for pairwise and network meta-analysis of randomized controlled trials. Med Decis Mak. 2013;33(5):607–17.
23. Dias S, Sutton AJ, Welton NJ, Ades AE. Evidence synthesis for decision making 3: heterogeneity–subgroups, meta-regression, bias, and bias-adjustment. Med Decis Mak. 2013;33(5):618–40.
24. Tan SH, Cooper NJ, Bujkiewicz S, Welton NJ, Caldwell DM, Sutton AJ. Novel presentational approaches were developed for reporting network meta-analysis. J Clin Epidemiol. 2014;67(6):672–80.
25. Moher D, Liberati A, Tetzlaff J, Altman DG. Preferred reporting items for systematic reviews and meta-analyses: the PRISMA statement. BMJ. 2009; 339:b2535.
26. Abdelaziz HK, Elkilany W, Khalid S, Sabet S, Saad M. Efficacy and safety of intracoronary verapamil versus sodium nitroprusside for the prevention of microvascular obstruction during primary percutaneous coronary intervention for ST-segment elevation myocardial infarction. Coron Artery Dis. 2017;28(1):11–6.
27. Akagi T, Sarazawa K, Inai Y, Kitagawa M, Takahashi N, Hamanaka I, et al. Continuous administration of nicorandil decreases QT dispersion during the chronic phase of acute myocardial infarction. Int Heart J. 2006;47(3):351–61.
28. Akturk IF, Yalcin AA, Biyik I, Sarikamis C, Caglar NT, Erturk M, et al. Effects of verapamil and adenosine in an adjunct to tirofiban on resolution and prognosis of noreflow phenomenon in patients with acute myocardial infarction. Minerva Cardioangiol. 2014;62(5):389–97.
29. Amit G, Cafri C, Yaroslavtsev S, Fuchs S, Paltiel O, Abu-Ful A, et al. Intracoronary nitroprusside for the prevention of the no-reflow phenomenon after primary percutaneous coronary intervention in acute myocardial infarction. A randomized, double-blind, placebo-controlled clinical trial. Am Heart J. 2006;152(5):887.e9–14.
30. Bai S, Fu X, Gu X, Wang Y, Li W, Fan Y, et al. Intracoronary administration of different doses of anisodamine in primary percutaneous coronary intervention: protective effect in patients with ST-segment elevation myocardial infarction. Coron Artery Dis. 2016;27(4):302–10.
31. Chen C, Fu X, Li W, Jia X, Bai S, Geng W, et al. Intracoronary administration of anisodamine and nicorandil in individuals undergoing primary percutaneous coronary intervention for acute inferior myocardial infarction: a randomized factorial trial. Exp Ther Med. 2015;10(3):1059–65.
32. Chen JL, Fu XH, Jiang YF, Fan WZ, Gu XS, Liu JJ, et al. Effect of urapidil on heart function and ventricular systolic synchrony in acute myocardial infarction patients with no-reflow phenomenon after percutaneous coronary intervention. Zhongguo Wei Zhong Bing Ji Jiu Yi Xue. 2008;20(4): 197–9.
33. Darahim K, Mahdy MM, Ryan MM, Khashaba AA, Thabet SS, Hassan OM, et al. Does high-dose intracoronary adenosine improve regional systolic left ventricular function in patients with acute myocardial infarction? Egypt Heart J. 2014;66(4):289–97.

34. Desmet W, Bogaert J, Dubois C, Sinnaeve P, Adriaenssens T, Pappas C, et al. High-dose intracoronary adenosine for myocardial salvage in patients with acute ST-segment elevation myocardial infarction. Eur Heart J. 2011;32(7): 867–77.
35. Fan WZ, Fu XH, Jiang YF, Gu XS, Wu WL, Li SQ, et al. Influence of intracoronary administration of anisodamine on no-reflow, ventricular function and systolic synchrony in acute myocardial infarction patients undergoing percutaneous coronary intervention. Zhonghua Xin Xue Guan Bing Za Zhi. 2007;35(10):908–13.
36. Fokkema ML, Vlaar PJ, Vogelzang M, Gu YL, Kampinga MA, de Smet BJ, et al. Effect of high-dose intracoronary adenosine administration during primary percutaneous coronary intervention in acute myocardial infarction: a randomized controlled trial. Circ Cardiovasc Interv. 2009;2(4):323–9.
37. Garcia-Dorado D, Garcia-del-Blanco B, Otaegui I, Rodriguez-Palomares J, Pineda V, Gimeno F, et al. Intracoronary injection of adenosine before reperfusion in patients with ST-segment elevation myocardial infarction: a randomized controlled clinical trial. Int J Cardiol. 2014;177(3):935–41.
38. Grygier M, Araszkiewicz A, Lesiak M, Janus M, Kowal J, Skorupski W, et al. New method of intracoronary adenosine injection to prevent microvascular reperfusion injury in patients with acute myocardial infarction undergoing percutaneous coronary intervention. Am J Cardiol. 2011;107(8):1131–5.
39. Hamza MA, Galal A, Suweilam S, Ismail M. Local intracoronary eptifibatide versus mechanical aspiration in patients with acute ST-elevation myocardial infarction. Int J Vasc Med. 2014;2014:294065.
40. Hendler A, Aronovich A, Kaluski E, Zyssman I, Gurevich Y, Blatt A, et al. Optimization of myocardial perfusion after primary coronary angioplasty following an acute myocardial infarction. Beyond TIMI 3 flow. J Invasive Cardiol. 2006;18(1):32–6.
41. Huang D, Qian J, Ge L, Jin X, Jin H, Ma J, et al. Restoration of coronary flow in patients with no-reflow after primary coronary intervention of acute myocardial infarction (RECOVER). Am Heart J. 2012;164(3):394–401.
42. Ji ZG, Han JM, Liu G, Liu KS. Effect of adenosine on ischemia-reperfusion injury during percutaneous coronary intervention. J Clin Rehabil Tissue Eng Res. 2007;11(51):10399–403.
43. Lee HC, An SG, Choi JH, Lee TK, Kim J, Kim JH, et al. Effect of intra-coronary nicorandil administration prior to reperfusion in acute ST segment elevation myocardial infarction. Circ J. 2008;72(9):1425–9.
44. Li Y, Li Q, Li F, Zong M, Miao G, Yang X, et al. Evaluation of short- and long-term efficacy of combined intracoronary administration of high-dose adenosine and tirofiban during primary percutaneous coronary intervention. Acta Cardiol Sin. 2016;32(6):640–8.
45. Marzilli M, Orsini E, Marraccini P, Testa R. Beneficial effects of intracoronary adenosine as an adjunct to primary angioplasty in acute myocardial infarction. Circulation. 2000;101(18):2154–9.
46. Miyazawa A, Ikari Y, Tanabe K, Nakajima H, Aoki J, Iijima R, et al. Intracoronary nicorandil prior to reperfusion in acute myocardial infarction. EuroIntervention. 2006;2(2):211–7.
47. Nameki M, Ishibashi I, Miyazaki Y, Sakai Y, Namikawa S, Kuriyama N, et al. Comparison between nicorandil and magnesium as an adjunct cardioprotective agent to percutaneous coronary intervention in acute anterior myocardial infarction. Circ J. 2004;68(3):192–7.
48. Nayel AE, Elabd AA, Fathalla H. Role of intracoronary injection of Na-nitroprusside in preventing no-reflow phenomenon in patients with STEMI during primary percutaneous coronary intervention. JACC Cardiovasc Interv. 2013;6(2):S7–8.
49. Nazir SA, McCann GP, Greenwood JP, Kunadian V, Khan JN, Mahmoud IZ, et al. Strategies to attenuate micro-vascular obstruction during P-PCI: the randomized reperfusion facilitated by local adjunctive therapy in ST-elevation myocardial infarction trial. Eur Heart J. 2016;37(24):1910–9.
50. Niccoli G, Rigattieri S, De Vita MR, Valgimigli M, Corvo P, Fabbiocchi F, et al. Open-label, randomized, placebo-controlled evaluation of intracoronary adenosine or nitroprusside after thrombus aspiration during primary percutaneous coronary intervention for the prevention of microvascular obstruction in acute myocardial infarction: the REOPEN-AMI study (intracoronary Nitroprusside versus adenosine in acute myocardial infarction). JACC Cardiovasc Interv. 2013;6(6):580–9.
51. Ota S, Nishikawa H, Takeuchi M, Nakajima K, Nakamura T, Okamoto S, et al. Impact of nicorandil to prevent reperfusion injury in patients with acute myocardial infarction: Sigmart multicenter angioplasty revascularization trial (SMART). Circ J. 2006;70(9):1099 104.
52. Pan W, Wang LF, Yu JH, Fan Y, Yang SS, Zhou LJ, et al. Intracoronary nitroprusside in the prevention of the no-reflow phenomenon in acute myocardial infarction. Chin Med J. 2009;122(22):2718–23.
53. Peng Y, Fu X, Li W, Geng W, Xing K, Ru L, et al. Effect of intracoronary anisodamine and diltiazem administration during primary percutaneous coronary intervention in acute myocardial infarction. Coron Artery Dis. 2014; 25(8):645–52.
54. Petronio AS, De Carlo M, Ciabatti N, Amoroso G, Limbruno U, Palagi C, et al. Left ventricular remodeling after primary coronary angioplasty in patients treated with abciximab or intracoronary adenosine. Am Heart J. 2005;150(5): 1015.
55. Qiao Z, Pu J, Ding S, Song W, Du Y, Shen J, et al. Effect of intracoronary verapamil on coronary flow, myocardial perfusion and clinical outcome during percutaneous coronary intervention for acute myocardial infarction. Chin J Intervent Cardiol. 2009;17(4):185–90.
56. Sai S, Fischer L, Shivkumar J, Shivkumar J, Vishnuarunachalam R. Impact of intracoronary administration of nitroprusside vs. nitroglycerine before balloon dilatation on slow reflow during percutaneous coronary intervention in patients with acute ST elevation myocardial infarction. J Am Coll Cardiol. 2011;57(14):E988.
57. Shinozaki N, Ichinose H, Hiramori S, Yahikozawa K, Hoshino K. Selective intracoronary administration of nitroprusside before balloon dilatation prevents slow reflow during percutaneous coronary intervention in patients with acute myocardial infarction. Am J Cardiol. 2010;105(9):32B.
58. Stoel MG, Marques KM, de Cock CC, Bronzwaer JG, von Birgelen C, Zijlstra F. High dose adenosine for suboptimal myocardial reperfusion after primary PCI: a randomized placebo-controlled pilot study. Catheter Cardiovasc Interv. 2008;71(3):283–9.
59. Sung GA, Tae IP, Ki WH, Choi JH, Tae KL, Han CL, et al. The effect of intra-coronary nicorandil prior to reperfusion in acute ST segment elevation myocardial infarction. Korean Circ J. 2008;38(2):95–100.
60. Taniyama Y, Ito H, Iwakura K, Masuyama T, Hori M, Takiuchi S, et al. Beneficial effect of intracoronary verapamil on microvascular and myocardial salvage in patients with acute myocardial infarction. J Am Coll Cardiol. 1997;30(5):1193–9.
61. Tong ZC, Li Q, Chen M, Miao GB, Wei Y, Li FO, et al. Efficacy comparison of combined intracoronary administration of high-dose adenosine and tirofiban versus intracoronary tirofiban during primary percutaneous coronary intervention in patients with acute myocardial infarction. Zhonghua Xin Xue Guan Bing Za Zhi. 2013;41(10):839–44.
62. Wang X, Ding Z, Chen J. Role of adenosine in primary percutaneous coronary intervention. J Clin Med In Pract. 2008;12(9):76–7.
63. Yamada K, Isobe S, Ishii H, Yokouchi K, Iwata H, Sawada K, et al. Impacts of nicorandil on infarct myocardium in comparison with nitrate: assessed by cardiac magnetic resonance imaging. Heart Vessel. 2016;31(9):1430–7.
64. Yang L, Mu L, Sun L, Qi F, Guo R. Effect of intracoronary nitroprusside injection on flow recovery during primary PCI in acute STEMI patients. Minerva Cardioangiol. 2017;65(2):111–8.
65. Yao DK, Jia SQ, Wang L, Li HW, Zhang YC, Wang YL, et al. Therapeutic effect of urapidil on myocardial perfusion in patients with ST-elevation acute coronary syndrome. Eur J Intern Med. 2009;20(2):152–7.
66. Zhao YJ, Fu XH, Ma XX, Wang DY, Dong QL, Wang YB, et al. Intracoronary fixed dose of nitroprusside via thrombus aspiration catheter for the prevention of the no-reflow phenomenon following primary percutaneous coronary intervention in acute myocardial infarction. Exp Ther Med. 2013; 6(2):479–84.
67. Elgendy IY, Huo T, Bhatt DL, Bavry AA. Is aspiration thrombectomy beneficial in patients undergoing primary percutaneous coronary intervention? Meta-analysis of randomized trials. Circ Cardiovasc Interv. 2015;8(7):e002258.
68. El Dib R, Spencer FA, Suzumura EA, Goma H, Kwong J, Guyatt GH, et al. Aspiration thrombectomy prior to percutaneous coronary intervention in ST-elevation myocardial infarction: a systematic review and meta-analysis. BMC Cardiovasc Disord. 2016;16(1):121.
69. Wei YY, Fu XH, Liu J. Effect of intra-coronary injection of anisodamine on the slow-reflow phenomenon in patients with acute myocardial infarction after percutaneous coronary intervention. Zhongguo Zhong Xi Yi Jie He Za Zhi. 2008;28(4):295–9.
70. Norby FL, Ren J. Anisodamine inhibits cardiac contraction and intracellular ca(2+) transients in isolated adult rat ventricular myocytes. Eur J Pharmacol. 2002;439(1–3):21–5.

71. Hottinger DG, Beebe DS, Kozhimannil T, Prielipp RC, Belani KG. Sodium nitroprusside in 2014: a clinical concepts review. J Anaesthesiol Clin Pharmacol. 2014;30(4):462–71.
72. Brogden RN, Benfield P. Verapamil: a review of its pharmacological properties and therapeutic use in coronary artery disease. Drugs. 1996;51(5): 792–819.
73. Wang A, Chen F, Xie Y, Guo Z, Yu Y. Protective mechanism of nicorandil on rat myocardial ischemia-reperfusion. J Cardiovasc Med (Hagerstown). 2012; 13(8):511–5.
74. Gregorini L, Marco J, Farah B, Bernies M, Palombo C, Kozakova M, et al. Effects of selective alpha1- and alpha2-adrenergic blockade on coronary flow reserve after coronary stenting. Circulation. 2002;106(23):2901–7.
75. Boengler K, Schulz R, Heusch G. Loss of cardioprotection with ageing. Cardiovasc Res. 2009;83(2):247–61.
76. Smits PC, Abdel-Wahab M, Neumann FJ, Boxma-de Klerk BM, Lunde K, Schotborgh CE, et al. Fractional flow reserve-guided multivessel angioplasty in myocardial infarction. N Engl J Med. 2017;376(13):1234–44.
77. Aksu T, Guler TE, Colak A, Baysal E, Durukan M, Sen T, et al. Intracoronary epinephrine in the treatment of refractory no-reflow after primary percutaneous coronary intervention: a retrospective study. BMC Cardiovasc Disord. 2015;15:10.

Relationship between plaque composition by virtual histology intravascular ultrasound and clinical outcomes after percutaneous coronary intervention in saphenous vein graft disease patients

Yin Liu[1†], Hai-Bo Wang[2†], Xiang Li[2†], Jian-Yong Xiao[1], Ji-Xiang Wang[1], Kathleen H. Reilly[3], Bo Sun[1] and Jing Gao[4*]

Abstract

Background: Plaque composition and morphologic characteristics identified by virtual histology intravascular ultrasound (VH-IVUS) can determine plaques at increased risk of clinical events following percutaneous coronary intervention (PCI) among coronary artery disease (CAD) patients. However, there have been few studies to investigate the relationship between plaque composition of saphenous vein graft (SVG) by VH-IVUS and clinical outcomes in patients with saphenous vein graft disease (SVGD) undergoing PCI. The purpose of this study is to determine whether plaque components and characteristics by VH-IVUS can predict major adverse cardiac events (MACEs) among SVGD patients undergoing PCI.

Methods/design: This is a prospective cohort study conducted in Tianjin Chest Hospital, China. Participants with SVGD referred for PCI will be invited to participate in this study, and will be followed up at 1, 6, 12, 24 and 36 months post-PCI to assess clinical outcomes.

The planned sample size is 175 subjects. We will recruit subjects with SVGD scheduled to receive PCI, aged 18–80 years, with a history of previous coronary artery bypass graft (CABG) surgery more than 1 year ago, and willing to participate in the study and sign informed consent.

The composite primary study endpoint is the incidence of MACEs after PCI for SVGD, including death from cardiac causes, non-fatal myocardial infarction, unplanned target lesion revascularization (TLR) and target vessel revascularization (TVR). The primary outcome analysis will be presented as Kaplan-Meier estimates and the primary outcome analysis will be carried out using a Cox proportional hazards regression model.

Discussion: Once the predictive values of plaque components and characteristics by VH-IVUS on subsequent clinical outcomes are determined among SVGD patients undergoing PCI, an innovative prediction tool of clinical outcomes for SVGD patients undergoing PCI will be created, which may lead to the development of new methods of risk stratification and intervention guidance.

(Continued on next page)

* Correspondence: heart201707@163.com; gaojing2088@163.com
†Yin Liu, Hai-Bo Wang and Xiang Li contributed equally to this work.
[4]Cardiovascular Institute, Tianjin Chest Hospital, No.261 Tai er zhuang RoadJinnan District, Tianjin 300222, People's Republic of China
Full list of author information is available at the end of the article

(Continued from previous page)

Keywords: Saphenous vein graft disease, Virtual histology intravascular ultrasound, Percutaneous coronary intervention, Major adverse cardiac events

Background

Coronary artery bypass graft (CABG) surgery is a widely used surgical procedure to treat coronary artery disease (CAD). Saphenous vein grafts (SVGs) are commonly used in CABG due to the advantage of availability, although the patency rates of SVGs are lower than that for arterial grafts [1–3]. However, about 40–50% of the SVGs will be occluded within 10 to 15 years after CABG surgery [1, 4, 5]. Newly developed atherosclerosis is the major reason for long-term poor prognosis [3]. SVG disease (SVGD), defined as a stenosis of 50% or more of the SVGs excluding distal anastomotic occlusion, has become an important cause of morbidity and mortality for CAD patients after CABG surgery [6, 7].

Both repeat CABG and percutaneous coronary intervention (PCI) are available treatment options for the management of SVGD [8–10]. Due to increased morbidity and mortality associated with patients undergoing repeat CABG, SVG PCI is the preferred therapeutic option to restore vessel patency and improve symptoms for patients with SVGD [11–13]. PCI in patients with prior CABG comprises up to 6% of the total PCI performed in the United States [14]. However, because of accelerated intimal proliferation and hyperplasia in venous conduits, SVG PCI is associated with increased risk of late failure and worse outcomes compared with native coronary artery interventions [15, 16]. Previous studies have shown that the incidence of major adverse cardiac events (MACEs) in patients who undergo bypass-graft PCI is significant higher than that in patients with native coronary artery PCI [17, 18]. It would be of particular interest to identify patients with poor prognosis after SVG PCI, which can be used for risk stratification and intervention guidance.

In recent years, intravascular ultrasound (IVUS) has been developed to identify vulnerable atherosclerotic plaques at high risk for coronary events. It was found that plaque characteristics (i.e., plaque burden, multiple plaque ruptures, lipid pool-like image and minimum luminal area) may be associated with no reflow phenomenon after PCI [19–22]. However, IVUS imposes limitations on identifying specific plaque components. Virtual histology-IVUS (VH-IVUS) is most widely used as it can assess both plaque composition and morphologic characteristics. VH-IVUS utilizes spectral and amplitude analysis of IVUS radiofrequency data to characterize plaque components, also suggesting the potential to identify vulnerable lesions [23, 24]. Moreover, several studies have demonstrated the independent relationship between VH-IVUS–defined plaque classification or plaque composition and MACEs [25, 26].

Considering similar pathophysiological mechanisms for CAD and SVGD, we hypothesized that plaque characteristics of SVG assessed by VH-IVUS might be associated with long-term clinical outcomes. However, data on plaque composition of SVG and its predictive values for clinical outcomes are still limited [27]. Thus, we sought to investigate the relationship between plaque composition of SVG by VH-IVUS and clinical outcome in SVGD patients undergoing PCI, which could identify morphologic features that are predictive of post-PCI MACEs.

Methods and design

Study design and setting

The study is a prospective cohort study conducted in Tianjin Chest Hospital, Tianjin city, China. Patients with SVGD referred for PCI are invited to participate in the study and VH-IVUS is performed in culprit SVG before and after PCI. Patients are recruited consecutively by surgeons at the Cardiology Department of Tianjin Chest Hospital. These subjects will be followed up at 1, 6, 12, 24 and 36 months post-PCI to assess clinical outcomes. The flow diagram of the study and the detailed study procedures are illustrated in Fig. 1.

Participants

The patients to be included in the study should meet all of the following criteria: (1) aged 18–80 years; (2) a history of previous CABG surgery more than 1 year ago; (3) diagnosed as SVGD which is defined as at least one SVG ≥50% diameter stenosis; (4) plans for receiving PCI using drug-eluting stents; (5) willing to participate in the study and sign informed consent.

Patients will be excluded from the study if any of the following criteria is met: (1) acute myocardial infarction within the previous 7 days; (2) having any contraindication to aspirin, clopidogrel, heparin or stainless steel; (3) impaired renal or hepatic function; (4) history of cerebral stroke or ischemic cerebrovascular disease within 3 months; (5) history of gastrointestinal bleeding or hemoptysis in the previous 4 weeks; (6) pregnant or breastfeeding; (7) vasculitis or other non-atherosclerotic CAD; (8) other major illnesses that would expose the participant to unexpected risk: hematologic disorder, malignancy, etc.

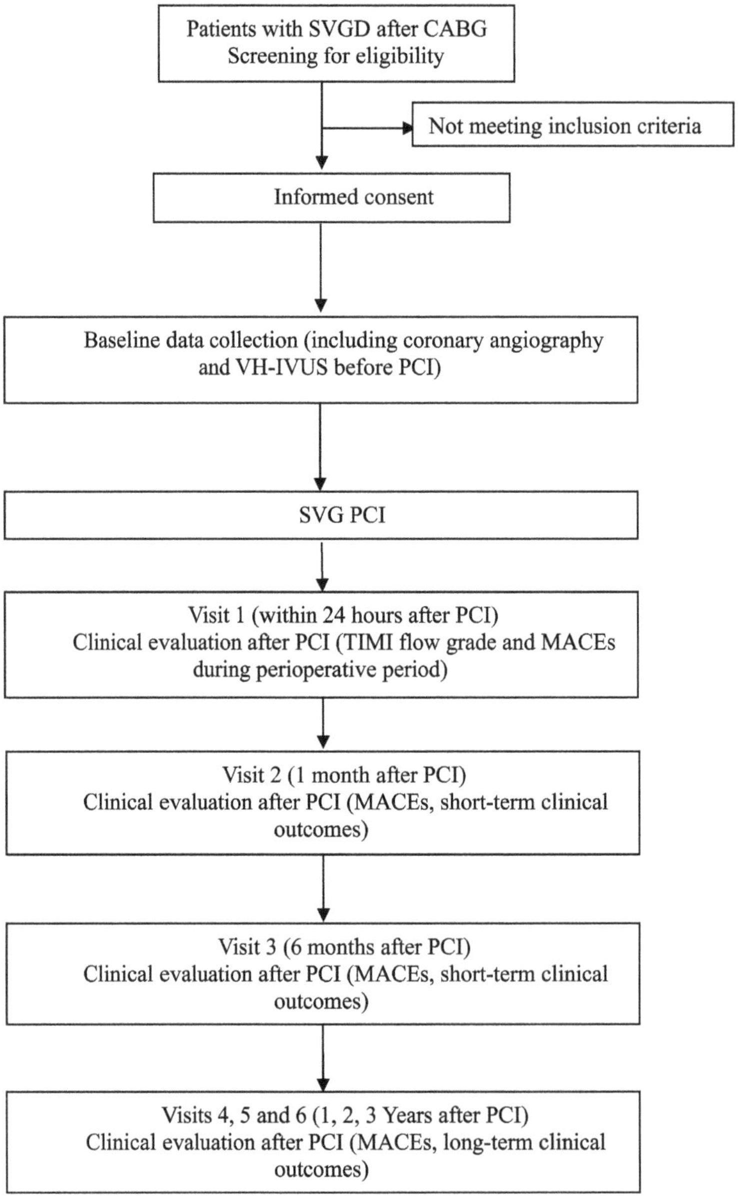

Fig. 1 Study flow chart

Participants can withdraw from the study at any time without any adverse outcome on subsequent treatment; the reasons for withdrawal will be recorded. The investigator can also exclude a participant from the study for reasons including serious adverse events or poor compliance with research protocol.

Evaluation of the coronary angiography

Coronary angiography is performed using angiography system with a flat-panel detector (Philips Allura Xper FD10, Philips Healthcare, Netherlands) according to the Judkins technique. Angiography of the in situ coronary artery is performed with 6F catheters through radial or femoral access, while Judkins R (JR) 4.0 is used as the first choice catheters for SVG angiography. The location of SVG is roughly determined according to previous CABG surgery procedure and it is displayed in at least two different projections. The presence of significant stenosis (≥50%) in at least one SVG is defined as SVGD.

VH-IVUS examination and plaque classification

After administration of heparin (100 U/Kg) and glyceryl trinitrate (100–200 μg), VH-IVUS is performed in SVG and other main coronary arteries before and after PCI. Data is obtained using a 20-MHz, 3.5-French EagleEye phased-array Gold catheter (Volcano Corporation, Rancho Cordova,

California, USA) with motorized pullback (0.5 mm per second) from the most distal safe position to guide the catheter. The IVUS grey-scale and Virtual histology analyses are performed offline using the Volcano Image Analysis Software (version 3.0.394,Volcano Corporation, USA) and are not used for PCI guidance or subsequent management. Spectral and amplitude analyses of IVUS backscattered radiofrequency are performed by two experienced interventional cardiologists without knowledge of subsequent clinical events. Angiographic qualitative assessment and quantitative measurements are obtained for SVG. Quantitative IVUS measurements include cross-sectional areas (CAS) of the lumen, the external elastic membrane (EEM), and the plaque and media (EEM CAS minus lumen CAS), lesion length, plaque burden (plaque and media CAS divided by EEM CAS), and plaque volume. Qualitative IVUS assessments include plaque rupture (intraplaque cavity that communicated with the lumen with an overlying residual fibrous cap fragment) and characterization of lesions. On the basis of radiofrequency IVUS, plaque components and morphology are classified into the following four types: fibrous tissue (FT), fibrofatty (FF), necrotic core (NC), and dense calcium (DC). A lesion on IVUS imaging is defined as a plaque burden ≥40% in at least 3 consecutive frames. Consistent with published VH-IVUS classifications [25, 28], such lesions are classified as one of the following: 1) fibrotic plaque, mainly fibrous tissue with < 10% confluent NC, < 10% confluent DC, and < 15% FF; 2) fibrocalcific plaque (FCa), mainly fibrous tissue with > 10% confluent DC but < 10% confluent NC; 3) pathologic intimal thickening (PIT), not meeting FCa plaque definitions and predominantly fibrous tissue; 4) fibroatheroma, > 10% confluent NC, including thick-cap fibroatheroma (ThCFA) and thin-cap fibroatheroma (TCFA).

Baseline assessment and follow-up

After receiving written informed consent, clinical staff will collect demographic and clinical characteristics from all participants. Medical records will be reviewed and related clinical information will be extracted. The data to be collected at baseline include demographic characteristics, medical history (diabetes mellitus, hypertension, hyperlipaemia, stroke, arrhythmia, previous myocardial infarction, PCI or CABG surgery, and medicines for cardiovascular disease), physical examination, clinical presentation (vital signs at hospital admission, onset time of chest pain, duration of chest pain, cardiac function with Killip classification), and smoking history. Cardiac color ultrasound, coronary angiogram, pre- and post-PCI VH-IVUS and 18 lead ECG will be done and used for checking inclusion/exclusion criteria. In addition, blood samples will be collected for laboratory testing, including routine blood, blood biochemistry, fasting glucose, coagulation function, homocysteine, cardiac damage markers (lactic dehydrogenase, creatine kinase, B-type natriuretic peptide, hydroxybutyrate dehydrogenase, troponin H, myoglobin), and inflammatory factors.

Eligible participants will be hospitalized for PCI treatment. In the therapy phase, patients will receive PCI for SVGD using drug-eluting stents. Operation notes (operation date, bleeding volume, medication), thrombolysis in myocardial infarction (TIMI) flow, corrected TIMI frame count (CTFC) and adverse events will be recorded in detail.

All subjects will be followed up at 1, 6, 12, 24 and 36 months after surgery, with MACEs and adverse events assessment collected at each time by clinic visits or telephone interview.

Study endpoints

The composite primary study endpoint is the incidence of MACEs after PCI for SVGD, including death from cardiac causes, non-fatal myocardial infarction, angina pectoris, target vessel revascularization (TVR) and hospitalization for heart failure.

Secondary endpoints are defined as: (1) the occurrence of the slow/no reflow, which is defined as thrombolysis in myocardial infarction (TIMI) grade 0, 1, or 2 flow within 24 h after SVG-PCI, despite successful treatment of the vessel obstruction; (2) myocardial infarction is defined as the onset of chest pain in combination with new, typical changes in the electrocardiogram and biochemical evidence of myocardial necrosis; (3)TVR is defined as a new revascularization procedure in the target vessel; (4)successful reperfusion is defined as TIMI flow grade 3 and less than 50% residual stenosis of SVG.

Sample size

We expect CAS of plaque and media 2.9 ± 1.7 mm^2 among patients with MACEs and 1.9 ± 1.5 mm^2 among patients without MACEs. It is estimated that the incidence of MACEs is 20% in 3 years after PCI for SVGD. Assuming a 20% drop-out rate, a total of 175 participants are required to provide 80% power, with a two-sided type I error of 0.05.

Statistical analysis

Analyses will be made using SAS statistical software (version 9.3) by researchers at the Peking University Clinical Research Institute. Continuous variables will be expressed as mean ± standard deviation or median ± interquartile range (IQR), and t-test or Wilcoxon rank sum test will be used to compare the difference between groups. For categorical variables, the chi-square test/ Fisher's exact test will be performed. Time-to-event data (MACEs in 3 year after PCI) will be presented as Kaplan-Meier estimates and the primary outcome analysis will be carried out using univariate and multivariate Cox proportional hazards regression models. The ideal cut-off of quantitative indexes of VH-IVUS and the diagnostic accuracy will be determined by the receiver-operating characteristic curve (ROC). A p-value < 0.05 will be considered statistically significant in all analyses.

Trial status

The first participant was enrolled in July 2017. As of August 2018, 67 participants have been enrolled and recruitment is ongoing in Tianjin Chest Hospital, China. Treatment and follow-up of all participants are planned to continue until December 2021.

Discussion

It has been indicated that plaque anatomy and composition identified by VH-IVUS is a predictor of long-term clinical outcomes in patients undergoing PCI. However, there have been few studies investigating the relationship between plaque composition of SVG by VH-IVUS and clinical outcome in SVGD patients undergoing PCI. PCI is a widely performed surgical procedure for SVGD patients. Considering the higher risk in conducting PCI among SVGD patients, it is necessary to explore the cardiovascular factors predicting the clinical outcome of PCI, which can be used for risk stratification and intervention guidance. In this prospective cohort study, we will identify atherosclerotic plaque components and characteristics in SVGD patients undergoing PCI and predict the long-term clinical outcomes identified with VH-IVUS.

Multiple novel intravascular imaging technologies have been developed to help identify high risk plaque characteristics in predicting cardiovascular adverse events [22, 29, 30]. Young Joon Hong et al. investigated the relationship between intravascular IVUS findings and the no-reflow phenomenon after PCI for SVGD [22]. But IVUS has limited value for identifying specific plaque components [31]. Computed tomography (CT) is routinely used for coronary angiography and can identify high risk features of plaques. Daniel R. Obaid et al. found that plaque components and classifications based on CT could not reliably classify plaques and identify TCFA [30]. With the highest spatial resolution, optical coherence tomography (OCT) has emerged as an important imaging modality for intracoronary evaluation [32]. The direct comparison between VH-IVUS and OCT by Brown et al. found that both VH-IVUS and OCT could identify advanced coronary plaques and that combined VH-IVUS/OCT was better than either alone [33]. However, OCT has a low signal penetration through lipid or necrotic core, and cannot adequately acquire images of the whole vessels with large lumen diameter or large necrotic core [29, 34]. This presents a problem for imaging of large vessels including vein grafts. The presence of macrophages, foam cells, microcalcifications, or hemosiderin, often co-existent with the necrotic core, could be adverse to accurate OCT assessment of lipidic plaque [29, 34]. VH-IVUS, which has become clinically available, can assess both plaque morphology and tissue characteristics using spectral and amplitude analysis of backscattered radiofrequency ultrasound signal. With different plaque components exhibiting a defined spectrum, VH-IVUS can classify atherosclerotic plaque into four types: FT, FF, NC, and DC [35, 36]. The radiofrequency signal is mathematically transformed into a color-coded representation, including lipid, fibrous tissue, calcification, and necrotic core [37]. Thus, VH-IVUS can identify atherosclerotic plaques exactly like histopathology.

Some meta-analysis studies have found that the relationship between absolute volume of NC components on VH-IVUS imaging and distal embolization after PCI in acute coronary syndrome (ACS) patients [35, 38]. Previous studies have demonstrated that TCFA, plaque burden, and minimum luminal area are associated with MACEs among ACS patients undergoing PCI [25, 26]. The VIVA (VH-IVUS in Vulnerable Atherosclerosis) Study showed that VH-IVUS TCFA was associated with nonrestenotic and total MACEs on individual plaque or whole patient analysis [26]. It was reported by the Providing Regional Observations to Study Predictors of Events in the Coronary Tree (PROSPECT) study that plaque burden > 70%, minimum luminal area < 4 mm^2, and VH-IVUS TCFA were the independent predictors of nonculprit lesion–related events. However, there are limited studies investigating the associations of degenerative lesions or plaque components of SVGD with clinical outcomes using VH-IVUS. Man-Hong Jim et al. sought to report the VH-IVUS findings in degenerative aortocoronary SVG lesions and correlate plaque compositions with clinical characteristics [39]. Lesions with a plaque burden ≥70% was found to be positively correlated with FF tissue, but negatively correlated with DC [39]. However, it is a cross-sectional study, the temporary relationship between VH-IVUS findings and clinical characteristics cannot be determined. As far as the authors know, there is currently no study exploring the relationship between VH-IVUS defined atherosclerotic plaque components and clinical outcomes in SVGD patients undergoing PCI.

The current study is subject to several limitations. This is an observational cohort study, confounding effects cannot be ruled out entirely. However, the multivariate Cox proportional regression model will be used to determine the independent effects of VH-IVUS findings on long-term clinical outcomes after adjusting for the impact of baseline characteristics. Second, participants with SVGD who are enrolled in a single center (Cardiovascular Institute, Tianjin Chest Hospital) may not represent the population in China. However, we speculate that the relationship between VH-IVUS findings and clinical outcomes should persist in other SVGD patients undergoing PCI, but with varying magnitudes of association. Third, although VH-IVUS is a widely used method in clinical setting, VH-IVUS has some technological limitations. VH-IVUS TCFA is not equivalent to histopathologic definitions and VH-IVUS tend to over-estimate TCFA compared with histology.

Conclusion

The proposed prospective cohort study aims to investigate whether plaque characteristics and components of culprit SVG lesion assessed by VH-IVUS could predict subsequent clinical outcome after PCI among SVGD patients. Once our hypothesis is confirmed, an innovative prediction tool of clinical outcomes can be created, which may lead to the development of new methods of risk stratification and intervention guidance.

Abbreviations

ACS: Acute coronary syndrome; CABG: coronary artery bypass grafting; CAD: coronary artery disease; CAS: cross-sectional areas; CT: Computed tomography; CTFC: Corrected TIMI frame count; DC: dense calcium; EEM: external elastic membrane; FCa: fibrocalcific plaque; FF: fibrofatty; FT: fibrous tissue; IVUS: intravascular ultrasound; MACEs: major adverse cardiac events; NC: necrotic core; OCT: Optical coherence tomography; PCI: percutaneous coronary intervention; PIT: Pathologic intimal thickening; PROSPECT: Providing Regional Observations to Study Predictors of Events in the Coronary Tree; ROC: Receiver-operating characteristic curve; SVGD: saphenous vein grafts disease; SVGs: saphenous vein grafts; TCFA: Thin-cap fibroatheroma; ThCFA: Thick-cap fibroatheroma; TIMI: Thrombolysis in myocardial infarction; TLR: target lesion revascularization; TVR: target vessel revascularization; VH-IVUS: virtual histology intravascular ultrasound

Acknowledgements

The authors thank all of the study participants for their great effort. Furthermore, we wish to thank the research staffs for their efforts in the study.

Funding

This research was funded by the Key Project of Scientific and Technological Support Plan of Tianjin in 2016 (No.:16YFZCSY00800) and the Key Project of Healthcare Industry of Tianjin in 2015 (No.: 15KG128). However, study sponsor doesn't involve in any activities related with study except monitoring.

Authors' contributions

YL, JG, XL, HBW, ZGG, JYX, JXW, KHR and BS developed the protocol for this project. GJ and YL were the principal investigators and managed the protocol. ZGG and JYX were responsible for data collection and management. JXW and BS were responsible for epidemiological investigations and laboratory testing. XL, HBW and KHR performed all statistical analysis. YL, JG, XL, HBW, ZGG, JYX, JXW, KHR and BS were involved in the initial draft of the manuscript and writing it. JG, HBW and KHR assisted with writing and editing of the manuscript. The manuscript was amended based on comments from all authors. All authors read and approved the final manuscript.

Competing interests

The authors declare that they have no competing interests.

Author details

[1]Department of Cardiology, Tianjin Chest Hospital, No.261 Tai er zhuang RoadJinnan District, Tianjin 300222, People's Republic of China. [2]Peking University Clinical Research Institute, Xueyuan Rd 38#, Haidian Dist, Beijing 100191, People's Republic of China. [3]Independent Consultant, New York City, NY, USA. [4]Cardiovascular Institute, Tianjin Chest Hospital, No.261 Tai er zhuang RoadJinnan District, Tianjin 300222, People's Republic of China.

References

1. Parang P, Arora R. Coronary vein graft disease: pathogenesis and prevention. Can J Cardiol. 2009;25(2):e57–62.
2. Yayla C, Canpolat U, Akyel A, Yayla KG, Yilmaz S, Acikgoz SK, Ozcan F, Turak O, Dogan M, Yeter E, et al. Association between platelet to lymphocyte ratio and saphenous vein graft disease. Angiology. 2016;67(2):133–8.
3. Gaudino M, Puskas JD, Di Franco A, Ohmes LB, Iannaccone M, Barbero U, Glineur D, Grau JB, Benedetto U, D'Ascenzo F, et al. Three arterial grafts improve late survival: a meta-analysis of propensity-matched studies. Circulation. 2017;135(11):1036–44.
4. Owens CD. Adaptive changes in autogenous vein grafts for arterial reconstruction: clinical implications. J Vasc Surg. 2010;51(3):736–46.
5. Barbero U, Iannaccone M, d'Ascenzo F, Barbero C, Mohamed A, Annone U, Benedetto S, Celentani D, Gagliardi M, Moretti C, et al. 64 slice-coronary computed tomography sensitivity and specificity in the evaluation of coronary artery bypass graft stenosis: a meta-analysis. Int J Cardiol. 2016;216:52–7.
6. Demircelik B, Cakmak M, Nazli Y, Gurel OM, Akkaya N, Cetin M, Cetin Z, Selcoki Y, Kurtul A, Eryonucu B. Adropin: a new marker for predicting late saphenous vein graft disease after coronary artery bypass grafting. Clin Invest Med. 2014;37(5):E338–44.
7. Akpinar I, Sayin MR, Gursoy YC, Karabag T, Kucuk E, Buyukuysal MC, Aydin M, Haznedaroglu IC. Plateletcrit. A platelet marker associated with saphenous vein graft disease. Herz. 2014;39(1):142–8.
8. Harskamp RE, Lopes RD, Baisden CE, de Winter RJ, Alexander JH. Saphenous vein graft failure after coronary artery bypass surgery: pathophysiology, management, and future directions. Ann Surg. 2013;257(5):824–33.
9. Levine GN, Bates ER, Blankenship JC, Bailey SR, Bittl JA, Cercek B, Chambers CE, Ellis SG, Guyton RA, Hollenberg SM, et al. 2011 ACCF/AHA/SCAI guideline for percutaneous coronary intervention: executive summary: a report of the American College of Cardiology Foundation/American Heart Association task force on practice guidelines and the Society for Cardiovascular Angiography and Interventions. Circulation. 2011;124(23): 2574–609.
10. D'Ascenzo F, Barbero U, Moretti C, Palmerini T, Della Riva D, Mariani A, Omede P, DiNicolantonio JJ, Biondi-Zoccai G, Gaita F. Percutaneous coronary intervention versus coronary artery bypass graft for stable angina: meta-regression of randomized trials. Contemp Clin Trials. 2014;38(1):51–8.
11. Lee MS, Park SJ, Kandzari DE, Kirtane AJ, Fearon WF, Brilakis ES, Vermeersch P, Kim YH, Waksman R, Mehilli J, et al. Saphenous vein graft intervention. JACC Cardiovasc Interv. 2011;4(8):831–43.
12. Yap CH, Sposato L, Akowuah E, Theodore S, Dinh DT, Shardey GC, Skillington PD, Tatoulis J, Yii M, Smith JA, et al. Contemporary results show repeat coronary artery bypass grafting remains a risk factor for operative mortality. Ann Thorac Surg. 2009;87(5):1386–91.
13. Morrison DA, Sethi G, Sacks J, Henderson WG, Grover F, Sedlis S, Esposito R. Investigators of the Department of Veterans Affairs Cooperative Study AWESOME: percutaneous coronary intervention versus repeat bypass surgery for patients with medically refractory myocardial ischemia: AWESOME randomized trial and registry experience with post-CABG patients. J Am Coll Cardiol. 2002;40(11):1951–4.
14. Brilakis ES, Rao SV, Banerjee S, Goldman S, Shunk KA, Holmes DR Jr, Honeycutt E, Roe MT. Percutaneous coronary intervention in native arteries versus bypass grafts in prior coronary artery bypass grafting patients: a report from the National Cardiovascular Data Registry. JACC Cardiovasc Interv. 2011;4(8):844–50.
15. de Vries MR, Simons KH, Jukema JW, Braun J, Quax PH. Vein graft failure: from pathophysiology to clinical outcomes. Nat Rev Cardiol. 2016;13(8):451–70.
16. Brilakis ES, O'Donnell CI, Penny W, Armstrong EJ, Tsai T, Maddox TM, Plomondon ME, Banerjee S, Rao SV, Garcia S, et al. Percutaneous coronary intervention in native coronary arteries versus bypass grafts in patients with prior coronary artery bypass graft surgery: Insights From the Veterans Affairs Clinical Assessment, Reporting, and Tracking Program. JACC Cardiovasc Interv. 2016;9(9):884–93.
17. Roffi M, Mukherjee D, Chew DP, Bhatt DL, Cho L, Robbins MA, Ziada KM, Brennan DM, Ellis SG, Topol EJ. Lack of benefit from intravenous platelet glycoprotein IIb/IIIa receptor inhibition as adjunctive treatment for percutaneous interventions of aortocoronary bypass grafts: a pooled analysis of five randomized clinical trials. Circulation. 2002;106(24):3063–7.

18. Redfors B, Genereux P, Witzenbichler B, McAndrew T, Diamond J, Huang X, Maehara A, Weisz G, Mehran R, Kirtane AJ, et al. Percutaneous coronary intervention of saphenous vein graft. Circ Cardiovasc Interv. 2017;10(5).
19. Ohshima K, Ikeda S, Kadota H, Yamane K, Izumi N, Ohshima K, Hamada M. Impact of culprit plaque volume and composition on myocardial microcirculation following primary angioplasty in patients with ST-segment elevation myocardial infarction: virtual histology intravascular ultrasound analysis. Int J Cardiol. 2013;167(3):1000–5.
20. Iijima R, Shinji H, Ikeda N, Itaya H, Makino K, Funatsu A, Yokouchi I, Komatsu H, Ito N, Nuruki H, et al. Comparison of coronary arterial finding by intravascular ultrasound in patients with "transient no-reflow" versus "reflow" during percutaneous coronary intervention in acute coronary syndrome. Am J Cardiol. 2006;97(1):29–33.
21. Tanaka A, Kawarabayashi T, Nishibori Y, Sano T, Nishida Y, Fukuda D, Shimada K, Yoshikawa J. No-reflow phenomenon and lesion morphology in patients with acute myocardial infarction. Circulation. 2002;105(18):2148–52.
22. Hong YJ, Jeong MH, Ahn Y, Kang JC, Mintz GS, Kim SW, Lee SY, Kim SY, Pichard AD, Satler LF, et al. Intravascular ultrasound findings that are predictive of no reflow after percutaneous coronary intervention for saphenous vein graft disease. Am J Cardiol. 2012;109(11):1576–81.
23. Zhao XY, Wang XF, Li L, Zhang JY, Du YY, Yao HM. Plaque characteristics and serum pregnancy-associated plasma protein a levels predict the no-reflow phenomenon after percutaneous coronary intervention. J Int Med Res. 2013;41(2):307–16.
24. Raichlin E, Bae JH, Kushwaha SS, Lennon RJ, Prasad A, Rihal CS, Lerman A. Inflammatory burden of cardiac allograft coronary atherosclerotic plaque is associated with early recurrent cellular rejection and predicts a higher risk of vasculopathy progression. J Am Coll Cardiol. 2009;53(15):1279–86.
25. Yun KH, Mintz GS, Farhat N, Marso SP, Taglieri N, Verheye S, Foster MC, Margolis MP, Templin B, Xu K, et al. Relation between angiographic lesion severity, vulnerable plaque morphology and future adverse cardiac events (from the providing regional observations to study predictors of events in the coronary tree study). Am J Cardiol. 2012;110(4):471–7.
26. Calvert PA, Obaid DR, O'Sullivan M, Shapiro LM, McNab D, Densem CG, Schofield PM, Braganza D, Clarke SC, Ray KK, et al. Association between IVUS findings and adverse outcomes in patients with coronary artery disease: the VIVA (VH-IVUS in vulnerable atherosclerosis) study. JACC Cardiovasc Imaging. 2011;4(8):894–901.
27. Wood FO, Badhey N, Garcia B, Abdel-karim AR, Maini B, Banerjee S, Brilakis ES. Analysis of saphenous vein graft lesion composition using near-infrared spectroscopy and intravascular ultrasonography with virtual histology. Atherosclerosis. 2010;212(2):528–33.
28. Maehara A, Cristea E, Mintz GS, Lansky AJ, Dressler O, Biro S, Templin B, Virmani R, de Bruyne B, Serruys PW, et al. Definitions and methodology for the grayscale and radiofrequency intravascular ultrasound and coronary angiographic analyses. JACC Cardiovasc Imaging. 2012;5(3 Suppl):S1–9.
29. Iannaccone M, Quadri G, Taha S, D'Ascenzo F, Montefusco A, Omede P, Jang IK, Niccoli G, Souteyrand G, Yundai C, et al. Prevalence and predictors of culprit plaque rupture at OCT in patients with coronary artery disease: a meta-analysis. Eur Heart J Cardiovasc Imaging. 2016;17(10):1128–37.
30. Obaid DR, Calvert PA, Gopalan D, Parker RA, Hoole SP, West NE, Goddard M, Rudd JH, Bennett MR. Atherosclerotic plaque composition and classification identified by coronary computed tomography: assessment of computed tomography-generated plaque maps compared with virtual histology intravascular ultrasound and histology. Circ Cardiovasc Imaging. 2013;6(5):655–64.
31. Pu J, Mintz GS, Brilakis ES, Banerjee S, Abdel-Karim AR, Maini B, Biro S, Lee JB, Stone GW, Weisz G, et al. In vivo characterization of coronary plaques: novel findings from comparing greyscale and virtual histology intravascular ultrasound and near-infrared spectroscopy. Eur Heart J. 2012;33(3):372–83.
32. Niccoli G, Giubilato S, Di Vito L, Leo A, Cosentino N, Pitocco D, Marco V, Ghirlanda G, Prati F, Crea F. Severity of coronary atherosclerosis in patients with a first acute coronary event: a diabetes paradox. Eur Heart J. 2013; 34(10):729–41.
33. Brown AJ, Obaid DR, Costopoulos C, Parker RA, Calvert PA, Teng Z, Hoole SP, West NE, Goddard M, Bennett MR. Direct comparison of virtual-histology intravascular ultrasound and optical coherence tomography imaging for identification of thin-cap Fibroatheroma. Circ Cardiovasc Imaging. 2015; 8(10):e003487.
34. Mintz GS. Optical coherence tomography and virtual-histology intravascular ultrasound: strange bedfellows? ... Or not? Circ Cardiovasc Imaging. 2015; 8(10):e004045.
35. Ding S, Xu L, Yang F, Kong L, Zhao Y, Gao L, Wang W, Xu R, Ge H, Jiang M, et al. Association between tissue characteristics of coronary plaque and distal embolization after coronary intervention in acute coronary syndrome patients: insights from a meta-analysis of virtual histology-intravascular ultrasound studies. PLoS One. 2014;9(11):e106583.
36. Vince DG, Dixon KJ, Cothren RM, Cornhill JF. Comparison of texture analysis methods for the characterization of coronary plaques in intravascular ultrasound images. Comput Med Imaging Graph. 2000;24(4):221–9.
37. Kawasaki M, Takatsu H, Noda T, Ito Y, Kunishima A, Arai M, Nishigaki K, Takemura G, Morita N, Minatoguchi S, et al. Noninvasive quantitative tissue characterization and two-dimensional color-coded map of human atherosclerotic lesions using ultrasound integrated backscatter: comparison between histology and integrated backscatter images. J Am Coll Cardiol. 2001;38(2):486–92.
38. Claessen BE, Maehara A, Fahy M, Xu K, Stone GW, Mintz GS. Plaque composition by intravascular ultrasound and distal embolization after percutaneous coronary intervention. JACC Cardiovasc Imaging. 2012;5(3 Suppl):S111–8.
39. Jim MH, Hau WK, Ko RL, Siu CW, Ho HH, Yiu KH, Lau CP, Chow WH. Virtual histology by intravascular ultrasound study on degenerative aortocoronary saphenous vein grafts. Heart Vessel. 2010;25(3):175–81.

Permissions

All chapters in this book were first published in CD, by BioMed Central; hereby published with permission under the Creative Commons Attribution License or equivalent. Every chapter published in this book has been scrutinized by our experts. Their significance has been extensively debated. The topics covered herein carry significant findings which will fuel the growth of the discipline. They may even be implemented as practical applications or may be referred to as a beginning point for another development.

The contributors of this book come from diverse backgrounds, making this book a truly international effort. This book will bring forth new frontiers with its revolutionizing research information and detailed analysis of the nascent developments around the world.

We would like to thank all the contributing authors for lending their expertise to make the book truly unique. They have played a crucial role in the development of this book. Without their invaluable contributions this book wouldn't have been possible. They have made vital efforts to compile up to date information on the varied aspects of this subject to make this book a valuable addition to the collection of many professionals and students.

This book was conceptualized with the vision of imparting up-to-date information and advanced data in this field. To ensure the same, a matchless editorial board was set up. Every individual on the board went through rigorous rounds of assessment to prove their worth. After which they invested a large part of their time researching and compiling the most relevant data for our readers.

The editorial board has been involved in producing this book since its inception. They have spent rigorous hours researching and exploring the diverse topics which have resulted in the successful publishing of this book. They have passed on their knowledge of decades through this book. To expedite this challenging task, the publisher supported the team at every step. A small team of assistant editors was also appointed to further simplify the editing procedure and attain best results for the readers.

Apart from the editorial board, the designing team has also invested a significant amount of their time in understanding the subject and creating the most relevant covers. They scrutinized every image to scout for the most suitable representation of the subject and create an appropriate cover for the book.

The publishing team has been an ardent support to the editorial, designing and production team. Their endless efforts to recruit the best for this project, has resulted in the accomplishment of this book. They are a veteran in the field of academics and their pool of knowledge is as vast as their experience in printing. Their expertise and guidance has proved useful at every step. Their uncompromising quality standards have made this book an exceptional effort. Their encouragement from time to time has been an inspiration for everyone.

The publisher and the editorial board hope that this book will prove to be a valuable piece of knowledge for researchers, students, practitioners and scholars across the globe.

List of Contributors

Jonas Emil Sabroe, Per Thayssen, Lisbeth Antonsen, Mikkel Hougaard, Knud Nørregaard Hansen and Lisette Okkels Jensen
Department of Cardiology, Odense University Hospital, Sdr. Boulevard 29, 5000 Odense, Denmark

Mathias Wolfrum, Gregor Fahrni, Giovanni Luigi de Maria, Rajesh K. Kharbanda and Adrian P. Banning
Oxford Heart Centre, Oxford University Hospitals, Headley Way, Oxford OX39DU, UK

Guido Knapp
Department of Statistics, TU University Dortmund, Dortmund, Germany

Nick Curzen
University Hospital Southampton NHS Foundation Trust, Southampton, UK

Georg M. Fröhlich
Department of Cardiology, Charité Universitätsmedizin Berlin (Campus Benjamin Franklin), Berlin, Germany

Min Meng, Bei Gao, Xia Wang, Ri-na Sa and Bin Ge
Department of Pharmacy, Gansu Provincial Hospital, Donggang West Road No. 204, Lanzhou, Gansu 730000, China

Zheng-gang Bai
Evidence-Based Medicine Center, Lanzhou University, Lanzhou, Gansu 730000, China

Juho Viikilä
Department of Cardiology, Päijät-Häme Central Hospital, Keskussairaalankatu 7, 15850 Lahti, Finland

Tuomo Nieminen, Ilkka Tierala and Mika Laine
Department of Cardiology, Helsinki University Central Hospital, Helsinki, Finland

Pravesh Kumar Bundhun and Feng Huang
Institute of Cardiovascular Diseases, the First Affiliated Hospital of Guangxi Medical University, Nanning, Guangxi 530021, People's Republic of China

Chandra Mouli Yanamala
Department of Internal Medicine, EALING Hospital, University of Buckingham, Uxbridge road, Southall, UB1 3HW London, UK

Ge Li-Sha
Department of Pediatric, Second Affiliated Hospital of Wenzhou Medical University, Wenzhou 325000, China

Chen Peng and Li Yue-Chun
Department of Cardiology, Second Affiliated Hospital of Wenzhou Medical University, 109 Xueyuan Road, Wenzhou, Zhejiang, China

Pravesh Kumar Bundhun and Wei-Qiang Huang
Institute of Cardiovascular Diseases, the First Affiliated Hospital of Guangxi Medical University, Nanning, Guangxi 530021, People's Republic of China

Abhishek Rishikesh Teeluck and Akash Bhurtu
Guangxi Medical University, Nanning, Guangxi 530027, People's Republic of China

Tetsuya Nomura, Taku Kato, Hiroshi Kubota, Daisuke Miyawaki, Ryota Urata, Takeshi Sugimoto, Yusuke Higuchi, Natsuya Keira and Tetsuya Tatsumi
Department of Cardiovascular Medicine, Nantan General Hospital, 25, Yagi-Ueno, Yagi-cho, Nantan City, Japan

Ming Gao, Yi Cheng, Yang Zheng, Weihua Zhang, Lin Wang and Ling Qin
The Cardiovascular Center, the First Hospital of Jilin University, 71 Xinmin Street, Changchun 130021, China

Yi Cheng
Laboratory for Cardiovascular Diseases, Institute of Translational Medicine, the First Hospital of Jilin University, Changchun, China
Key Laboratory for Cardiovascular Mechanism of Traditional Chinese Medicine, the First Hospital of Jilin University, Changchun, China

Jian-wei Zhang and Yu-jie Zhou
Department of Cardiology, Beijing Anzhen Hospital, Capital Medical University, Beijing Institute of Heart Lung and Blood Vessel Disease, the Key Laboratory of Remodeling-related Cardiovascular Disease, Ministry of Education, Beijing 100029, China

See W Low
Department of Cardiovascular Diseases, University of Arizona South Campus, 2800 E Ajo Way, Tucson, AZ 85713, USA

Justin Z Lee
Department of Internal Medicine, University of Arizona, 1501 N Campbell Ave, RM 6336, Tucson, AZ 85724, USA

Kwan S Lee
3950 S Country Club Road, Suite 200, Tucson, AZ 85714, USA

Pravesh Kumar Bundhun
Institute of Cardiovascular Diseases, the First Affiliated Hospital of Guangxi Medical University, Nanning, Guangxi 530027, People's Republic of China

Chakshu Gupta
Guangxi Medical University, Nanning, Guangxi 530027, People's Republic of China

Guang Ma Xu
Department of Cardiology, The People's Hospital of Guangxi Zhuang Autonomous Region, Nanning, Guangxi 530021, People's Republic of China

Zrinko Prskalo, Ivica Brizić, Darko Markota and Ivica Markota
Department of Cardiology, University Hospital Mostar, Bijeli Brijeg bb, 88 000 Mostar, Bosnia and Herzegovina

Monika Tomic
Department of Nephrology, University Hospital Mostar, Mostar, Bosnia and Herzegovina

Mladen Boban
Department of Pharmacology, University of Split, Split, Croatia

Boris Starcevic
Department of Cardiology, University Hospital Dubrava, Zagreb, Croatia

Motoki Kubo, Toru Miyoshi, Yuko Ohno, Kazufumi Nakamura and Hiroshi Ito
Department of Cardiovascular Medicine, Okayama University Graduate School of Medicine, Dentistry and Pharmaceutical Sciences, Okayama, Japan

Hiroki Oe
Center of Ultrasonography, Okayama University Graduate School of Medicine, Dentistry and Pharmaceutical Sciences, Okayama, Japan

Pravesh Kumar Bundhun and Wei-Qiang Huang
Institute of Cardiovascular Diseases, the First Affiliated Hospital of Guangxi Medical University, Nanning, Guangxi 530027, People's Republic of China

Girish Janoo and Abhishek Rishikesh Teeluck
Guangxi Medical University, Nanning, Guangxi 530027, People's Republic of China

Karen-leigh Edward, John Stephenson and Jo-Ann Giandinoto
Australian Catholic University and St Vincent's Private Hospital Melbourne Ltd, Locked Bag 4115 MDC, Fitzroy 3065, Australia

Karen-leigh Edward and John Stephenson
University of Huddersfield, Huddersfield, United Kingdom

Andrew Wilson, Robert Whitbourn, Jack Gutman and Andrew Newcomb
University of Melbourne and St Vincent's Hospital Melbourne, Melbourne, Australia

Pravesh Kumar Bundhun and Wei-Qiang Huang
Institute of Cardiovascular Diseases, the First Affiliated Hospital of Guangxi Medical University, Nanning, Guangxi 530027, People's Republic of China

Manish Pursun
Guangxi Medical University, Nanning, Guangxi 530027, People's Republic of China

Wei-Qiang Huang
Institute of Cardiovascular Diseases, the First Affiliated Hospital of Guangxi Medical University, Nanning, Guangxi 530021, People's Republic of China

Hyung Joon Joo, Han Saem Jeong, Hyungdon Kook, Seung Hun Lee, Jae Hyoung Park, Soon Jun Hong, Cheol Woong Yu and Do-Sum Lim
Department of Cardiology, Cardiovascular Center, Korea University Anam Hospital, 126-1, 5ka, Anam-dong, Sungbuk-ku, Seoul 136-705, Republic of Korea

Johannes Wild, Tommaso Gori, Thomas Münzel and Philip Wenzel
Center for Cardiology - Cardiology I, University Medical Center Mainz, Langenbeckstrasse 1, 55131 Mainz, Germany

Tommaso Gori, Thomas Münzel and Philip Wenzel
German Center for Cardiovascular Research (DZHK) - Partner site Rhine-Main, University Medical Center Mainz, Langenbeckstrasse 1, 55131 Mainz, Germany

Thomas Münzel and Philip Wenzel
Center for Thrombosis and Hemostasis, University Medical Center Mainz, Langenbeckstrasse 1, 55131 Mainz, Germany

Tan Xu, Youqin Zhan, Nan Lu, Zhuoqiao He and Xuerui Tan
Department of Cardiology, First Affiliated Hospital of Shantou University Medical College, Changping Road NO.57, Shantou, Guangdong 515041, China

Xi Su
Department of Cardiology, Wuhan Asian Heart Hospital, Wuhan, Hubei 430022, China

Tuncay Kırıs and Aykan Çelik
Department of Cardiology, Izmir Katip Celebi University, Ataturk Training and Research Hospital, 35360 Izmir, Turkey

Eyüp Avcı
Department of Cardiology, Balikesir University Faculty of Medicine, 10345 Balikesir, Turkey

Wataru Takagi, Masayuki Doi, Keisuke Okawa, Kazumasa Nosaka, Tomoyuki Nishibe and Naoaki Matsuo
Department of Cardiology, Kagawa Prefectural Central Hospital, Takamatsu, Japan

Toru Miyoshi and Hiroshi Ito
Department of Cardiovascular Medicine, Okayama University Graduate School of Medicine, Dentistry and Pharmaceutical Sciences, 2-5-1 Shikata-cho, Okayama 700-8558, Japan

Satoshi Hirohata
Department of Medical Technology, Okayama University Graduate School of Health, Okayama, Japan

Marco Albanese, Korhan Alpaslan, Peter Merguet and Wolfgang Schöls
Herzzentrum Duisburg, Gerrickstr. 21, D-47137 Duisburg, Germany

Taoufik Ouarrak and Steffen Schneider
Stiftung Institut für Herzinfarktforschung, Bremserstraße 79 - Haus, MD-67063 Ludwigshafen a. Rh, Germany

Marco Albanese
Klinik für Kardiologie und Angiologie, Herzzentrum Duisburg, Gerrickstr. 21, 47137 Duisburg, Germany

Marco Albanese
Herzzentrum Hirslanden Zentralschweiz, Klinik St. Anna, St. Anna Str. 32, CH-6006 Luzern, Switzerland

Xiaowei Niu
The First School of Clinical Medicine, Lanzhou University, Tianshui South Road, No. 222, Lanzhou, Gansu 730000, China

Jingjing Zhang
Baiyin Second People's Hospital, Gongyuan Road, No. 509, Baiyin, Gansu 730900, China

Ming Bai, Yu Peng and Zheng Zhang
Department of Cardiology, the First Hospital of Lanzhou University, Donggang West Road, No. 1, Lanzhou, Gansu 730000, China

Shaobo Sun
Key Lab of Prevention and Treatment for Chronic Disease, Gansu University of Chinese Medicine, Dingxi East Road, No. 35, Lanzhou, Gansu 730000, China

Yin Liu, Jian-Yong Xiao, Ji-Xiang Wang and Bo Sun
Department of Cardiology, Tianjin Chest Hospital, No.261 Tai er zhuang RoadJinnan District, Tianjin 300222, People's Republic of China

Hai-Bo Wang and Xiang Li
Peking University Clinical Research Institute, Xueyuan Rd 38#, Haidian Dist, Beijing 100191, People's Republic of China

Kathleen H. Reilly
Independent Consultant, New York City, NY, USA

Jing Gao
Cardiovascular Institute, Tianjin Chest Hospital, No.261 Tai er zhuang Road Jinnan District, Tianjin 300222, People's Republic of China

Index

M

N

O

P

R

S

T

U

V

www.ingramcontent.com/pod-product-compliance
Lightning Source LLC
Chambersburg PA
CBHW082044190326
41458CB00010B/3455
9781632419279